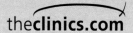

RADIOLOGIC CLINICS
OF NORTH AMERICA

Genitourinary Tract Imaging

Guest Editors

MICHAEL A. BLAKE, MRCPI, FFR(RCSI), FRCR

MANNUDEEP K. KALRA, MD

January 2008 • Volume 46 • Number 1

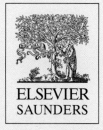

**ELSEVIER
SAUNDERS**

An imprint of Elsevier, Inc

PHILADELPHIA LONDON TORONTO MONTREAL SYDNEY TOKYO

W.B. SAUNDERS COMPANY
A Division of Elsevier Inc.

1600 John F. Kennedy Boulevard • Suite 1800 • Philadelphia, Pennsylvania 19103-2899

http://www.theclinics.com

RADIOLOGIC CLINICS OF NORTH AMERICA Volume 46, Number 1
January 2008 ISSN: 0033-8389; ISBN-13: 978-1-4160-5119-0; ISBN-10: 1-4160-5119-8

Editor: Barton Dudlick

Reprints: For copies of 100 or more, of articles in this publication, please contact the Commercial Reprints Department, Elsevier Inc., 360 Park Avenue South, New York, New York 10010-1710. Tel.: (+1) 212-633-3813; Fax: (+1) 212-462-1935; E-mail: reprints@elsevier.com.

The ideas and opinions expressed in *Radiologic Clinics of North America* do not necessarily reflect those of the Publisher does not assume any responsibility for any injury and/or damage to persons or property arising out of or related to any use of the material contained in this periodical. The reader is advised to check the appropriate medical literature and the product information currently provided by the manufacturer of each drug to be administered to verify the dosage, the method and duration of administration, or contraindications, It is the responsibility of the treating physician or other health care professional, relying on independent experience and knowledge of the patient, to determine drug dosages and the best treatment for the patient. Mention of any product in this issue should not be construed as endorsement by the contributiors, editors, or the Publisher of the productor manufacturers' claims.

Radiologic Clinics of North America (ISSN 0033-8389) is published bimonthly in January, March, May, July, September, and November by Elsevier Inc., 360 Park Avenue South, New York, NY 10010-1710. Business and editorial offices: 1600 John F. Kenedy Boulevard, Suite 1800, Philadelphia, Pennsylvania 19103-2899. Customer Service Office: 6277 Sea Harbor Drive, Orlando, FL 32887-4800. Periodicals postage paid at New York, NY, and additional mailing offices. Subscription prices are USD 290 per year for US individuals, USD 431 per year for US institutions, USD 142 per year for US students and residents, USD 339 per year for Canadian individuals, USD 530 per year of Canadian institutions, USD 394 per year for international individuals, USD 530 per year for international institutions, and USD 192 per year for Canadian and foreign students/residents. To receive student and resident rate, orders must be accompanied by name of affiliated institution, date of term, and the signature of program/residency coordinatior on institution letterhead. Orders will be billed at individual rate until proof of status is received. Foreign air speed delivery is included in all Clinics subscriptionprices. All prices are subject to change without notice. **POSTMASTER:** Send address changes to *Radiologic Clinics of North America,* Elsevier Journals Customer Service, 6277 Sea Harbor Drive, Orlando, FL 32887-4800. **Customer Service: 1-800-654-2452 (US). From outside of the US, call (+1) 407-563-6020. Fax: 407-363-9661. E-mail: JournalsCustomerService-usa@elsevier.com.**

Radiologic Clinics of North America also published in Greek Paschalidis Medical Publications, Athens, Greece.

Radiologic Clinics of North America is covered in *Index Medicus, EMBASE/Excerpta Medica, Current Contents/Life Sciences, Current Contents/Clinical Medicine, RSNA Index to Imaging Literature, BIOSIS, Science Citation Index,* and *ISI/BIOMED.*

Printed in the United States of America.

GENITOURINARY TRACT IMAGING

GUEST EDITORS

MICHAEL A. BLAKE, MRCPI, FFR(RCSI), FRCR
Assistant Professor of Radiology, Harvard Medical School; and Department of Radiology, Division of Abdominal Imaging and Intervention, Massachusetts General Hospital, Boston, Massachusetts

MANNUDEEP K. KALRA, MD
Clinical Fellow, Department of Radiology, Massachusetts General Hospital, Boston, Massachusetts

CONTRIBUTORS

MICHAEL A. BLAKE, MRCPI, FFR(RCSI), FRCR
Assistant Professor of Radiology, Harvard Medical School; and Department of Radiology, Division of Abdominal Imaging and Intervention, Massachusetts General Hospital, Harvard Medical School, Boston, Massachusetts

GILES W. BOLAND, MD
Associate Professor of Radiology, Harvard Medical School; and Department of Radiology, Division of Abdominal Imaging and Intervention, Massachusetts General Hospital, Boston, Massachusetts

NEAL C. DALRYMPLE, MD
Department of Radiology, University of Texas Health Science Center at San Antonio, San Antonio, Texas

FIONA M. FENNESSY, MD, PhD
Assistant Professor of Radiology, Harvard Medical School; and Department of Radiology, Brigham and Women's Hospital, Boston, Massachusetts

ALAN J. FISCHMAN, MD, PhD
Division of Nuclear Medicine, Department of Radiology, Massachusetts General Hospital; and Professor of Radiology, Harvard Medical School, Boston, Massachusetts

JURGEN J. FÜTTERER, MD, PhD
Department of Radiology, University Medical Centre Nijmegen, Nijmegen, the Netherlands

DEBRA A. GERVAIS, MD
Associate Division Head, Division of Abdominal Imaging and Interventional Radiology, Department of Radiology, Massachusetts General Hospital; and

Associate Professor of Radiology, Harvard Medical School, Boston, Massachusetts

WEI HE, MD
Division of Nuclear Medicine, Department of Radiology, Massachusetts General Hospital; and Harvard Medical School, Boston, Massachusetts

STIJN W.T.P.J. HEIJMINK, MD
Department of Radiology, University Medical Centre Nijmegen, Nijmegen, the Netherlands

NAGARAJ-SETTY HOLALKERE, MD
Fellow in Radiology, Harvard Medical School; and Department of Radiology, Division of Abdominal Imaging and Intervention, Massachusetts General Hospital, Boston, Massachusetts

BOBBY KALB, MD
Department of Radiology, Emory University School of Medicine, Atlanta, Georgia

MANNUDEEP K. KALRA, MD
Clinical Fellow, Department of Radiology, Massachusetts General Hospital, Boston, Massachusetts

MICHAEL M. MAHER, MD, FRCSI, FFR(RSCI), FRCR
Professor, Departments of Radiology, Cork University Hospital, Wilton; and Mercy University Hospital and University College Cork, Cork, Ireland

DIEGO R. MARTIN, MD, PhD
Professor of Radiology and Director of MRI, Department of Radiology, Emory University School of Medicine, Atlanta, Georgia

SEAN E. McSWEENEY, MB, MRCSI, FFR(RSCI)
Departments of Radiology, Cork University
Hospital, Wilton; and Mercy University Hospital
and University College Cork, Cork, Ireland

PAUL R. MORRISON, MSc
Department of Radiology, Harvard Medical School,
Brigham and Women's Hospital, Boston,
Massachusetts

PETER R. MUELLER, MD
Division Head, Division of Abdominal Imaging
and Interventional Radiology, Department of
Radiology, Massachusetts General Hospital; and
Professor of Radiology, Harvard Medical School,
Boston, Massachusetts

OWEN J. O'CONNOR, MD, MRCSI
Departments of Radiology, Cork University
Hospital, Wilton; and Mercy University Hospital
and University College Cork, Cork, Ireland

SRINIVASA R. PRASAD, MD
Department of Radiology, University of Texas
Health Science Center at San Antonio, San Antonio,
Texas

DUSHYANT V. SAHANI, MD
Director of CT, Department of Radiology, Division
of Abdominal Imaging and Intervention,
Massachusetts General Hospital; and Associate
Professor, Harvard Medical School, Boston,
Massachusetts

KHALIL SALMAN, MD
Department of Radiology, Emory University School
of Medicine, Atlanta, Georgia

PUNEET SHARMA, PhD
Department of Radiology, Emory University School
of Medicine, Atlanta, Georgia

ANAND K. SINGH, MD
Research Fellow, Department of Radiology,
Division of Abdominal Imaging and Intervention,
Massachusetts General Hospital, Boston,
Massachusetts

SARABJEET SINGH, MBBS, MMST
Research Fellow, Department of Radiology,
Massachusetts General Hospital, Boston,
Massachusetts

J. ROAN SPERMON, MD, PhD
Department of Urology, University Medical Centre
Nijmegen, Nijmegen, the Netherlands

VENKATESWAR R. SURABHI, MD
Department of Radiology, University of Texas
Health Science Center at San Antonio, San Antonio,
Texas

CLARE M. TEMPANY, MD
Professor of Radiology, Harvard Medical School;
and Department of Radiology, Brigham and
Women's Hospital, Boston, Massachusetts

KEMAL TUNCALI, MD
Instructor in Radiology, Harvard Medical School;
and Department of Radiology, Brigham and
Women's Hospital, Boston, Massachusetts

RAUL N. UPPOT, MD
Assistant Radiologist, Division of Abdominal
Imaging and Interventional Radiology, Department
of Radiology, Massachusetts General Hospital; and
Instructor of Radiology, Harvard Medical School,
Boston, Massachusetts

JOHN R. VATOW, PhD
Department of Radiology, Emory University School
of Medicine, Atlanta, Georgia

GENITOURINARY TRACT IMAGING

Volume 46 · Number 1 · January 2008

Contents

reduced morbidity and mortality. Elucidation of specific oncologic pathways in renal cell carcinomas has led to the development of molecularly targeted therapies. The critical role of cross-sectional imaging techniques in the diagnosis, surveillance, and management of patients who have renal masses continues to expand.

Hematuria may have a number of causes, of which the more common are urinary tract calculi, urinary tract infection, urinary tract neoplasms (including renal cell carcinoma and urothelial tumors), trauma to the urinary tract, and renal parenchymal disease. This article discusses the current status of imaging of patients suspected of having urologic causes of hematuria. The role of all modalities, including plain radiography, intravenous urography or excretory urography, retrograde pyelography, ultrasonography, and multidetector computed tomography (MDCT) in evaluation of these patients is discussed. The article highlights the current status of MDCT urography in imaging of patients with hematuria, and discusses various-often controversial-issues, such as optimal protocol design, accuracy of the technique in imaging of the urothelium, and the significant issue of radiation dose associated with MDCT urography.

The male reproductive system encompasses several organs: the testes, ejaculatory ducts, seminal vesicles, prostate, and penis. The function of this system is to accomplish reproduction. Diagnostic imaging modalities, such as ultrasound, CT, MR imaging, and positron emission tomography (PET), are increasingly used to evaluate the male reproductive tract. The purpose of this review is to provide an overview of the use of imaging techniques in the male reproductive tract and to discuss current trends and future directions in prostate and testicular imaging. This review focuses on the prostate and scrotum.

MR imaging-guided interventions are well established in routine patient care in many parts of the world. There are many approaches, depending on magnet design and clinical need, based on MR imaging providing excellent inherent tissue contrast without ionizing radiation risk for patients. MR imaging- guided minimally invasive therapeutic procedures have advantages over conventional surgical procedures. In the genitourinary tract, MR imaging guidance has a role in tumor detection, localization, and staging and can provide accurate image guidance for minimally invasive procedures. The advent of molecular and metabolic imaging and use of higher strength magnets likely will improve diagnostic accuracy and allow targeted therapy to maximize disease control and minimize side effects.

GOAL STATEMENT

The goal of the *Radiologic Clinics of North America* is to keep practicing radiologists and radiology residents up to date with current clinical practice in radiology by providing timely articles reviewing the state of the art in patient care.

ACCREDITATION

The *Radiologic Clinics of North America* is planned and implemented in accordance with the Essential Areas and Policies of the Accreditation Council for Continuing Medical Education (ACCME) through the joint sponsorship of the University of Virginia School of Medicine and Elsevier. The University of Virginia School of Medicine is accredited by the ACCME to provide continuing medical education for physicians.

The University of Virginia School of Medicine designates this educational activity for a maximum of 15 *AMA PRA Category 1 Credits*™. Physicians should only claim credit commensurate with the extent of their participation in the activity.

The American Medical Association has determined that physicians not licensed in the US who participate in this CME activity are eligible for 15 *AMA PRA Category 1 Credits*™.

Credit can be earned by reading the text material, taking the CME examination online at http://www.theclinics.com/home/cme, and completing the evaluation. After taking the test, you will be required to review any and all incorrect answers. Following completion of the test and evaluation, your credit will be awarded and you may print your certificate.

FACULTY DISCLOSURE/CONFLICT OF INTEREST

The University of Virginia School of Medicine, as an ACCME accredited provider, endorses and strives to comply with the Accreditation Council for Continuing Medical Education (ACCME) Standards of Commercial Support, Commonwealth of Virginia statutes, University of Virginia policies and procedures, and associated federal and private regulations and guidelines on the need for disclosure and monitoring of proprietary and financial interests that may affect the scientific integrity and balance of content delivered in continuing medical education activities under our auspices.

The University of Virginia School of Medicine requires that all CME activities accredited through this institution be developed independently and be scientifically rigorous, balanced and objective in the presentation/discussion of its content, theories and practices.

All authors/editors participating in an accredited CME activity are expected to disclose to the readers relevant financial relationships with commercial entities occurring within the past 12 months (such as grants or research support, employee, consultant, stock holder, member of speakers bureau, etc.). The University of Virginia School of Medicine will employ appropriate mechanisms to resolve potential conflicts of interest to maintain the standards of fair and balanced education to the reader. Questions about specific strategies can be directed to the Office of Continuing Medical Education, University of Virginia School of Medicine, Charlottesville, Virginia.

The authors/editors listed below have identified no financial or professional relationships for themselves or their spouse/partner:
Michael A. Blake, MRCPI, FFR(RCSI), FRCR (Guest Editor); Giles W. Boland, MD; Neal C. Dalrymple, MD; Barton Dudlick (Acquisitions Editor); Fiona M. Fennessy, MD, PhD; Alan J. Fischman, MD, PhD; Jurgen J. Fütterer, MD, PhD; Wei He, MD; Stijn W.T.P.J. Heijmink, MD; Nagaraj-Setty Holalkere, MD; Mannudeep K. Kalra, MD (Guest Editor); Michael M. Maher, MD, FRCSI, FRR(RCSI), FRCR; Sean E. McSweeney, MB, MRCSI, FFR(RCSI); Paul R. Morrison, MSc; Owen J. O'Connor, MD, MRCSI; Srinivasa R. Prasad, MD; Khalil Salman, MD; Puneet Sharma, PhD; Anand K. Singh, MD; Sarabjeet Singh, MBBS, MMST; Jesse Roan Spermon, MD, PhD; Venkateswar R. Surabhi, MD; Kemal Tuncali, MD; Raul N. Uppot, MD; and John R. Votaw, PhD.

The authors/editors listed below have identified the following financial or professional relationships for themselves or their spouse/partner:
Debra A. Gervais, MD is an independent contractor and serves on the Speaker's bureau for Covidien (formerly Valleylab).
Bobby Kalb, MD has received a Bracco Clinical Translational Body MRI Training Award.
Diego R. Martin, MD, PhD performs investigator initiated research for Siemens Medical Systems, General Electric, Bracco Diagnostics, and Berlex.
Peter R. Mueller, MD is a consultant for Cook.
Dushyant V. Sahani, MD has a research agreement with GE Healthcare, and serves as a speaker for Bracco Diagnostics.
Clare M. Tempany, MD is an independent contractor for NIH and a consultant for Insightec, Inc.

Disclosure of Discussion of Non-FDA Approved Uses for Pharmaceutical and/or Medical Devices:
The University of Virginia School of Medicine, as an ACCME provider, requires that all authors identify and disclose any "off label" uses for pharmaceutical and medical device products. The University of Virginia School of Medicine recommends that each physician fully review all the available data on new products or procedures prior to clinical use.

TO ENROLL

To enroll in the *Radiologic Clinics of North America* Continuing Medical Education program, call customer service at 1-800-654-2452 or sign up online at http://www.theclinics.com/home/cme. The CME program is available to subscribers for an additional annual fee USD 205.

RADIOLOGIC CLINICS OF NORTH AMERICA

Radiol Clin N Am 46 (2008) xi–xii

Preface

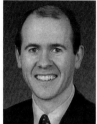
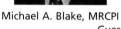
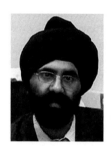

Michael A. Blake, MRCPI   Mannudeep K. Kalra, MD
Guest Editors

Michael A. Blake, MRCPI, FFR(RCSI), FRCR
Department of Radiology
Massachusetts General Hospital
55 Fruit Street
Boston, MA 02114, USA

E-mail address:
mblake2@partners.org (M.A. Blake)

Mannudeep K. Kalra, MD
Department of Radiology
Massachusetts General Hospital
55 Fruit Street
Boston, MA 02114, USA

E-mail address:
mkalra@partners.org (M.K. Kalra)

Recent technical advances and novel discoveries, both of benefits and, indeed, of adverse effects, combine to make this an exciting but challenging time for genitourinary (GU) imaging. All GU modalities have benefited from technological developments, although some more than others; for example, the intravenous pyelogram yielding much of its former preeminent role to CT. However, all radiation-based modalities must now contend with much more stringent expectations of radiation dose optimization. Technologic advances are helping to meet some of these issues, as Drs. Kalra, Singh, and Blake discuss in their article entitled "CT of the Urinary Tract: Turning Attention to Radiation Dose." MR imaging faces new challenges too, including the recent discovery of the association between certain gadolinium agents in the setting of renal failure and the systemic condition of nephrogenic systemic fibrosis. This challenge is discussed along with the many other important MR considerations and developments in the articles devoted to MR imag-

ing, including the one focusing on "Magnetic Resonance Nephrourography: Current and Developing Techniques" by Drs. Kalb, Votaw, Salman, Sharma, and Martin.

Nuclear medicine procedures are also constantly in evolution, and are finding greater and greater applications in nephrology and urology. Radionuclide imaging of the GU tract has become an invaluable asset to clinicians in the evaluation of renal parenchyma and urologic abnormalities. This role is highlighted by Drs. He and Fischman in their "Nuclear Imaging in the Genitourinary Tract: Recent Advances and Future Directions" article. Developments in imaging have helped fuel the increasingly impressive contribution of interventional radiology to the optimal management of patients who have GU system disorders. Drs. Uppot, Gervais, and Mueller provide their overview of the current status of GU intervention.

The small size of the adrenal gland belies its critical importance in medicine. Imaging of the

doi:10.1016/j.rcl.2008.02.001

adrenal gland has made tremendous strides in the last decade as new technologies continue to evolve. Drs. Blake, Holalkere, and Boland emphasize the pertinent anatomic and physiologic imaging principles that underpin both the current major adrenal imaging modalities as well as the promising new techniques that are becoming available. Drs. Singh and Sahani demonstrate how, with the many advances in imaging modalities along with upgrades in image postprocessing, meticulous renal donor selection and early detection of renal transplant complications are now possible. The critical role of cross-sectional imaging techniques in the diagnosis, surveillance, and management of patients with renal masses also continues to expand as Drs. Prasad, Dalrymple, and Surabhi discuss in "Cross-Sectional Imaging Evaluation of Renal Masses."

Drs. O'Connor, McSweeney, and Maher review the role of all radiologic modalities in their article "Imaging of Hematuria." They highlight the current status of multidetector computed tomography urography (MDCTU) in imaging of patients who have hematuria and discuss various, often controversial issues such as optimal protocol design, accuracy of the technique in imaging of the urothelium, and again the significant issue of

radiation dose associated with MDCTU. Drs. Fütterer, Heijmink, and Spermon, in "Imaging the Male Reproductive Tract: Current Trends and Future Directions," provide an overview of the use of imaging techniques in the male reproductive tract. They discuss current trends and future directions in prostate and testicular imaging, including the development of lymph node imaging with ultra small iron-oxide particles. The issue concludes with Dr. Fennessy and colleagues Tuncali, Morrison, and Tempany sharing their insight into the applications of MR GU intervention in their review "MR Imaging-Guided Interventions in the Genitourinary Tract: An Evolving Concept."

Overall, this issue on genitourinary tract imaging focuses on the current state-of-the-art radiology of the GU system. We are very grateful to our distinguished GU imaging experts for their important contributions, which highlight the current trends and future directions in genitourinary tract imaging. We are also very thankful to Elsevier for giving us this opportunity, to all of the *Radiologic Clinics of North America* staff who assisted us, and, in particular, to Barton Dudlick, Beth Howley, and Theresa Collier for all of their generous help and support.

RADIOLOGIC
CLINICS
OF NORTH AMERICA

Radiol Clin N Am 46 (2008) 1–9

ELSEVIER
SAUNDERS

CT of the Urinary Tract: Turning Attention to Radiation Dose

Mannudeep K. Kalra, MD*, Sarabjeet Singh, MBBS, MMST,
Michael A. Blake, MRCPI, FFR(RCSI), FRCR

- CT: revolutionary evolution
- Radiation risks
- Management of radiation dose
  *Appropriateness of CT in imaging
  the urinary tract*
- *Standardization of CT protocols
  for urinary tract evaluation*
- Education
- Summary
- References

Imaging plays an important role in the evaluation of patients who have genitourinary tract ailments. Ultrasonography, CT, and MR imaging are now the chief workhorses for urinary tract imaging. Enhanced by remarkable improvements in both hardware and software within the last decade, CT has become the imaging modality of choice for a variety of urinary pathologies (although MR imaging continues to challenge some of these applications). Positron emission tomography (PET)-CT recently has emerged as an important modality for imaging of female genital tract malignancies, although its applications in the urinary tract are still limited. The benefits of these advances have been undeniable [1,2], but controversies have emerged over the possible overuse of these imaging modalities. In particular, concerns involve over rising costs and radiation risks, particularly with CT scanning [3].

In the past decade, developments in CT technology have changed the way urinary tract imaging is performed. The risks of radiation dose to the patient associated with CT scanning should not be ignored, however. This article reviews the issues surrounding the radiation dose to patients associated with CT imaging of the urinary tract.

CT: revolutionary evolution

From step-and-shoot conventional CT scanners, the introduction first of helical CT technology and then of multidetector-row CT scanners in the late 1990s and early 2000s brought about changes in imaging of the urinary tract. The introduction of multidetector-row CT scanners has two notable effects: improved scan coverage and enhanced temporal resolution [2]. Although the improvements in temporal resolution with multidetector-row CT scanners have had greatest effect on cardiac and vascular imaging, these improvements also have made it possible to evaluate the entire urinary tract in a short, single breath-hold. Faster scanners help minimize motion and stair-step artifacts and allow acquisition of a well-timed multiphase CT volume data for high-quality three-dimensional reformats [4]. In addition, the improvement in the detector configurations used for multidetector-row CT scanners permits acquisition of 4 to up to 320 slices per rotations. The United States Food and Drug Administration (FDA) has approved 4-slice through single- and dual-source 64-slice multidetector-row CT scanners for clinical purposes; other scanners are confined mainly to research applications and

Department of Radiology, Massachusetts General Hospital, 55 Fruit St., Boston, MA 02114, USA
* Corresponding author. 25 New Chardon St., Suite 400, Boston, MA 02114.
E-mail address: mkalra@partners.org (M.K. Kalra).

0033-8389/08/$ – see front matter © 2008 Elsevier Inc. All rights reserved.   doi:10.1016/j.rcl.2008.01.002
radiologic.theclinics.com

await data demonstrating their safety and clinical relevance. These scanners image a wider area of interest per gantry rotation at isotropic resolution, mainly through their improved z-axis resolution over conventional step-and-shoot and single-slice helical predecessors. Thus, thinner slices can be acquired over the entire area of interest in a single breath-hold for fewer partial-volume average artifacts and superior three-dimensional reformats.

Some multidetector-row CT systems also have a wider gantry aperture and higher gantry table capacity to accommodate patients weighing more than 500 pounds or 250 kg [5,6]. These scanners allow the imaging of morbidly obese patients, who are difficult to assess with earlier CT scanners and with other available imaging techniques such as ultrasound and MR imaging.

For imaging obese patients, the recently introduced dual-source multidetector-row CT may offer some advantages. The system uses data acquired simultaneously from two x-ray tubes and two detector arrays mounted orthogonally on a single gantry system. The use of two x-ray tubes at their full power $(80 + 80 = 160 \text{ kW})$ may help improve image quality by reducing noise and streak artifacts from photon starvation in the patient with a large body habitus. Indeed, preliminary phantom studies suggest that dual-source CT may help in imaging of obese patients [6]. The ability to combine the attenuation data from two x-ray sources into one image dataset improves the temporal resolution for the system by about twofold. It is unclear at present, however, how this development will affect urinary tract imaging.

In addition, the two x-ray tubes in dual-source CT scanners also can be used at two different tube potentials (kilovoltage or kVp [kilovolt, peak]), which offer opportunities for tissue characterization with dual energy [7]. Although dual kVp CT has been assessed and used for more than a decade, the opportunity of simultaneously acquiring differential energy CT images is new and has attracted renewed attention. Dual-energy CT has been used in prior studies for characterization of liver lesions, quantification of fatty liver, and characterization of pulmonary nodules [8–10]. There now are some initial data on the role of dual-energy or kVp imaging in urinary tract CT [11,12]. Accurate determination of the chemical composition of urinary stones is still in an experimental stage, with most data coming from phantom studies using dual-energy CT technique. Prior studies with single-slice helical CT showed that dual-energy CT can help differentiate composition of uric acid, struvite, and calcium oxalate stones [13]. In a recent anthropomorphic phantom model with multiple stone types, it was reported that dual-energy CT

could discriminate uric acid stones from other stone types accurately [11]. Although these phantom studies offer some evidence that dual-energy CT can characterize the type of renal calculi, it remains to be seen whether dual-energy CT will be helpful in clinical settings for characterizing renal stones or for differentiating simple benign renal cysts from more ominous, enhancing renal lesions.

At least two vendors have released plans for development of the 256- and 320-slice multidetector-row CT scanners. These scanners offer 12- to 16-cm coverage per gantry rotation, which suggests that the entire kidney or pelvis can be scanned in about 0.5 second or less. As with the dual-source CT, the use of these scanners in urinary tract evaluation has not been assessed specifically. It is expected that these scanners will help in acquiring entire-organ imaging in subsecond durations, thus making possible entire-organ perfusion studies with extended coverage. Prospective studies will be needed to assess if these scanners will have any role in imaging patients who have urinary tract diseases, particularly those who have renal masses and complex arteriovenous malformations.

CT perhaps is the most rapidly evolving imaging modality. In this rapid evolutionary process, however, in which the development of technology precedes the definition of clinical applications, few prospective studies have been performed to assess the appropriate indications for CT use and the associated radiation dose.

Radiation risks

Radiation scientists and physicists have used data from the Hiroshima and Nagasaki atomic explosions to support the belief that the linear nonthreshold theory for radiation-induced carcinogenesis is valid also at the low radiation doses associated with CT scanning [1,14,15]. These investigators contend that CT scanning will contribute to a greater incidence of cancer in the future. Others, however, disagree about the applicability of such data to CT scanning [16–18]. They point out that, whereas the data from atomic explosions reflect a single exposure, patients are exposed to effects of cumulative radiation doses from repeat or follow-up CT scanning. Also, they contend that biologic response to particulate exposure from the former atomic explosions may not be similar to the response to x-ray exposure from CT scanning. A prime argument is that the benefits of CT scanning may far outweigh the potential risk of radiation-induced cancer.

Although a prospective, controlled study of the risks of CT radiation versus the benefits of the clinical information derived from CT scanning might provide an answer to these concerns, such a study would be difficult to perform. Much attention therefore has turned toward the overuse of CT scanning in modern clinical practice. There are no formal studies, but proponents of the linear nonthreshold theory argue that almost one third of all CT studies in the United States lack appropriate indications [1]. Thus, until a consensus is achieved about what does and does not constitute an appropriate indication for CT scanning in the context of a particular patient's age, gender, clinical complaints, and available practical therapeutic and management options, most governmental and nongovernmental authorities and scientific organizations agree that radiology departments must keep the radiation dose associated with CT scanning at a level that is as low as reasonably achievable (ALARA) [19–21]. This safeguard is especially important because, although CT scans represent only 10% of all radiology examinations, more than two thirds of the total radiation dose from all medical diagnostic procedures comes from CT examinations [22,23].

Management of radiation dose

Having justified the need for continued surveillance and optimization of the radiation dose associated with CT scanning, the discussion now turns to the management of the radiation dose of CT scanning. The discussion looks at three aspects of management: appropriateness, standardization, and education.

Appropriateness of CT in imaging the urinary tract

Henry David Thoreau, an American author and philosopher of the nineteenth century, stated "If a man is alive, there is always *danger* that he may die, though the danger must be allowed to be less in proportion as he is dead-and-alive to begin with. A man sits as many risks as he runs." Radiologists and physicians need to understand how this quotation relates to evaluating the benefits and risks for given clinical indications before proceeding with CT scanning.

Rising health care costs and increasing radiation doses from CT have given rise to concerns about over- and inappropriate use of CT in modern medical practice [1]. Although there are no generalizable scientific data on the extent of its overuse, some authors claim that about 30% to 50% of all CT examinations are medically unnecessary [1,24]. Others have used natural language processing software to assess the yield of radiology reports for important findings [25]. These authors state that about 25% of CT reports do not have significant findings. Their database, however, was limited to radiology reports from a single institution. Furthermore, the natural language processing software does not account for CT examinations that are performed to rule out conditions as opposed to rule in or confirm lesions. In some circumstances, CT examinations that these software programs label "negative for important findings" are as important as those labeled "positive for important findings."

Although there are no actual tracking or monitoring systems in place for measuring the actual use of CT, inferences about the use of CT scanning in the United States can be drawn from surveys such as those performed by FDA as part of the Nationwide Evaluation of X-ray Trends in 2000 and 2001. According to this survey, about 58 million CT studies were performed in the United States in the year 2000. Although these numbers are estimated and projected, they clearly highlight the burden of radiation dose from CT.

Efforts must be directed toward determining the appropriateness of the indications for CT examinations [26]. The American College of Radiology has proposed guidelines to assist radiologists and physicians determine the appropriateness of radiology examinations for different indications, including those for urinary tract evaluation [26]. Recent reports also have suggested that decision-support programs can assist physicians and radiologists in ordering radiology examinations [27,28]. Initial clinical experience using an intranet radiology order entry with a decision-support program suggested a decrease in low-utility examinations from 6% to 2% [28].

Likewise, attention must be paid to the appropriateness of the clinical indications for CT examinations of the urinary tract (Box 1). In particular, close attention must be paid to the frequent use of CT for evaluation or follow-up of benign and non–life-threatening urinary tract lesions.

Standardization of CT protocols for urinary tract evaluation

Factors that may contribute to the delivery of high radiation doses from CT evaluation of the urinary tract include the replacement of conventional radiography with CT, the need for multiple follow-up CT studies, and the need for multiphase CT protocols.

Replacement of conventional radiography

Multidetector CT scanning has replaced conventional radiography for the evaluation of patients who have acute flank pain and urinary tract calculi because of its greater sensitivity and accuracy in the detection, localization, characterization, follow-up, assessment of treatment response, and prediction of stone burden. CT, however, is associated with much higher radiation doses than conventional

Urinary colic
Hematuria
Urinary tract calculi

- Detection
- Stone burden
- ? Stone type
- Treatment decisions

Urinary tract infections

- Complications
- Nonresponsive
- Xanthogranulomatous pyelonephritis
- Emphysematous pyelonephritis
- Renal or perirenal infection

Urinary tract neoplasm

- Detection
- Characterization
- Staging
- Posttreatment follow-up—recurrent or residual lesions
- Planning nephron-sparing surgery
- Image-guided ablation procedure

Congenital anomalies
Renal donor imaging
Renal artery stenosis
Urinary tract trauma

radiography. Likewise, in many institutions CT has largely replaced intravenous urography for the evaluation of patients who have hematuria, although, again, it is associated with greater radiation dose.

Need for multiple follow-up CT studies

Katz and colleagues [29] have reported that patients who have nephrolithiasis are at a greater risk of having follow-up CT studies, leading to potentially high cumulative effective doses. In this study, the mean effective doses for a single-stone protocol study using single-row helical CT and multidetector-row CT scanners were 6.5 and 8.5 mSv, respectively. In this study about 4% of patients had three or more CT examinations with cumulative radiation doses between 19.5 and 153.7 mSv.

Need for multiphase CT

With the exception of stone protocol CT, most CT protocols for urinary tract evaluation are multiphase acquisitions with two to four phases. If all scan parameters are held identical, a four-phase CT exposes patients to a fourfold higher radiation dose. CT scanning for evaluation of renal masses and hematuria and for renal donors usually is performed using multiphase protocols, increasing the radiation dose substantially.

These considerations make it important to standardize CT protocols for urinary tract evaluation. Protocols must be standardized with an understanding of the image quality needed for a given clinical indication and the effect of different modifiable scan parameters on image quality and radiation dose (Box 2). The basic principles for image quality and management of radiation dose in CT scanning for urinary tract evaluation are the same as for those for other regions of the body.

The two most important determinants of image quality related to the radiation dose are image noise or graininess and image contrast. Image noise is inversely related to radiation dose. In general, images obtained at lower radiation doses have greater image noise; images obtained with higher radiation doses have less noise. The increased noise of images obtained with low-radiation-dose CT can affect the ability to differentiate low-contrast lesions and to evaluate subtle characteristics of lesions [19]. On the other hand, the imaging of high-contrast lesions such as kidney stones or the evaluation of structures with high contrast such as contrast-enhanced blood vessels or ureters generally is not compromised excessively by the high image noise obtained with low-radiation-dose CT.

The foremost consideration in the management of CT-associated radiation dose is the realization that children are at much greater risk from CT radiation than adults and elderly persons [19,24]. Therefore, greater priority must be given to

Tube current: most commonly used parameter to adjust radiation dose

- Manual selection of fixed tube current
- Automatic exposure control

    Angular modulation
    Longitudinal or z-axis modulation
    Combined modulation
    ECG-controlled modulation (for cardiac CT)

Tube potential
Scan length
Number of phases acquired
Pitch, table speed, and detector configuration
Gantry rotation time
Prospective reconstructed section thickness
Reconstruction kernel
Noise-reduction filters
Shields: in-plane and out-of-plane shields for dose reduction

optimizing the radiation dose in children. Adult protocols must never be used in pediatric CT, because at a given radiation dose children are at much higher risk of cancer than adults. Efforts must be directed first toward assessing the appropriateness of a CT examination for the clinical indication and the availability of other non–radiation-based imaging tests to answer the clinical query. Finally, attempts must be made to reduce radiation dose for children by modifying scan parameters so that, regardless of the clinical indication, they receive less radiation dose than adults. For children the radiation dose can be reduced by using lower tube current and by using CT protocols with fewer phases.

Fortunately, CT vendors have taken the call for radiation dose reduction seriously and have put efforts into optimizing the dose while maintaining and improving applications of their systems [19,30]. In modern CT scanners better detector configurations, scanner speed, automatic exposure control techniques, prepatient x-ray beam collimation, noise-reduction filters, and prepatient bow tie and other physical x-ray beam filters have been developed and deployed to reduce the radiation dose [19].

To improve the image quality of low-radiation-dose CT, noise-reduction filters also have been used [31–36]. These noise-reduction filters are postprocessing software that manipulate and decrease image noise. Thus filters help convert low-radiation-dose images with greater noise so that they resemble images with less image noise. Although initial noise-reduction filters compromised image contrast and sharpness [32], more recent three-dimensional nonlinear noise-reduction filters reduce image noise without sacrificing image contrast or lesion conspicuity [36]. Noise-reduction filters can be applied to noisier images either at the CT console or in the network between CT console and picture archiving and communication system workstations [31].

Among scan parameters, adjustment of tube current has been the cornerstone for most studies of radiation-dose optimization, including those related to urinary tract CT. A 50% reduction in tube current implies a 50% reduction in radiation dose, provided that the other scanning parameters and scan length are kept constant. Tube current can be adjusted either manually or by an automatic exposure control. For manual adjustment of the tube current, the operator selects a fixed tube current according to the clinical indication or patient size. Radiation dose is directly proportional to the applied tube current if all other scanning parameters are kept constant. Thus, the use of lower tube current is associated with a lower radiation dose; higher tube current entails the use of a higher radiation dose. Prior studies have reported significant reductions in radiation dose with the use of lower tube current for scanning, particularly for renal calculi [36–38]. The use of weight- or size-based tube current for optimizing the radiation dose in abdominal CT also has been described [39]. On the other hand, Kalra and colleagues [37] used automatic exposure control to optimize the radiation dose for CT scanning of the urinary tract. This technique modulates tube current to a specified image quality for the given patient size and body region being scanned. Compared with fixed tube current scanning, automatic exposure control resulted in a 43% to 66% reduction in radiation dose for the stone protocol CT.

The use of low kVp or tube potential also can reduce the radiation dose associated with CT scanning. CT scanning at lower kVp has been used for children, in whom, because of their small size, acceptable image quality can be obtained with even a low-energy x-ray beam. Lower kVp CT also is helpful in the evaluation of renal donors undergoing renal CT angiography. Caution must be used in reducing the tube potential in adults, particularly in those with large body habitus, because increased image noise and streak artifacts can adversely affect the diagnostic acceptability of the study.

Scan length is another important determinant of radiation dose to patients undergoing CT scanning. Radiation dose is directly proportional to the scan length. Studies have shown that most technologists have a tendency to extend the scan beyond the intended or desired body region of interest, thereby increasing the radiation dose to patient [40]. Therefore, close attention must be paid to avoid extending the scan unnecessarily beyond the region of interest.

Another important aspect of urinary tract imaging related to the CT radiation dose is the prevalence of multiphase protocols. Except for protocols for urinary calculi, most renal protocols involve the acquisition of two or more phases. Efforts must be made to reduce the number of phases or to adapt scan parameters for one or more phases to reduce radiation dose. Again, the appropriateness of clinical indications for multiphase protocols should monitored closely to reduce the radiation dose from such protocols.

Knowledge of scanning parameters and available technology can help in tailoring radiation dose for specific protocols. Literature on radiation-dose reduction is available for three urinary tract CT protocols: evaluation of urinary tract calculi, hematuria (CT urography), and renal donors. The next sections review protocol-specific strategies for optimizing radiation dose.

Stone protocol CT

As stated earlier, high-contrast stones generally can be assessed on low-dose CT images with greater image noise. Therefore, several strategies have been used to reduce the radiation dose of stone protocol CT without sacrificing the conspicuity of urinary tract calculi. Adjusting tube current is the most commonly reported method for optimizing the radiation dose in stone protocol CT. Kim and colleagues [36] have reported that for renal calculi, CT can be performed with 81% dose, at 50 mAs instead of 260 mAs, without loss of conspicuity of renal calculi larger than 2 mm. In a recent publication, Poletti and colleagues [38] found no difference in conspicuity of renal calculi greater than or equal to 3 mm between 30 and 180 mAs CT images in patients with a body mass index of less than 30 kg/m^2. In larger patients, however, they noticed some decrease in the ability to detect renal calculi. The radiation dose for urinary calculi evaluation with standard-dose CT has been reported to be between 4.3 and 16.1 mSv [41]. With low-dose protocols, the radiation dose was decreased to 0.5 to 2.82 mSv in different studies [41]. Kluner and colleagues [41] also have reported that with use of 120 kVp, tube current as low as 10 mAs, and beam pitch of 1.43:1, the radiation dose can be reduced to 0.5 mSv for men and 0.7 mSv for women, equivalent to that of kidney-urinary-bladder radiography. Kalra and colleagues [37] also have reported a reduction in radiation dose of up to 66% with use of z-axis automatic exposure control compared with standard-dose CT performed with fixed tube current. Unlike manually selected tube current, automatic exposure control helps tailor low-dose protocols individually to patient size and body region, thus avoiding suboptimal image quality in patients who have large body habitus.

Thus, the use of nonoverlapping pitch, lower tube current, and low-radiation-dose settings in automatic exposure control techniques can help reduce the radiation dose associated with stone protocol CT.

CT urography

Higher radiation doses are associated with CT urography than with stone protocol CT, primarily because more than one phase is acquired for CT urography. Often up to four phases are acquired for CT urography studies, including noncontrast, corticomedullary, nephrographic, and excretory phases. If scanning parameters are not modified for the individual phases, the radiation dose can be four times greater than that associated with standard single-phase abdominal-pelvic CT.

Some studies have reported that a two-phase CT urography protocol can provide the information needed for the evaluation of patients who have hematuria [1,42,43]. These protocols include acquisition of a noncontrast CT phase to assess for urinary calculi and calcifications and a mixed nephrographic and excretory phase to assess renal parenchyma and urothelium. These protocols employ a split bolus of contrast media. After acquisition of images in the noncontrast phase, a small bolus of intravenous contrast agent is administered. Five to 10 minutes later a larger bolus of contrast agent is administered. Scanning starts 100 seconds after the administration of the second contrast bolus. In this way, a single postcontrast phase provides information that usually is acquired from two phases: the initial, smaller bolus provides information about the excretory phase, and the later, larger bolus provides information about the nephrographic phase [1,43]. The incidence of urothelial cancer in patients who have hematuria and who are less than 40 years old is lower; therefore, if urinary calculus is seen on an initial noncontrast CT, the postcontrast CT can be avoided, allowing a further, significant reduction in radiation dose [1,43].

Compared with three- or four-phase protocols, a two-phase CT urography can result in substantial dose reduction. Thus in multiphase CT protocols, attempts must be made to reduce the number of phases as well as to modify scanning parameters for the individual phases. For the noncontrast phase, the radiation dose must be reduced in stone protocol CT. In addition, for three- or four-phase CT protocols, dose reduction can be achieved by restricting the scan length to the region of interest (eg, scanning only the upper abdomen or the kidneys for the corticomedullary and nephrographic phases and scanning from the kidneys to the bladder for the excretory phase).

Renal donor imaging

As in CT urography, most CT protocols described for renal donor evaluation also involve high radiation doses because they comprise multiple phases (ie, noncontrast, arterial, venous, and excretory phases). Thus, studies on reducing radiation dose in renal donor protocol CT have concentrated mainly on reducing the number of phases. For example, Kawamoto and colleagues [44] and Namasivayam and colleagues [45] have reported that the venous phase can be omitted safely from the renal donor protocol, because most normal and anomalous renal venous anatomy can be assessed on arterial-phase images. Likewise, the noncontrast phase can be omitted because significant calculus disease can be appreciated on postcontrast images. A single localizer radiograph acquired after the venous phase can replace the excretory phase for assessment of the collecting system, ureters, and bladder.

Namasivayam and colleagues [46] have reported that renal donors can be assessed with a single phase acquired after administration of intravenous contrast agent. The authors described split-bolus contrast injection for simultaneous arterial and venous enhancement. For this protocol, Namasivayam and colleagues [47] also used 80 kVp to reduce the radiation dose further and to increase the differences in attenuation between arterial and venous structures. The excretory phase was replaced by a localizer radiograph acquired a few minutes after acquisition of the dynamic image data.

MR angiography can provide the information needed for evaluation of renal donors. Although MR angiography has a tremendous advantage over CT in terms of lack of radiation exposure, there presently are concerns about inadequate visualization of small anomalous vascular structures and urinary calculi with MR imaging.

Education

In recent years, heightened awareness and concerns about the radiation dose associated with CT scanning has affected the radiology and physics communities. In the United States, the major annual meetings of the Radiological Society of North America, the American Association of Physicists in Medicine, the American Roentgen Ray Society, and the Society of Pediatric Radiology have taken the lead in organizing and encouraging the presentation of educational seminars and scientific papers regarding the radiation dose associated with CT scanning. The recently convened American College of Radiology Blue Ribbon Panel on Radiation Dose in Medicine emphasized the need to increase further the knowledge of radiation dose issues in the radiology community [26]. The panel recommended several measures to enhance and enforce radiation-dose optimization, particularly in collaboration with referring physicians.

Presently, there is no active program to educate radiology residents or radiologists in interpreting images acquired at lower radiation doses. Such programs might pave the way for greater confidence among radiologists for lower-radiation-dose CT imaging.

Summary

In summary, CT has replaced radiography and intravenous urography for most applications and is preferred to ultrasound and MR imaging for the evaluation of several urinary tract abnormalities. Integration of anatomic CT information with functional information from PET scans in hybrid PET/CT scanners has enhanced its stature in oncologic imaging further. Concerns remain, however, about the increasing use of CT and the risks of the collective radiation dose to the patients. Radiologists, along with all other responsible parties, must strive to optimize the radiation dose necessary for adequate imaging of patients who have urinary tract indications for CT.

References

[1] Maher MM, Kalra MK, Rizzo S, et al. Multidetector CT urography in imaging of the urinary tract in patients with hematuria. Korean J Radiol 2004;5(1):1–10.

[2] Kalra MK, Maher MM, D'Souza R, et al. Multidetector computed tomography technology: current status and emerging developments. J Comput Assist Tomogr 2004;28(Suppl 1):S2–6.

[3] Brenner DJ, Hall EJ. Computed tomography—an increasing source of radiation exposure. N Engl J Med 2007;357(22):2277–84.

[4] Maher MM, Kalra MK, Sahani DV, et al. Techniques, clinical applications and limitations of 3D reconstruction in CT of the abdomen. Korean J Radiol 2004;5(1):55–67.

[5] Flohr TG, Schoepf UJ, Ohnesorge BM. Chasing the heart: new developments for cardiac CT. J Thorac Imaging 2007;22(1):4–16.

[6] Kalra MK, Schmidt B, Suess C, et al. Comparison of single and dual source 64-channel MDCT scanners for evaluation of large patients: a phantom study. Radiological Society of North America; 2005. Available at: http://rsna2005.rsna.org/rsna2005/V2005/conference/event_display.cfm?em_id=4425786. Accessed November 30, 2007.

[7] Johnson TR, Krauss B, Sedlmair M, et al. Material differentiation by dual energy CT: initial experience. Eur Radiol 2007;17(6):1510–7.

[8] Raptopoulos V, Karellas A, Bernstein J, et al. Value of dual-energy CT in differentiating focal fatty infiltration of the liver from low-density masses. AJR Am J Roentgenol 1991;157(4):721–5.

[9] Wang B, Gao Z, Zou Q, et al. Quantitative diagnosis of fatty liver with dual-energy CT. An experimental study in rabbits. Acta Radiol 2003;44(1):92–7.

[10] Bhalla M, Shepard JA, Nakamura K, et al. Dual kV CT to detect calcification in solitary pulmonary nodule. J Comput Assist Tomogr 1995;19(1):44–7.

[11] Primak AN, Fletcher JG, Vrtiska TJ, et al. Noninvasive differentiation of uric acid versus non-uric acid kidney stones using dual-energy CT. Acad Radiol 2007;14(12):1441–7.

[12] Scheffel H, Stolzmann P, Frauenfelder T, et al. Dual-energy contrast-enhanced computed tomography for the detection of urinary stone disease. Invest Radiol 2007;42(12):823–9.

[13] Deveci S, Coşkun M, Tekin MI, et al. Spiral computed tomography: role in determination of chemical compositions of pure and mixed urinary stones—an in vitro study. Urology 2004;64(2):237–40.

[14] Pierce DA, Preston DL. Radiation-related cancer risks at low doses among atomic bomb survivors. Radiat Res 2000;154(2):178–86.

[15] Preston DL, Pierce DA, Shimizu Y, et al. Effect of recent changes in atomic bomb survivor dosimetry on cancer mortality risk estimates. Radiat Res 2004;162(4):377–89.

[16] Cohen BL. Cancer risk from low-level radiation. AJR Am J Roentgenol 2002;179(5):1137–43.

[17] Upton AC. Low-dose radiation: risks vs benefits. Postgrad Med 1981;70(6):34–7.

[18] Olivieri G. Adaptive response and its relationship to hormesis and low dose cancer risk estimation. Hum Exp Toxicol 1999;18(7):440–2.

[19] Kalra MK, Maher MM, Toth TL, et al. Strategies for CT radiation dose optimization. Radiology 2004;230(3):619–28.

[20] Rehani MM, Berry M. Radiation doses in computed tomography. The increasing doses of radiation need to be controlled. BMJ 2000; 320(7235):593–4.

[21] Paterson A, Frush DP. Dose reduction in paediatric MDCT: general principles. Clin Radiol 2007; 62(6):507–17.

[22] Wiest PW, Locken JA, Heintz PH, et al. CT scanning: a major source of radiation exposure. Semin Ultrasound CT MR 2002;23(5):402–10.

[23] Mettler FA Jr, Wiest PW, Locken JA, et al. CT scanning: patterns of use and dose. J Radiol Prot 2000;20(4):353–9.

[24] Frush DP. Pediatric CT: practical approach to diminish the radiation dose. Pediatr Radiol 2002; 32(10):714–7.

[25] Dreyer KJ, Kalra MK, Maher MM, et al. Application of recently developed computer algorithm for automatic classification of unstructured radiology reports: validation study. Radiology 2005; 234(2):323–9.

[26] Amis ES Jr, Butler PF, Applegate KE, et al. American College of Radiology. American College of Radiology white paper on radiation dose in medicine. J Am Coll Radiol 2007;4(5):272–84.

[27] Khorasani R. Clinical decision support in radiology: what is it, why do we need it, and what key features make it effective? J Am Coll Radiol 2006; 3(2):142–3.

[28] Rosenthal DI, Weilburg JB, Schultz T, et al. Radiology order entry with decision support: initial clinical experience. J Am Coll Radiol 2006; 3(10):799–806.

[29] Katz SI, Saluja S, Brink JA, et al. Radiation dose associated with unenhanced CT for suspected renal colic: impact of repetitive studies. AJR Am J Roentgenol 2006;186(4):1120–4.

[30] Kalra MK, Maher MM, Toth TL, et al. Techniques and applications of automatic tube current modulation for CT. Radiology 2004;233(3): 649–57.

[31] Kalra MK, Forsberg A, Shepard JA, et al. Radiation dose reduction. Noise reduction image filters can help. Radiological Society of North America; 2007. Available at: http://rsna2007.rsna.org/ rsna2007/V2007/conference/event_display.cfm? em_id=5010830. Accessed November 30, 2007.

[32] Kalra MK, Maher MM, Blake MA, et al. Detection and characterization of lesions on low-radiation-dose abdominal CT images postprocessed with noise reduction filters. Radiology 2004; 232(3):791–7.

[33] Kalra MK, Maher MM, Sahani DV, et al. Low-dose CT of the abdomen: evaluation of image improvement with use of noise reduction filters pilot study. Radiology 2003;228(1):251–6.

[34] Kalra MK, Wittram C, Maher MM, et al. Can noise reduction filters improve low-radiation-dose chest CT images? Pilot study. Radiology 2003;228(1):257–64.

[35] Rizzo SM, Kalra MK, Schmidt B, et al. CT images of abdomen and pelvis: effect of nonlinear three-dimensional optimized reconstruction algorithm on image quality and lesion characteristics. Radiology 2005;237(1):309–15.

[36] Kim BS, Hwang IK, Choi YW, et al. Low-dose and standard-dose unenhanced helical computed tomography for the assessment of acute renal colic: prospective comparative study. Acta Radiol 2005; 46(7):756–63.

[37] Kalra MK, Maher MM, D'Souza RV, et al. Detection of urinary tract stones at low-radiation-dose CT with z-axis automatic tube current modulation: phantom and clinical studies. Radiology 2005;235(2):523–9.

[38] Poletti PA, Platon A, Rutschmann OT, et al. Low-dose versus standard-dose CT protocol in patients with clinically suspected renal colic. AJR Am J Roentgenol 2007;188(4):927–33.

[39] Frush DP, Soden B, Frush KS, et al. Improved pediatric multidetector body CT using a size-based color-coded format. AJR Am J Roentgenol 2002; 178(3):721–6.

[40] Kalra MK, Maher MM, Toth TL, et al. Radiation from "extra" images acquired with abdominal and/or pelvic CT: effect of automatic tube current modulation. Radiology 2004;232(2):409–14.

[41] Kluner C, Hein PA, Gralla O, et al. Does ultra-low-dose CT with a radiation dose equivalent to that of KUB suffice to detect renal and ureteral calculi? J Comput Assist Tomogr 2006;30(1): 44–50.

[42] Chow LC, Kwan SW, Olcott EW, et al. Split-bolus MDCT urography with synchronous nephrographic and excretory phase enhancement. AJR Am J Roentgenol 2007;189(2):314–22.

[43] Kalra MK, Maher MM, Sahani DV, et al. Current status of multidetector computed tomography urography in imaging of the urinary tract. Curr Probl Diagn Radiol 2002;31(5):210–21.

[44] Kawamoto S, Lawler LP, Fishman EK. Evaluation of the renal venous system on late arterial and venous phase images with MDCT angiography in potential living laparoscopic renal donors. AJR Am J Roentgenol 2005;184(2):539–45.

[45] Namasivayam S, Kalra MK, Waldrop SM, et al. Multidetector row CT angiography of living

related renal donors: is there a need for venous phase imaging? Eur J Radiol 2006;59(3):442–52.

[46] Namasivayam S, Kalra M, Waldrop S, et al. Single phase mesenteric MDCT angiography using a split-bolus contrast injection technique: comparison with biphasic MDCT protocol using single bolus contrast injection. Radiological Society of North America; 2006. Available at: http://rsna2006.rsna.org/rsna2006/V2006/conference/event_display.cfm?em_id=4440796. Accessed November 30, 2007.

[47] Namasivayam S, Kalra M, Baumgarten D, et al. Evaluation of low tube potential (kVp) technique for MDCT angiography of renal donors. Radiological Society of North America; 2006. Available at: http://rsna2006.rsna.org/rsna2006/V2006/conference/event_display.cfm?em_id=4440931. Accessed November 30, 2007.

RADIOLOGIC
CLINICS
OF NORTH AMERICA

Radiol Clin N Am 46 (2008) 11–24

Magnetic Resonance Nephrourography: Current and Developing Techniques

Bobby Kalb, MD, John R. Votaw, PhD, Khalil Salman, MD, Puneet Sharma, PhD, Diego R. Martin, MD, PhD*

- Normal kidney
- MR nephrourography—structure
- MR nephrourography—function
- Imaging techniques
  Gadolinium-enhanced renal perfusion-distribution imaging
- Image analysis
- Calculation of single-kidney renal blood flow
- Calculation of single-kidney glomerular filtration rate

  Gadolinium systemic model, analysis of arterial curve
  Gadolinium kidney model, analysis of kidney curve
- Clinical applications
  Congenital anomalies and obstruction
  The transplanted kidney
- Limitations
- Summary
- References

The MR imaging techniques used for liver are well suited for renal analysis. A useful imaging protocol includes a combination of (1) breath-hold T2-weighted single-shot echo-train coronal and axial images, with at least one plane performed with fat suppression; (2) T1-weighted gradient echo (GRE) precontrast axial and coronal fat-suppressed images; and (3) T1-weighted gadolinium-enhanced arterial capillary– and delayed-phase images. T1-weighted imaging using newer three-dimensional (3D) GRE sequences (eg, 3D volumetric interpolated breath-hold examination [VIBE], T1-weighted fast acquisition multiple excitation [FAME], or 3D T1-weighted high resolution isotropic volume examination [THRIVE]), combined with gadolinium enhancement, has improved spatial resolution for resolving masses and vascular anatomy. T2-like imaging using breath-hold balanced echo true free-induction with steady-state precession (TFISP) imaging may provide additional information for urographic evaluation of the collecting system, with urine having high signal on such images. Additionally, acquisition of pre- and postcontrast 3D GRE images performed with identical field of view, resolution, and slice parameters allows the precontrast images to be used as a subtraction mask. The resultant image shows only areas of increased signal caused by gadolinium enhancement. This technique may be useful for determining vascularity and tumor within a high-signal protein- or blood-containing renal lesion.

Normal kidney

The advantages of MR multiplanar imaging are exploited by combining axial and coronal imaging, allowing optimal visualization of the renal

Bobby Kalb was supported in part by a Bracco Clinical Translational Body MRI Training Award.
Department of Radiology, Emory University School of Medicine, Building A, Suite AT622, Atlanta, GA 30322, USA
* Corresponding address.
E-mail address: dmartin@emory.edu (D.R. Martin).

doi:10.1016/j.rcl.2008.01.001

pelvis and poles (Fig. 1). The use of dynamic gadolinium-enhanced T1 imaging combined with rapid acquisition may be referred to as "functional MR nephrourography" (MRNU).

MR nephrourography—structure

In the past, obtaining both structural and functional data of the kidneys has not been possible without compromise involving one or both of these areas. With increasingly rapid image acquisition, however, MRNU offers the ability to capture simultaneously exquisite anatomic detail and physiologic data in parameters that have not been previously possible, even with traditional nuclear medicine techniques.

To obtain structural and functional renal data simultaneously, several imaging sequences are needed. T2-weighted images offer excellent morphologic evaluation of the kidneys and collecting system. The intrinsic signal characteristics of T2-bright urine contrast well with isointense urothelium, allowing the identification of filling defects within the collecting system. Distension of the urinary

system with the administration of furosemide has been shown to be helpful [1], although many clinically significant abnormalities of the collecting system, especially the bladder, often can be identified even with minimal distension because of the intrinsic contrast resolution on T2-weighted sequences. The relative contribution of T2-weighted images may be increased in patients who have significantly impaired renal function, because the visibility of the collecting system does not depend completely on the excretion of contrast material, a requirement of gadolinium-chelate–enhanced imaging.

In addition, with the use of relatively motion-insensitive T2-weighted half-Fourier acquisition single-shot turbo spin-echo (HASTE) sequences, high-quality images of the kidneys can be obtained even in free-breathing patients. Pulse sequences that use steady-state magnetization, such as TFISP, also can demonstrate the morphology of the collecting system in the absence of excretion. Like T2-weighted HASTE sequences, TFISP has excellent in-plane motion insensitivity and may display collecting system morphology in a nondistended

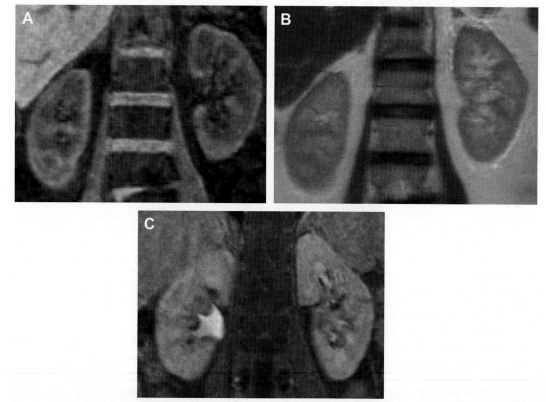

Fig. 1. (A) On T1 imaging, normal cortico-medullary differentiation (CMD) is seen with the cortex slightly brighter than skeletal muscle and the medulla relatively dark. Inherent CMD usually is best shown on T1 fat-suppressed images. (B) On T2 imaging, CMD is reversed relative to T1 imaging, with brighter-signal medulla, and lower-signal cortex. Gadolinium enhancement in the arterial-capillary phase (20-second delay) shows enhancement of the cortex. (C) Delayed gadolinium-enhanced interstitial-phase images show filling in of the medulla and subsequent excretion of contrast into the renal pelvis.

system better than single-shot T2-weghted images, although this advantage should be balanced against a drop in contrast resolution compared with T2-weighted sequences. A disadvantage of two-dimensional (2D) T2-weighted images is the inability to reconstruct the images in a volume format. Volume-acquired 3D T2-weighted images, however, may be acquired to generate a maximum-intensity projection (MIP) dataset that can demonstrate collecting system morphology in a rotating manner from multiple-projection reconstructions, similar to the MIP reconstructions often used in vascular imaging [2]. Multiple projection reconstructions provide a powerful anatomic overview of the collecting system helpful for referring clinical services. Disadvantages of the 3D technique are a significant increase in data acquisition time compared with single-slice T2-weighted HASTE and loss of the motion insensitivity inherent in the 2D technique. Respiratory gating with a 2D navigation system can be used but at the expense of further increases in the total acquisition time for all the slices.

3D GRE contrast-enhanced T1-weighted sequences are another mainstay of MR nephrourography. Although T2-weighted images provide excellent contrast resolution and morphologic data, postcontrast 3D GRE images can provide functional data in addition to complementary views of tissue contrast. Precontrast T1-weighted images are ideal for displaying hemorrhage and proteinaceous debris. Dynamic contrast-enhanced images at varying time points allow the identification of neoplastic processes involving either the renal parenchyma or the urothelium. For example, early contrast-enhanced images clearly demonstrate enhancement of the urothelium against a background of dark urine before the excretion of gadolinium. This inherent contrast differential allows identification of enhancing tumors within the renal pelvis, ureters, or bladder, even in the setting of poorly functioning kidneys with diminished excretion. Tumor visibility is enhanced with the routine use of fat suppression, causing the surrounding retroperitoneal fat to become dark. This technique has the effect of allowing enhancing tissues to fill the available gray-scale values, allowing easier depiction of urothelial neoplastic processes (Fig. 2). Use of a 3D volume acquisition with thin partitions allows the initial coronal data to be reformatted into additional imaging planes as desired to enhance lesion detection further. Disadvantages to the 3D T1-weighted technique include sensitivity to motion, which can degrade images significantly in a free-breathing patient. Additional techniques to shorten the acquisition time (eg, increased parallel processing acceleration) can reduce these detrimental effects but at the cost of a decreased

signal-to-noise ratio. Contrast enhancement of the collecting system is dependent on renal excretion, which may be reduced markedly with severe renal disease. This problem is not unique to MR imaging, however, and is encountered in both nuclear renal scintigraphy and CT urography. Thus MR imaging provides still another advantage by having alternative contrast strategies using T2-weighted imaging to visualize the collecting system even when the kidney's excretory function may be severely impaired.

In addition to morphologic imaging, 3D GRE images are the critical sequences necessary for the quantitative evaluation of renal function with MR imaging. Advances in parallel processing and in undersampling and underfilling of k-space have reduced imaging times so that a coronal volume of images through the kidneys can be acquired in 0.9 seconds with these techniques. Repeated T1-weighted GRE acquisitions through the kidneys every second during the administration of intravenous gadolinium allows the calculation of differential glomerular filtration rate (GFR) and renal blood flow (RBF) for each kidney.

MR nephrourography—function

The clinical management of patients who have kidney diseases is somewhat limited by the lack of readily available noninvasive methods to test and follow renal function, to diagnose causes of renal dysfunction, or to monitor treatment response. Among the most commonly used tests for evaluation of renal function are measurement of serum creatinine level, endogenous creatinine clearance, and urinalysis for measurement of proteinuria. These indirect measures of renal GFR and loss of filtration integrity are insensitive and nonspecific and do not supply information that would differentiate the right kidney from the left [3]. Accurate 24-hour urine collections are challenging generally, and it is particularly difficult to ensure accuracy in younger patients.

There remains a clinical need for a sensitive and noninvasive in vivo imaging method that can be performed quickly and safely to provide regionally specific functional information about the kidney and to facilitate repeated evaluation, especially when there is a need for monitoring the progression of disease or the response to a treatment. Although nuclear medicine methods such as renal scintigraphy [4,5] have been used for determining renal function, these techniques suffer from low spatial resolution and do not provide detailed analysis of both structure and function. Furthermore, Technetium-99m mercaptoacetyltriglycine (MAG-3), commonly used in nuclear renal imaging, is an agent actively excreted by the renal tubules, and the rate of excretion does not measure the GFR. The use of radioactive tracers,

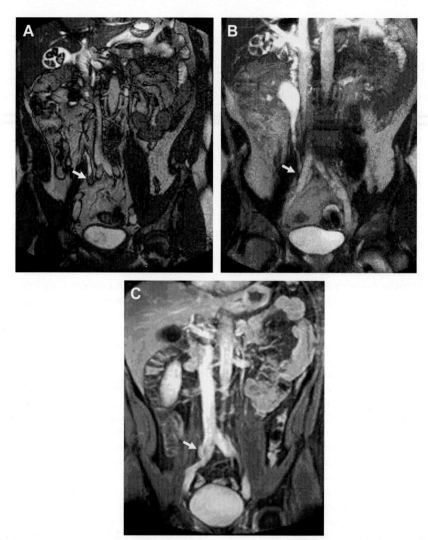

Fig. 2. Coronal TFISP image (*A*) demonstrating isointense soft tissue within the distal right ureter (*arrow*) contrasted against high-signal urine, again seen with (*B*) a MIP reconstruction of the TFISP images. (*C*) This filling defect corresponds exactly to a focal area of enhancement (*arrow*) demonstrated on the coronal 3D GRE sequence, confirming the presence of tumor and not stone or clot, neither of which would demonstrate enhancement. Surgical pathology returned a diagnosis of transitional cell carcinoma.

particularly in monitoring applications where the study will be repeated, raises the concern of radiation risk [6,7]. This concern is particularly important when dealing with younger or pregnant patients. Dynamic CT imaging has been used [8], but it also involves undesirable risks from ionizing radiation. In the setting of acute renal disease, or in patients who have risk factors such as diabetes mellitus, CT may be dangerous because it uses potentially nephrotoxic iodinated contrast agents [9].

Advantages of MR imaging include the ability to achieve scans with higher temporal resolution than obtained with CT and nuclear scans and with higher spatial resolution than obtained with nuclear scans, without the exposure to ionizing radiation

that occurs with CT and nuclear scans. Important measures of renal function can be related to RBF and GFR. From these parameters the filtration fraction can be determined. Recently, the potential of gadolinium-enhanced dynamic MR imaging, or MRNU, of the kidney has emerged as having the capacity to measure GFR [10–14]. This method uses rapid "snapshots" of the kidney at different time points following administration of a gadolinium-chelate paramagnetic contrast agent, combining mathematical modeling of tracer kinetics to determine RBF [10] and GFR [13,15]. There has been development and evolving validation of gadolinium-chelate perfusion MR imaging techniques for the evaluation of GFR, relying on its behavior as a filtered agent without active excretion or uptake from the renal tubules.

Several methods have been developed for estimating the GFR from dynamic nuclear medicine data, but all are hampered by the poor counting statistics of such dynamic studies and the problem of accounting for the extrarenal component of the signal. Recently, several groups have applied the methods developed for nuclear medicine to dynamic MR imaging data acquired in conjunction with an injection of the contrast agent gadolinium-diethylenetriamine pentaacetic acid. In applying these techniques to MR imaging data, several issues must be addressed. First, although nuclear medicine measures the activity, and hence the concentration, of the contrast agent directly, in MR imaging the contrast agents change signal by altering the relaxation times of the tissue, producing a linear relationship with the concentration over only a limited range of concentrations. Second, the exact relationship between the signal and concentration depends on the flip angle used, and because the flip angle varies across the slice in 2D studies, time-consuming corrections are required for 2D data, making these unsuitable for routine clinical applications. Third, to obtain an adequate signal-to-noise ratio, it generally is necessary to use surface array coils for the reception of the signal, which in turn can lead to local variations in signal intensity that complicate the analysis of the data. One approach that the present authors have advocated [10] addresses these problems by using a slow injection of contrast over 10 seconds to limit the arterial concentration, by using a 3D technique and discarding the outer slices to ensure a uniform flip angle, and by using the precontrast signal to correct for spatial variations in the signal intensity.

Calculation of the individual RBF and GFR from gadolinium-enhanced MRNU can be coupled with measurement of the individual kidney volumes (cortex plus medulla). This technique makes it possible to determine RBF and GFR in proportion to a unit measure of kidney volume that can be expressed, for example, as RBF or GFR per milliliter of kidney. This value may provide an additional functional parameter for monitoring renal dysfunction and response to interventions, which previously was not possible in the clinical setting (Fig. 3). Potential applications range across the full spectrum of renal diseases.

Imaging techniques

Gadolinium-enhanced renal perfusion-distribution imaging

Both 2D and 3D GRE techniques have been proposed to capture the critical period when the infused gadolinium arrives in the renal artery. The principle that has been adopted is that the blood flow to the kidney can be determined in the first few seconds as the gadolinium contrast agent perfuses the renal parenchyma; the GFR then can be measured by measuring the total amount of gadolinium agent within the entire kidney parenchyma as a function of time with the data collected up to the point of urinary excretion. The strength of 2D techniques is that a turbo-flash sequence can be implemented providing a fast acquisition method that is relatively insensitive to motion, as has been used to evaluate cardiac perfusion. A limitation of this approach is that volumetric determination of total kidney signal and volume is less accurate. Using 3D GRE provides volumetric data for more accurate evaluation of total kidney signal and volume. A challenge has been to acquire 3D GRE with a sufficiently short acquisition time to provide the necessary temporal resolution demanded from the kinetic modeling. Volumetric GRE also is more motion sensitive. The present authors have approached this problem by using 3D GRE with a high degree of acceleration to achieve the necessary short acquisition time and to reduce motion sensitivity. Use of surface coils with parallel processing inherently corrects for coil element sensitivity profile and helps overcome the problem of positional changes in signal intensities within the field of view.

The authors have adopted a technique to achieve a long infusion period combined with a minimal gadolinium concentration. The objectives are to produce a more uniform arterial gadolinium concentration over the period of data collection and to maintain the gadolinium concentration at the lowest detectable level, to minimize susceptibility effects. They administer the gadolinium agent using a dual-syringe power injector at a dose of 0.1 mmol/kg diluted into a total volume of 60 mL with normal saline and injected at a rate of 0.6 mL/s. Renal perfusion imaging is performed during the first pass using a coronal 3D GRE technique with fat saturation and centric-radial k-space acquisition using a 430-mm^2 field of view, 96 matrix (60% scan percentage, reconstructed to 256), recovery time/echo time/flip angle of 3.7/1.7ms/ 30°, 30 slices at a 2.8-mm slice thickness, 120 k-lines/segment, and a sensitivity encoding factor of 3. These parameters result in an acquisition time of 0.9 seconds per dynamic scan. The resultant images have an acceptable signal-to-noise ratio and provide adequate spatial resolution. A benefit of this highly accelerated acquisition time is that the imaging may be performed during normal breathing with negligible motion-related image deterioration.

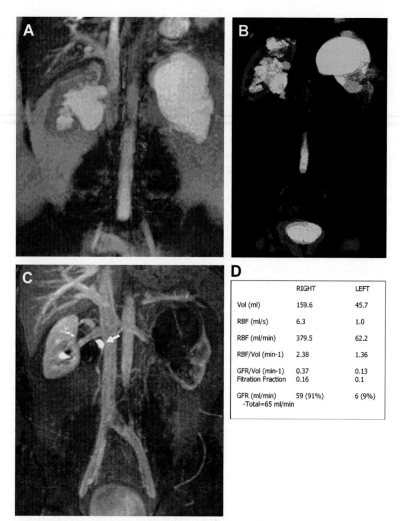

	RIGHT	LEFT
Vol (ml)	159.6	45.7
RBF (ml/s)	6.3	1.0
RBF (ml/min)	379.5	62.2
RBF/Vol (min-1)	2.38	1.36
GFR/Vol (min-1)	0.37	0.13
Fitration Fraction	0.16	0.1
GFR (ml/min) -Total=65 ml/min	59 (91%)	6 (9%)

Fig. 3. A 52-year-old man who presented with unexplained bilateral hydronephrosis based on ultrasound examination. (*A*) Coronal TFISP MIP shows what appears to be bilateral hydronephrosis affecting the pelvis and calyces, moderate on the right and severe on the left side. (*B*) Colorization of the coronal MIP image is possible using readily available commercial image postprocessing software. In this case, it incrementally accentuates the severely dilated collecting system of the left kidney, including interconnecting dilated calyces and pelvis. (*C*) The right kidney calyces are mildly blunted. Coronal post-gadolinium contrast-enhanced 3D GRE MIP shows no detectable excretion of contrast after 10 minutes. There is excretion from the right kidney and filling of the bladder. This image shows that the major calyces and the pelvis are compressed and thinned, and the proximal ureter (*arrow*) is draped over the medial border of the fluid filled structure shown on the coronal TFISP images. These findings are in keeping with large peripelvic cysts. (*D*) The summary of quantitative information derived from the gadolinium-enhanced MRNU shows that the function of the right kidney is within expected limits, but the left kidney is markedly impaired, with the loss of approximately two thirds of the left renal parenchyma volume as compared with the right kidney. This study shows that the MRNU provides a unique array of structural and functional information that is important for an accurate diagnosis and for optimized management.

Image analysis

Proposals for modeling the kinetics have ranged from the simple two-compartment analysis, based on the Patlak-Rutland model [13,16,17], to more complex models that range to seven compartments [15]. The authors have adopted a model that takes into consideration the blood, interstitial, and filtered tubular compartments in keeping with a three-compartment model. They believe that a three-compartment model provides sufficient sophistication to account for the major regions of gadolinium distribution and have been able to validate their belief empirically by showing excellent fit between the measured and the predicted values in a variety of disease states.

The relative signal from within each kidney is calculated to determine the signal contribution from the contrast agent perfusion. The bulk kidney signal represents the total amount of gadolinium agent present in the kidney per unit time. The three dynamic signal-intensity time courses (aorta, right kidney, and left kidney) are evaluated. They have modeled three compartments (blood, extracellular space, and glomerular filtration), as described later. An assumption required for the analysis discussed here is that the measured increased signal within an image voxel, either within the feeding artery or within the kidney parenchyma, is proportional to the amount of gadolinium within the respective voxel. They have performed phantom studies to show that maintaining the low gadolinium administration rate maintains the blood concentration within a range that retains a mostly linear relationship between the gadolinium concentration and the increase in signal intensity over background [10].

Each total perfused kidney volume (cortex and medulla) can be segmented using a semiautomatic algorithm based on user-defined intensity thresholds (**Fig.** 4), morphologic erosion/dilation, and region growing steps [10,18]. Renal pelvis, pelvic vessels, and adjacent soft tissues are excluded from the renal segments. Additionally, a dynamic signal-intensity mask is created in the descending aorta to serve as the input function. These segmented binary masks of the kidneys and aorta are applied to the images at each time point and are adjusted for position changes related to respiration. Positional correction to account for respiration can be performed manually or by motion-tracking software. The authors have found that for images acquired during restful breathing in regions of

interest around the kidney, and particularly in transplanted kidneys where motion is inherently negligible, motion-corrected results often are not significantly different from the uncorrected results.

The output from the perfusion masks is a time course of signal intensity in the aorta and each kidney. Summing the number of pixels in the kidney mask and multiplying by the voxel size provides the perfused kidney volume, *V*.

The mean signal intensity for the renal volumes is calculated for each 0.9-second scan. Relative signal values are determined by the formula $(S_t - S_0) / S_0$, where S_t is the signal at time t and S_0 is the mean precontrast signal, calculated from the mean of at least three unenhanced precontrast images. The relative signal is used both to isolate the signal contribution from the contrast agent perfusion and to help eliminate residual signal variations that may result from imperfect coil spatial sensitivity corrections or other field inhomogeneities.

Calculation of single-kidney renal blood flow

Fick's first law of diffusion states that the rate of uptake of gadolinium within the kidney is equal to the blood flow through the organ times the arterial-venous difference in the concentration of the tracer (gadolinium signal in this application). In

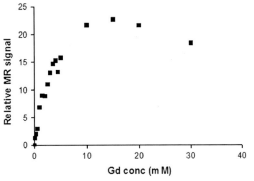

Fig. 5. The MR signal response of the 3D GRE perfusion sequence as a function of gadolinium concentration (Gd conc), as determined with an array of gadolinium-doped plasma phantoms. Signal intensities were measured after the fifth dynamic scan to ensure the system was in steady state, as expected with in vivo conditions. There is an apparent region of linearity between MR signal intensity and gadolinium concentration below approximately 3.5 mM, allowing the simple use of physiologic models, such as the two-compartment model, for describing changes in tracer concentrations. Beyond the linearity threshold, the relationship between signal and gadolinium concentration is no longer predictable, and the kinetic model cannot be used. This phenomenon occurs primarily because of T1 and T2* effects of the imaged species, in addition to effects of sequence parameters such as the flip angle.

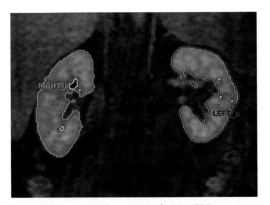

Fig. 4. Representative coronal 3D GRE contrast-enhanced image showing manually placed segmentation of right (*green*) and left (*red*) kidney. The last image just before appearance of contrast spillage into the pelvic collecting system is used for this process to ensure inclusion of the entire renal parenchyma.

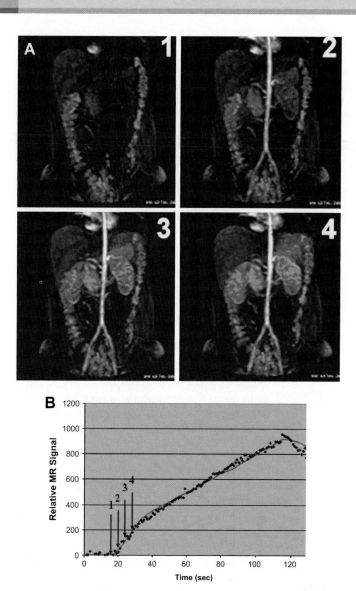

Fig. 6. (*A*) Selected dynamic coronal MIP series of contrast enhanced 3D GRE 0.9-second scans with a 430-mm² field of view, 96 matrix (reconstructed to 256), recovery time/echo time/flip angle of 3.7/1.7ms/30°, 30 slices at 2.8-mm slice thickness, acquired in a freely breathing subject just before the arrival of contrast in the aorta and kidneys (1), followed by sample points (2–4) within the first 7 seconds from the time contrast has arrived showing progressive enhancement of the kidneys. (*B*) The relative MR signal from the left kidney from each 0.9-second scan is shown as an individual point in relation to the time of acquisition. The points indicated by numbered arrows (1–4) indicate the acquisition time and measured renal signal of the corresponding MIP image shown in panel A. The solid line represents the curve calculated using Eq. 2. The first 10 seconds of data fit Eq. 1 and were used to calculate "F," a parameter in Eq. 2 (see text). The first few seconds of data are acquired from the time contrast arrives within the kidney until the time contrast exits the kidney in the renal vein. The degree of calculated curve fit to the measured data serves as indirect support for the assumptions made in the kinetic modeling.

this approach, data collection must focus on the kidney images acquired before venous drainage of gadolinium from the kidney. Hence, the RBF may be determined from Eq. 1:

$$C_T(t)V = F \int_0^t C_a(s - t_d)ds \qquad \text{Eq.1}$$

where C_T is the measured gadolinium tissue concentration in the whole kidney, V is the kidney volume, F is the blood flow into the kidney, C_a is the measured gadolinium concentration in the artery supplying the kidney, and t_d is the time difference between when the gadolinium is measured in the artery and the kidney. It is recognized that in application, V is the volume of the kidney region of interest, and C_T is the average pixel intensity inside this region. Thus VC_T is proportional to the total

amount of gadolinium in the kidney. This approach has been described in detail [10].

Calculation of single-kidney glomerular filtration rate

Gadolinium systemic model, analysis of arterial curve

Assuming the equilibration of gadolinium is fast relative to the clearance, then clearance of gadolinium through the kidney can be considered a first-order concentration-driven process (Fig. 5). Under these conditions, gadolinium clears exponentially from the system with a characteristic half-life related to the GFR. Hence, gadolinium concentration at the measurement point after injection of a very short bolus at the input point is expected to have the general shape known as the point spread function:

$$y_g(t) = \begin{cases} a_1 e^{-p_1(t-t_c)^2} & t \leq t_c \\ (a_1 - a_2)e^{-p_2(t-t_c)^2} + a_2 e^{-p_3(t-t_c)} & t > t_c \end{cases}$$

where the a represents amplitude, p the rate constant, and t_c is the time of the peak. The amount of dispersion is characterized by the width of the peak at half of its height (full width half maximum, FWHM). Equation parameters are determined by minimizing the error-weighted chi-square function using Powell's method. The error was assumed to be fractional (ie, 12% of the value) and was determined by fitting a single exponential to the tail of the aorta curve and taking the standard deviation about the fit value. The tail (long after the injection has stopped) of the aorta curve is affected by the clearance rate of gadolinium from the blood and is well described by a single exponential function.

Gadolinium kidney model, analysis of kidney curve

The general shape of the curve of gadolinium concentration in the kidney over time was modeled with three phases. The first phase is a rapid increase in concentration occurring after gadolinium enters the kidney but before any gadolinium appears in the renal vein. This process is proportional to the amount of blood flowing into the kidney. The second phase lasts until the end of the infusion. During this phase, the gadolinium concentrations in the blood and extracellular space are in quasi-equilibrium, with the blood concentration being greater. Both concentrations increase because the constant infusion is adding gadolinium to the system faster than it is being cleared via the kidney. The third phase begins at the end of infusion and lasts until gadolinium appears in the ureter (the end of the study). After a short transient in this phase, there is a greater concentration in the blood, and gadolinium continues to accumulate in the kidney (Fig. 6). A mathematical model of gadolinium in the renal system has been elaborated [19].

Briefly, the gadolinium concentration throughout the kidney at time t is modeled with the following time-dependent coupled equations:

$$\frac{\partial C_a(x,t)}{\partial t} = -\frac{F}{A}\frac{\partial C_a(x,t)}{\partial x} - K_1 C_a(x,t) + \frac{k_2 V_e}{LA}C_e(x,t)$$

$$\frac{\partial C_e(x,t)}{\partial t} = K_1 \frac{LA}{V_e} C_a(x,t) - (k_2 + k_3)C_e(x,t)$$

$$\frac{\partial C_t(x,t)}{\partial t} = k_3 \frac{V_e}{V_t} C_e(x,t)$$

V_e and V_t represent the total volumes of the interstitial and tubular portions of the kidney. All concentrations are zero at time $t = 0$. The input condition, $C_a(0,t)$, is the measured curve from the descending aorta (after a suitable shift for the transit time between the descending aorta and kidney measurements). These equations were solved numerically by finite differencing using a two-step Lax-Wendroff method. As a quality-control step, the accuracy of the solution is verified by dividing the time step size (dt) in half and checking that the solution does not change. Because the MR imaging signal is a global kidney signal, the calculated values must be summed over the entire kidney. Hence, the measured data are identified to be

$$MRI(t) = \int_0^L \left(LAC_a(x,t) + V_e C_e(x,t) + V_t C_t(x,t) \right) dx$$

Eq.2

The parameters of interest, F, k_1, k_2, k_3, are adjusted using Powell's algorithm until the model estimate (Eq. 2) matches the measured value in

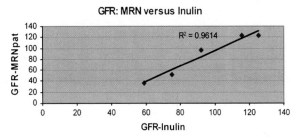

GFR: MRN versus Inulin

Fig. 7. Correlation plot between GFR measured concurrently by inulin and by MRNU technique in five patients. The GFR ranged from normal to moderately impaired by chronic renal disease. The inulin study results in a total GFR for both kidneys. The MRNU GFR results are shown as the sum of individually calculated GFR measurements for each kidney. The correlation shows good linear least squares fit. There is an apparent persistent offset with the MRNU technique showing a lower GFR value for each patient. The reason for this apparent bias remains the focus of continued investigation.

the region of interest as closely as possible (least squares difference). Then blood flow into the kidney, F, is obtained. The GFR is the amount of blood that flows into the kidney multiplied by fraction of the blood that enters the tubules (Fk_3).

Measurement accuracy

Measurement of RBF using the MRNU technique has been compared with phase-contrast imaging, and the results show no significant differences between the methods [20].

Different methods have been used to compare MRNU-derived GFR measurements against different standards of reference, including GFR determined by scintigraphic [18] and iothalamate [21] clearance methods. The authors also have compared their MRNU technique with the inulin clearance method. Although not used routinely because of its expense and complexity, inulin clearance generally is accepted as the reference standard for measuring GFR,. The authors' findings show high correlation with GFR measured concurrently by

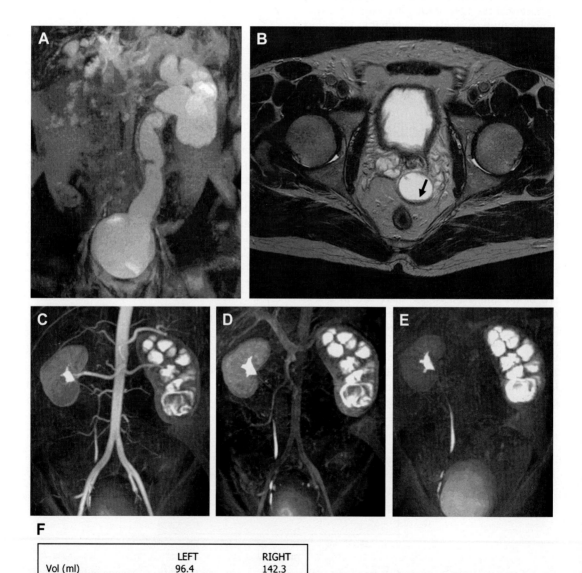

	LEFT	RIGHT
Vol (ml)	96.4	142.3
RBF (ml/s)	6.722	7.810
RBF (ml/min)	403.32	468.63
RBF/Vol (min-1)	4.18	3.29
GFR/Vol (min-1)	0.50	0.56
HCT	43.10	

the inulin clearance technique (Fig. 7). In this example, five patients who had normal to moderately impaired renal function were studied first by MRNU and immediately afterwards by the inulin technique.

Clinical applications

Congenital anomalies and obstruction

There has been considerable clinical experience in the use of MRNU in the analysis of congenital anomalies of the urinary tract. Congenital anomalies of the urinary tract are common in young children, with a frequency of between 1:650 and 1:1000, and are one of the major causes of renal insufficiency and renal failure. An initial diagnosis commonly is made on an antenatal ultrasound scan, but the complete postnatal evaluation requires both anatomic and functional information. Currently ultrasound is used to provide somewhat limited anatomic information, and a nuclear medicine test is used to obtain functional information. Combined MR anatomic and functional imaging may have a marked impact on the management of pediatric patients [2].

The differential renal function as measured by dynamic renal scintigraphy (DRS) is based on the integration of the tracer curve over a range of time points at which the tracer is assumed to be located predominately in the parenchyma. The spatial resolution of DRS studies is limited; fixed time limits are used because the exact location of the tracer cannot be confirmed by visual inspection of the images. Because DRS measurements are based on projection images of the whole kidney, they measure the

activity in the whole kidney but inadvertently may include the collecting system or adjacent soft tissues, such as spleen or liver. The MRNU approach provides high-resolution 3D volumes and avoids the limitations of the scintigraphic methods (Fig. 8). The methodology presented here makes a clear distinction between functioning and nonfunctioning tissue and accounts for the effects of cortical scarring or unusual morphology, such as seen in the polycystic or dysplastic kidneys often encountered in the pediatric population.

The ability to determine GFR as a function of renal volume provides additional potential application. Currently, GFR in children is indexed most often with body surface area [22,23]. Using functional MRNU, it is possible that normalizing GFR and RBF to the volume of renal parenchyma may provide more precise comparisons of the renal function of an obstructed kidney over time or between pediatric patients. It is hoped that this approach may yield a better understanding of patients at risk for progressive loss of renal function who may benefit from interventions and help determine the benefits of therapies.

The transplanted kidney

Repeated diagnostic imaging of a transplanted kidney often is needed to evaluate complications and to determine optimal intervention. Complications may be categorized as prerenal (vascular complications), renal (intrinsic parenchymal disease), and postrenal (obstruction). Currently, differentiation between different categories and disease entities requires a combination of multiple imaging modalities to evaluate both structure and function, using

Fig. 8. A 38-year-old man with ectopic insertion of the left ureter resulting in obstruction. (*A*) Coronal TFISP MIP shows severe left-side hydronephrosis and hydroureter to the level of the bladder. (*B*) Axial T2 fast spin-echo image at the level of the bladder shows that the severely distended distal ureter ectopically passes posterior to the seminal vesicle, where it narrows abruptly to a thin channel. Note the sedimentation (*arrow*) collecting along the dependent wall of the left ureter. Panels *C, D,* and–*E* show progressively delayed post-gadolinium coronal 3D GRE images. The collecting system is severely distended, the kidney size is enlarged overall, but the parenchyma and particularly the medullary component of the kidney appear thinned. (*F*) The summary of the quantitative analysis from the MRNU study. A concurrent MAG-3 nuclear study measured a differential function of 46% on the left and 54% on the right. The MRNU shows that the differential GFR is greater than that measured on MAG-3 and shows that the overall GFR is mildly impaired (stage 2 disease). This finding is in keeping with the mildly elevated creatinine level persistently measuring between 1.5 and 1.8 mg/dL during the time of these scans. The MAG-3 scan lacks the spatial resolution to evaluate the degree of loss in parenchyma in the left kidney and blurs together adjacent soft tissues such as the spleen. In the setting of obstruction, the kidney and the collecting system cannot be separated anatomically, and the capacitance of the severely dilated pelvis makes interpretation of clearance results challenging. The MR examination provides a comprehensive evaluation that includes determination of the cause of the obstruction. In the setting of urinary obstruction, therapeutic intervention depends on understanding both the cause of the disease and the degree of residual function of the affected kidney to evaluate the potential value of therapy. In this patient, the quantitative GFR for each kidney cannot be determined by the MAG-3 examination alone. The MRNU results suggest that this patient is dependent on both kidneys to achieve an acceptable combined GFR and that any improvements in left renal function may have significant impact.

CT, ultrasound, nuclear scintigraphy, and MR imaging to varying degrees. MRNU may offer a comprehensive analysis that provides a higher diagnostic yield than has been possible previously.

Prerenal causes of transplant dysfunction can be discerned with MR angiography techniques that already are widely in use. Intrinsic parenchymal disease is a diagnostic challenge with purely anatomic imaging, although it may be suggested by increased cortical T2 signal and loss of corticomedullary differentiation. Serial evaluation of GFR and RBF, however, can provide quantitative evaluation of

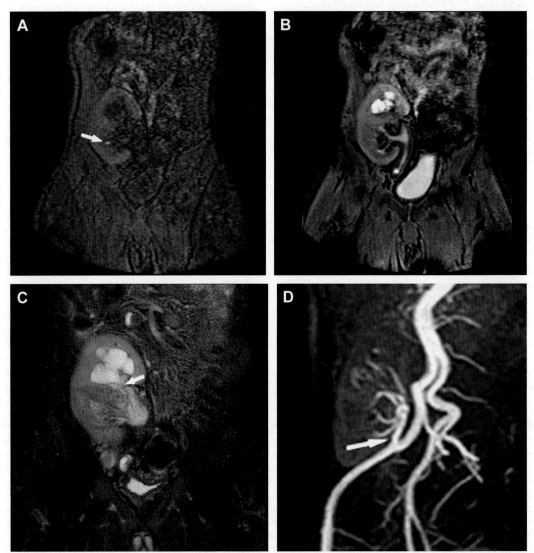

Fig. 9. Selected coronal images from an MRNU study in a patient who had undergone renal transplantation and who had impaired renal function initially misdiagnosed as caused by ureteric obstruction at the ureterovesical junction. Imaging was performed with 3D GRE over a 3-minute period during administration of low-dose gadolinium infusion. Images were acquired every 6 seconds. (*A*) A selected slice, reconstructed at 2-mm thickness, acquired 2.5 minutes from the time contrast first appeared in the renal artery, shows the first appearance of contrast at the tip of a lower pole papilla (*arrow*), representing a renal transit time at the upper limit of normal. (*B*) The upper-pole transit time was impaired at 5 minutes, and the upper-pole calyces fill later and show marked dilation 7 minutes after first arrival of contrast. (*C*) On a 9-minute image, the lower-pole calyces have normal configuration, and the upper-pole major calyx demonstrates stenosis (*arrow*). (*D*) Angiographic phase images can be viewed using MIP images and on an oblique coronal view show a normal renal transplant artery anastomosis (*arrow*). This complex case was delineated on MRNU after multiple attempts with ultrasound, scintigraphy, and biopsy failed to yield a comprehensive picture of the abnormalities.

transplant function, providing an earlier clue to acute or chronic rejection and potentially reducing the need for biopsy, which introduces its own complications. Postrenal causes of transplant dysfunction primarily involve obstruction of the collecting system (Fig. 9) and of venous outflow. The collecting system may be evaluated morphologically in excellent anatomic detail, even in the absence of contrast excretion (with the use of T2-weioghted images), allowing identification of an anatomic site of narrowing. Dynamic acquisition of images allows more precise evaluation of the contrast transit time into the collecting system than possible with nuclear medicine. Evaluation of the transplant renal vein usually is a trivial matter when employing 3D postcontrast VIBE or THRIVE sequences.

Limitations

Although MRNU is a robust technique offering a large amount of clinically useful data, there are a few limitations. The most significant is the relatively poor sensitivity of MR imaging of calcium [24], resulting from a combination of decreased proton density and increased T2 relaxation rates [25]. Large stones may be identified as hypointense filling defects within the collecting system on T2-weighted images, but smaller stones usually are invisible with MR imaging. The contribution of small stones to impaired renal function is uncertain, and the presence of small stones in a donor kidney is not a contraindication to renal transplantation [26]. If stone disease is a primary consideration in evaluation of the genitourinary system, low-dose unenhanced CT remains the modality of choice.

Another limitation to consider is the recent association between certain gadolinium agents, in the setting of renal failure and the systemic condition of nephrogenic systemic fibrosis (NSF) [27,28]. First described by Cowper and colleagues [20], NSF is a systemic disease presenting initially as thickening and hardening of the skin, possibly leading to permanent disability. Most cases have been associated with the use of gadodiamide [2], a linear-structure gadolinium agent that is more than 1 million times less stable than the most stable macrocyclic chelate in clinical use. Several case studies have reported the deposition of gadolinium within the soft tissues of patients who have NSF, and the disease may be secondary to deposition of toxic dissociated gadolinium within the soft tissues of patients who have renal failure [2]. The causes of NSF are multifactorial, but the common requirements for disease include severe renal disease (at least stage 4; GFR < 30 mL/min) and use of gadodiamide. Furthermore, there is a dose relationship

between the gadolinium agent and NSF [29,30], and the dose may be cumulative over multiple prior doses. Even in the presence of these factors, the rates of NSF are on the order of 2% to as high as 5% [29,31,32]. The authors believe that the risk of NSF may be minimized by the use of more stable gadolinium chelates and by a reduction in the cumulative lifetime dose in patients who have renal failure. These measures should allow the continued judicious use of contrast-enhanced MR imaging in this patient population. For each patient, the risk and benefits must be considered. For patients who have normal to moderately impaired renal function (stage 3; GFR of 30–59 mL/min), the clinical risk for NSF seems to be immeasurably small. Similarly, the risk of NSF with the use of usual doses of the more stable agents has remained immeasurably small, even in high-risk patients who have severe renal insufficiency (stage 4 or 5) or who are receiving dialysis.

Summary

MRNU is a powerful tool that makes it possible to obtain both structural and functional data within a single imaging examination that does not use ionization radiation, a significant benefit, especially in younger patients. The functional data available with MRNU allow renal physiology to be examined in ways that were not possible previously, including measurements of individual renal GFR and RBF and simultaneous measurement of individual renal perfused and functional volumes. Coupled with the exquisite soft tissue contrast provided by the standard MR images, MRNU can provide a comprehensive study that yields critical diagnostic information on structural diseases of the kidneys and collecting system, including congenital and acquired diseases, and also the full range of the causes of dysfunction in the transplanted kidney.

References

[1] Ergen FB, Hussain HK, Carlos RC, et al. 3D excretory MR urography: improved image quality with intravenous saline and diuretic administration. J Magn Reson Imaging 2007;25(4):783–9.

[2] Grattan-Smith JD, Jones RA. MR urography in children. Pediatr Radiol 2006;36(11):1119–32 [quiz: 1228–9].

[3] Lacour B. Creatinine and renal function. Nephrologie 1992;13(2):73–81 [in French].

[4] Russell CD, Dubovsky EV. Quantitation of renal function using MAG3. J Nucl Med 1991;32(11): 2061–3.

[5] Russell CD, Thorstad BL, Yester MV, et al. Quantitation of renal function with technetium-99m MAG3. J Nucl Med 1988;29(12):1931–3.

[6] Brenner DJ, Elliston CD. Estimated radiation risks potentially associated with full-body CT screening. Radiology 2004;232(3):735–8.

[7] Mayo JR, Aldrich J, Muller NL. Radiation exposure at chest CT: a statement of the Fleischner Society. Radiology 2003;228(1):15–21.

[8] Hackstein N, Buch T, Rau WS, et al. Split renal function measured by triphasic helical CT. Eur J Radiol 2007;61(2):303–9.

[9] McCullough P. Outcomes of contrast-induced nephropathy: experience in patients undergoing cardiovascular intervention. Catheter Cardiovasc Interv 2006;67(3):335–43.

[10] Martin DR, Sharma P, Salman K, et al. Individual kidney blood flow measured by contrast enhanced magnetic resonance first-pass perfusion imaging. Radiology 2008;246(1): 241–8.

[11] McDaniel BB, Jones RA, Scherz H, et al. Dynamic contrast-enhanced MR urography in the evaluation of pediatric hydronephrosis: part 2, anatomic and functional assessment of uteropelvic junction obstruction. AJR Am J Roentgenol 2005;185(6):1608–14.

[12] Jones RA, Perez-Brayfield MR, Kirsch AJ, et al. Dynamic contrast-enhanced MR urography in the evaluation of pediatric hydronephrosis: part 1, functional assessment. AJR Am J Roentgenol 2005;185(6):1598–607.

[13] Hackstein N, Kooijman H, Tomaselli S, et al. Glomerular filtration rate measured using the Patlak plot technique and contrast-enhanced dynamic MRI with different amounts of gadolinium-DTPA. J Magn Reson Imaging 2005; 22(3):406–14.

[14] Huang AJ, Lee VS, Rusinek H. Functional renal MR imaging. Magn Reson Imaging Clin N Am 2004;12(3):469–86 vi.

[15] Lee VS, Rusinek H, Bokacheva L, et al. Renal function measurements from MR renography and a simplified multicompartmental model. Am J Physiol Renal Physiol 2007;292(5): F1548–59.

[16] Peters AM. Graphical analysis of dynamic data: the Patlak-Rutland plot. Nucl Med Commun 1994;15(9):669–72.

[17] Hackstein N. Measurement of single kidney GFR using contrast enhanced GRE and Rutland-Patlak plot. J Magn Reson Imaging 2003;18: 14–25.

[18] Lee VS, Rusinek H, Noz ME, et al. Dynamic three-dimensional MR renography for the measurement of single kidney function: initial experience. Radiology 2003;227(1):289–94.

[19] Votaw JR, Martin DR. Modeling systemic and renal gadolinium chelate transport with MRI. Pediatric Radiology 2008;38:28–34.

[20] Cowper SE, Su LD, Bhawan J, et al. Nephrogenic fibrosing dermopathy. Am J Dermatopathol 2001;23(5):383–93.

[21] Hackstein N, Wiegand C, Rau WS, et al. Glomerular filtration rate measured by using triphasic helical CT with a two-point Patlak plot technique. Radiology 2004;230(1):221–6.

[22] Peters AM, Henderson BL, Lui D. Indexed glomerular filtration rate as a function of age and body size. Clin Sci (Lond) 2000;98(4):439–44.

[23] Hogg RJ, Furth S, Lemley KV, et al. National Kidney Foundation's Kidney Disease Outcomes Quality Initiative clinical practice guidelines for chronic kidney disease in children and adolescents: evaluation, classification, and stratification. Pediatrics 2003;111(6 Pt 1):1416–21.

[24] Kucharczyk W, Henkelman RM. Visibility of calcium on MR and CT: can MR show calcium that CT cannot? AJNR Am J Neuroradiol 1994; 15(6):1145–8.

[25] Henkelman M, Kucharczyk W. Optimization of gradient-echo MR for calcium detection. AJNR Am J Neuroradiol 1994;15(3):465–72.

[26] Martin G, Sundaram CP, Sharfuddin A, et al. Asymptomatic urolithiasis in living donor transplant kidneys: initial results. Urology 2007; 70(1):2–5 [discussion: 5–6].

[27] Grobner T. Gadolinium—a specific trigger for the development of nephrogenic fibrosing dermopathy and nephrogenic systemic fibrosis? Nephrol Dial Transplant 2006;21(4):1104–8.

[28] Thomsen HS, Morcos SK, Dawson P. Is there a causal relation between the administration of gadolinium based contrast media and the development of nephrogenic systemic fibrosis (NSF)? Clin Radiol 2006;61(11):905–6.

[29] Lauenstein TC, Salman K, Morreira R, et al. Nephrogenic systemic fibrosis: center case review. J Magn Reson Imaging 2007;26(5):1198–203.

[30] Collidge TA, Thomson PC, Mark PB, et al. Gadolinium-enhanced MR imaging and nephrogenic systemic fibrosis: retrospective study of a renal replacement therapy cohort. Radiology 2007; 245(1):168–75.

[31] Broome DR, Girguis MS, Baron PW, et al. Gadodiamide-associated nephrogenic systemic fibrosis: why radiologists should be concerned. AJR Am J Roentgenol 2007;188(2):586–92.

[32] Sadowski EA, Bennett LK, Chan MR, et al. Nephrogenic systemic fibrosis: risk factors and incidence estimation. Radiology 2007;243(1):148–57.

**ELSEVIER
SAUNDERS**

RADIOLOGIC
CLINICS
OF NORTH AMERICA

Radiol Clin N Am 46 (2008) 25–43

Nuclear Imaging in the Genitourinary Tract: Recent Advances and Future Directions

Wei He, MD, Alan J. Fischman, MD, PhD*

For almost 3 decades, noninvasive radionuclide procedures for the evaluation of renal disease have been important components of nuclear medicine practice [1–3]. With the introduction of new imaging agents and procedures, these techniques can provide valuable data on perfusion and function of individual kidneys. In general, these procedures are easy to perform and carry a low radiation burden, and sedation is not required. Moreover, radionuclide imaging of the genitourinary tract has become an invaluable asset to clinicians in the evaluation of renal parenchyma and urologic abnormalities [4].

Nuclear medicine procedures in addition to other modalities, such as CT, MR imaging, and ultrasound (US), constantly are evolving and finding greater and greater applications in nephrology and urology. The specific areas in which radionuclide techniques play a key role include measurement of renal function, assessment of obstruction,

Division of Nuclear Medicine, Department of Radiology, Massachusetts General Hospital, Harvard Medical School, 55 Fruit Street, Boston, MA 02114, USA
* Corresponding author.
E-mail address: fischman@pet.mgh.harvard.edu (A.J. Fischman).

doi:10.1016/j.rcl.2008.01.006

monitoring the function of renal transplants, evaluation of renovascular hypertension, detection of metastatic lesions from urologic neoplasms, and imaging of the acute scrotum.

To provide clinicians with a better understanding of the different techniques for management of renal disorders, the advantages and limitations of nuclear medicine applications in urologic disorders need to be assessed.

Camera-based radionuclide assessment of glomerular filtration rate using ^{99m}Tc-labeled diethylenetriamine pentaacetic acid

Glomerular filtration rate (GFR) is defined as the volume of plasma that is completely cleared of a particular substance by the kidneys in a unit of time [5]. Urologists and nephrologists consider this parameter the reference measurement of renal function in clinical practice [6]. The gold standard for determining GFR is measurement of the clearance of exogenous substances such as insulin, iohexol, ^{51}Cr-EDTA, ^{99m}Tc-labeled diethylenetriamine pentaacetic acid (DTPA), or ^{125}I-labeled iothalamate [7]. The classic method of measuring GFR in humans requires constant intravenous infusion of the compound and timed collections of urine and blood. Because GFR determinations by inulin or radioisotope studies on large numbers of patients are impractical, cumbersome, and expensive, clinicians frequently rely on GFR prediction equations [8]. Because DTPA complexes are stable, have low protein binding, are cleared by glomerular filtration, and are not acted on by the renal tubules, ^{99m}Tc-labeled DTPA was introduced as a renal scanning agent in the 1970s [9,10].

Techniques using gamma camera imaging with ^{99m}Tc-DTPA, without blood or urine sampling, were developed to measure each kidney's GFR in the form of a split renal function test rather than merely reporting total GFR compared with a standard creatinine clearance and blood and urine sampling methods. Although many methods are available for GFR measurement by camera-based renography [11–14], each depends on specific clinical requirements and capabilities. In the United States, the tracer used most widely for measuring GFR is ^{99m}Tc-DTPA. In 1982, Gates demonstrated that the uptake of ^{99m}Tc-DTPA by each kidney at 2 to 3 minutes after intravenous injection is directly proportional to GFR [15]. The scintigraphic method has the advantage of noninvasively providing information about individual kidney function. Because of its reliance on absolute gamma camera counts, however, scintigraphy has the disadvantages of requiring calibration on each imaging system and appropriate attenuation and background correction.

Shore and colleagues demonstrated that plasma concentration of tracer is directly proportional to dosage and inversely proportional to body size and could be determined with a gamma camera alone by analyzing the initial portion of the renogram without blood sampling [16]. Camera-based DTPA clearance measurements avoid the cumbersome nature, inconvenience, and incomplete urine collections associated with a 24-hour creatinine clearance and can be obtained easily at the time of DTPA renal scanning. The camera-based DTPA clearance approach is highly correlated with creatinine clearance and provides a simple, safe, and convenient test of kidney function [17,18]. Currently, sequential injections of ^{99m}Tc-DTPA and ^{99m}Tc-mercaptoacetyltriglycine (MAG3) during the same imaging session allow the calculation of GFR, derivation of renogram curves, and superior images [19].

Indications

Quantification of individual kidney GFR and definition of renal failure is useful especially for serial evaluations of renal function [20–24]. Protocols for radionuclide renography with DTPA and MAG3 provide a complete evaluation of renal function that is unique to nuclear medicine [25].

Pitfalls and limitations

The camera-based radionuclide assessment of GFR is not an accurate measurement but only an approximation [26]. Some studies report that it overestimates GFR compared with inulin or creatinine sampling methods [27–29]. The accuracy of camera-based GFR measurement is affected by kidney depth and background correction and the error of the estimate increases in patients who have poor renal function [30,31]. The higher cost of camera-based radionuclide assessment of GFR compared with biochemical tests limits its wide clinical use.

Future prospects

Because the diagnostic accuracy of camera-based methods still is being debated, many clinical centers have focused on exploring more accurate methods for estimating GFR. Recently, it was indicated that increasing the simplicity of the technique leads to an increased error of the estimate [32,33]. Blaufox [34] suggested that it is unnecessary to continue to try to refine and develop clearance methods at this time, and that the available techniques are more than adequate to satisfy most clinical needs. Current research has focused on performing GFR measurements and diuretic renography in the same imaging session [25,35].

Determination of glomerular filtration rate by CT and MR imaging

More recently, dynamic renal contrast material enhancement has been assessed to determine if renal functional information also might be determined with CT [36,37]. These studies have used specific models of dynamic renal enhancement to extract functional parameters, such as GFR. Hackstein and colleagues [38] demonstrated that the Patlak method functioned well for estimating single-kidney GFR in normal kidneys. Daghini and colleagues [39] used a pig model to estimate single-kidney GFR with dynamic contrast-enhanced CT scanning and demonstrated the promise of the technique for noninvasive estimation of human single-kidney GFR. One limitation of renal function measurement with these techniques is that a particular model may be violated in some instances, thus leading to inaccuracy.

MRI can be used to evaluate kidney function because gadopentetate dimeglumine, a contrast agent used in MRI, is cleared by glomerular filtration and neither secreted nor reabsorbed by renal tubules. Lee and colleagues [40] demonstrated that the low-dose, gadolinium-enhanced, magnetic resonance renographic single-kidney GFR index based on whole-kidney gadolinium uptake (averaged during 2–3 minutes) is comparable to radionuclide measurements based on ^{99m}Tc-DTPA clearance. By combining anatomic imaging and functional renography in a single setting, MR imaging has the potential to improve the diagnosis of renal dysfunction across a spectrum of diseases.

A single CT or MR imaging examination combining excellent morphologic and accurate functional information would provide a powerful noninvasive tool for renal diagnosis. The findings of recent studies have indicated the possibility of estimating another fundamental parameter of single-kidney renal function, the renal extraction or filtration fraction, with contrast-enhanced CT and MR imaging [41,42]. The possibility of determining single-kidney renal function with contrast-enhanced CT or MR imaging is a subject of considerable research [43].

Diuretic renography

Urinary tract obstruction may be defined as a restriction to the flow of urine that results in symptoms or threatens renal function [44]. Obstruction above and below the vesicoureteric junction presents different clinical management. The diagnosis and management of urinary tract obstruction are of importance in pediatric and adult urology. Obstructive uropathy is a functional

disturbance and, therefore, static imaging alone is unreliable for clinical evaluation [44,45]. Intravenous urography (IVU), US, CT, MR imaging and conventional radionuclide renography provide little information on dynamic function to differentiate obstructive from nonobstructive causes of hydroureteronephrosis [46].

Conventional radionuclide renography with the administration of a potent diuretic is defined as diuretic renography [47]. The basic principle of diuretic renography is that the prolonged retention of a tracer seen in a nonobstructed, dilated system is caused by a reservoir effect [48]. A diuretic produces prompt washout of activity in a dilated nonobstructed system. In contrast, the capacity to augment washout is much less, resulting in prolonged retention of tracer proximal to the obstruction. Diuretic renography is well accepted in routine clinical practice for differentiating a dilated unobstructed urinary system from a true stenotic dilatation in the upper urinary tract and for the follow-up of patients who have hydronephrosis [49–51]. The diuretic used routinely is furosemide, which acts at the luminal face of epithelial cells in the ascending limb of the loop of Henle, blocking active reabsorption of chloride and sodium [52]. Intravenous administration is required because the peak effect after oral ingestion may not occur for an hour or longer. The guidelines published by the Society of Nuclear Medicine and the European Nuclear Medicine Association recommend the use of furosemide at a dose of 1 mg/kg, up to a maximum of 20 mg in children and 40 mg in adults. The diuretic response is unpredictable in the first 4 to 6 weeks of life and adult levels of renal function are not attained until approximately 6 months of age. Patients should be well hydrated, especially infants because of immaturity of the kidneys and patient compliance. Children, infants, and older subjects who cannot void voluntarily must be catheterized.

The time of diuretic administration varies in different nuclear medicine laboratories. There are three different but validated approaches for the time of diuretic injection: 20 minutes or later after the radiopharmaceutical (F+20), 15 minutes before tracer injection (F−15), or combined F+20 and F−15 renography, which can be performed if the washout is complete after the first injection [53–55]. Recently, simultaneous injection of tracer and diuretic (F+0 renography) has been advocated in children and adults. Tripathi and colleagues [56] evaluated the feasibility of F+0 renography in the investigation of hydronephrosis and hydroureteronephrosis in infants and children. The sensitivity of the F+0 study to differentiate between renal obstruction and nonobstruction was 100%, specificity was 78%, and accuracy was 83%. Wong studied

72 patients who had sonographic diagnoses of hydronephrosis or hydroureteronephrosis using F+0 renography. The sensitivity was 88.9%, specificity was 94.1%, and accuracy was 91.7%, demonstrating that F+0 diuresis renography produced excellent diuretic responses in normal kidneys and is a valid method for the investigation of hydronephrosis and hydroureteronephrosis in infants and children [57].

The F+0 protocol first was introduced for pediatric patients to shorten the acquisition time and avoid the need for an additional venous puncture. Although Donoso and colleagues [58] showed that early furosemide injection might result in an acceleration of renal transit and consequent underestimation of the renal function on the side with a short transit time, most groups have demonstrated good clinical results; comparable to F+20 and F−15 protocols. Turkolmez and colleagues [53] found that the F+0 and F−15 protocols allow clarification in cases of equivocal F+20 studies, although the F+0 protocol was more practical and shorter. Liu and colleagues [59] demonstrated that the F+0 renal diuretic protocol is associated with a significantly lower rate of disruption because of voiding than the F−15 protocol, likely the result of the shorter period between diuretic administration and study termination, thereby resulting in less bladder distention and discomfort. Currently, a modified diuretic renography, termed "the well-tempered renogram," is a widely used test to detect obstruction of the kidney or ureter in infants [60].

^{99m}Tc- MAG3, ^{123}I-orthoiodohippurate (OIH), and ^{99m}Tc-DTPA all can be used in diuretic renography. ^{99m}Tc-MAG3 is the radiopharmaceutical for renography used and recommended most frequently ^{99m}Tc-MAG3 has high extraction by the kidneys, rapid clearance, low radiation dose, and tubular secretion. Renal uptake by ^{99m}Tc-MAG3 is 55% compared with 20% uptake by ^{99m}Tc-DTPA [61]. This higher extraction results in better images for qualitative and quantitative analysis and is of particular benefit in neonates who have immature renal function.

Indications for diuretic renography

Diuretic renography is the initial screening study in patients found on urography or US to have a dilated upper urinary tract without obvious cause. It also is used to determine the clinical significance of a known partial obstruction in patients who have pelvic tumors. Because it is well tolerated and easily repeatable, it is appropriate for pediatric patients.

Pitfalls and limitations

Several factors, such as patient hydration status, renal insufficiency, and collecting system volume, affect the response to diuretics. If a patient is not well hydrated, the response is suboptimal. The level of renal function is a major determinant of diuretic-induced flow rate [62]. Unfortunately, the criteria of renal function in response to diuretic renography are not well established. Moreover, urinary flow rates are not elevated significantly by increased doses of diuretics in patients who have renal insufficiency [63]. Some nonobstructed patients who have very large collecting systems have an indeterminate response because the increased flow may be insufficient to wash out the tracer accumulating in a dilated collecting system [64]. Thus, the results of diuretic renography are neither positive nor negative and interpretation of the diuretic renogram is subjective. In addition, some renal tubular disorders, such as acute tubular necrosis (ATN) or Fanconi's syndrome, may interfere with the normal response to diurectics, Effects of bladder filling also can increase the risk for a false-positive result. Vesicoureteric reflux (VUR) can cause an upward deflection on time-activity histogram.

Future prospects

There is a great deal of variation in the performance and interpretation of the test between different centers and standardization is needed to improve accuracy. Research into renography is not an active area at present but there are a few important contributions that may improve the clinical value of radionuclide renography. Most groups have demonstrated good clinical results with F+0 comparable to F+20 and F−15 protocols [65–67]. Recently, Garcia and colleagues [68] used a new software engine to justify the conclusions of an expert system for detecting renal obstruction on ^{99m}Tc-MAG3 scans.

Other imaging modalities

US provides the best evaluation of hydronephrosis for screening and follow-up and remains the first-line imaging study to demonstrate dilation [69,70]. It can miss the diagnosis when patients are dehydrated markedly, however, or when there is coexisting sepsis. Conventional IVU as a diagnostic modality has limitations in patients who have obstructive uropathy and impaired renal function. Magnetic resonance urography (MRU) and CT urography (CTU) provide more refined imaging of the upper urinary tract compared with IVU [71]. CTU with or without contrast is used in the diagnosis of ureteric obstruction and calculi. CTU can be combined with low-dose furosemide to accelerate passage of excreted contrast material. This obviates abdominal compression and may provide valuable information in chronic urolithiasis, especially if associated with a distorted urinary tract anatomy. Unfortunately, it is limited by its radiation burden and the nephrotoxicity of radiographic contrast media. T2-weighted MRU is excellent for visualizing a dilated urinary tract, even in nonexcreting kidneys. The combination of gadolinium and low-dose furosemide (5–10 mg) allows evaluating the whole upper urinary tract [72,73]. In general, MRU and CTU play an important role in identifying causes for obstruction but neither routinely provides functional data.

Clinical applications

Prenatal hydronephrosis

Fetal hydronephrosis can be classified as transient and physiologic hydronephrosis, which postnatally may resolve spontaneously. Persistent hydronephrosis might be caused by pelviureteric junction stenosis, VUR, megaureter, multicystic dysplastic, or dulex kidney. This condition can be detected during the second or third trimester of pregnancy [74].

Nonoperative management with close follow-up during the first 2 years of life is a safe and recommended approach for neonates who have primary bilateral ureteropelvic junction (UPJ)-type hydronephrosis and can prevent permanent loss of renal function [75]. Diuretic renography and sonography can be used to evaluate renal function and grading degree of hydronephrosis in the follow-up of patients who have prenatal hydronephrosis.

IVU and CT are not used routinely in children because of radiation exposure. Although MRU provides high-resolution anatomic information without exposure to ionizing radiation, its high cost, long procedure time, and requirement for sedation limit its use in initial diagnosis and follow-up.

Adult hydronephrosis

Adult hydronephrosis usually presents with flank pain, hematuria, or renal colic and usually is diagnosed by US and IVU. Sonography is advocated for first-line investigation when patients who have hydronephrosis present to an emergency department. The priority of imaging strategies should focus on early identification of hydronephrosis to prevent further deterioration. Sonography allows the rapid diagnosis of hydronephrosis and could become a screening tool of choice in clinical practice. Unenhanced CT can be used to confirm the diagnosis and localize the level of obstruction.

CT is an important modality for imaging the urinary tract; however, unenhanced CT has low sensitivity for the diagnosis of noncalculous hydronephrosis (27%–42%) [76]. Some preliminary studies have demonstrated that dynamic gadolinium-enhanced MRU is a useful noninvasive imaging method for distinguishing obstructive from nonobstructive dilated systems, particularly in patients who have hydronephrosis and reduced renal function. It may be helpful in pregnant women, children, and patients who have allergies to contrast media [77]. Although MRU has many advantages, high cost limits its routine clinical use. Because diuretic renography provides information about renal parenchymal function and can be used to evaluate urinary drainage, it can be used to select patients who may benefit from surgery [78]. Overall, diuretic renography remains the noninvasive functional study of choice in patients who have hydronephrosis resulting from apparent UPJ obstruction. An example of a normal renogram is shown in Fig. 1 and renograms acquired in patients who had suspected obstruction are illustrated in Figs. 2 and 3.

Angiotension-coverting enzyme inhibition renography

Angiotension-coverting enzyme inhibitors (ACEIs) block the conversion of angiotensin I to angiotensin II, preventing efferent vasoconstriction. Postglomerular resistance decreases and, thus, the transglomerular filtration pressure falls abruptly, leading to GFR decreases in the affected kidney, which can be detected by renal scintigraphy [79]. Captopril was the first ACEI used in the diagnosis of renovascular hypertension with renography [80]. Subsequently, because of its more rapid onset of action (5 minutes compare with 60 minutes with captopril), enalapril was introduced for ACEI renography [81]. ^{99m}Tc-labeled MAG3 and DTPA are the preferred imaging agents for ACEI renography. The available data suggest that these tracers give comparable results in patients who have normal renal function. MAG3 enables better detection of excretory parameters in patients who have renal impairment, however [80]. Because it is excreted exclusively by glomerular filtration, DTPA likely is a more sensitive tracer for ACEI renography than MAG3. Because chronic treatment with ACEIs can reduce the effectiveness of ACEI renography, treatment with ACEIs should be stopped before imaging, for 3 days with captopril and 5 days with enalapril and lisnopril. It also is desirable to halt treatment with diuretics and calcium channel blockers [82]. To improve the reliability of the test, furosemide frequently is administered before or 2 minutes after beginning ACEI renography [83]. The advantage of furosemide treatment is that it minimizes pelvicalyceal stasis, which can

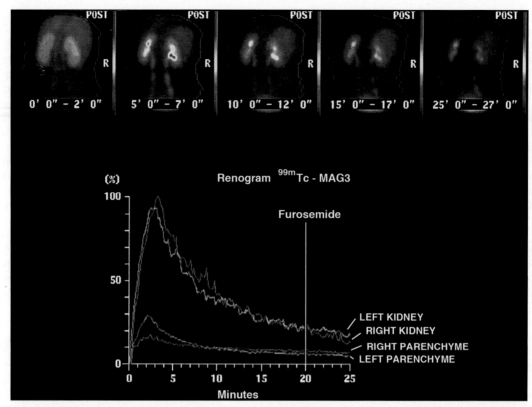

Fig. 1. Renal study with MAG3 in a subject who had normal kidney function. The upper row of images demonstrates rapid and symmetric clearance of the tracer. This is verified by the time-activity curves constructed from regions of interest drawn over the whole kidneys and the parenchyma. Furosemide injection had minimal effect in this individual. Split function was 50:50 (Right/Left).

affect the measurements and potentially lead to indeterminate or false-positive results. The disadvantage of furosemide treatment is volume depletion and a greater risk for severe hypotension [84]. Because of differences in protocols, interpretive criteria, and patient populations, it is difficult to assess the diagnostic accuracy of captopril renography precisely. Nonetheless, many investigations have reported that the sensitivity of ACEI renography ranges from 45% to 100%, most above 90% with DTPA, OIH, or MAG3 [85–89]. As demonstrated by Koyanagi and colleagues [90], the captopril test is more accurate for diagnosis of renovascular disease caused by renal artery stenosis (RAS) than renal artery aneurysm. Fig. 4 illustrates the appearance of the renogram in a patient who had RAS.

Indications

ACEI renography is a safe, noninvasive, sensitive, specific, and cost-effective test for excluding renovascular hypertension in patients who have normal or nearly normal renal function. It can be performed in patients who have moderate to high risk for renovascular hypertension; patients who have severe hypertension; or patients under age 30 or over age 55 who have abrupt or recent onset of hypertension, hypertension that is resistant to medical therapy, abdominal or flank bruits, unexplained azotemia, worsening renal function during therapy with ACEIs, end-organ damage, or occlusive disease in other vascular beds.

Pitfalls and limitations

In addition to controversies related to variation in technique, such as patient hydration, selection of tracer and ACEI, effect of medication, and use of diuretics, Blaufox and colleagues [91] and the Einstein/Cornell Collaborative Hypertension Group found that it is difficult to detect bilateral disease with the technique. Renal insufficiency frequently results in a nondiagnostic ACEI renogram. Overhydration may result in false-negative tests, whereas underhydration may result in a false-positive result. Moreover, an asymmetric small kidney with poor function often is unresponsive to the effects of captopril and, therefore, may be ipsilateral to RAS without typical diagnostic findings on a captopril renogram [84].

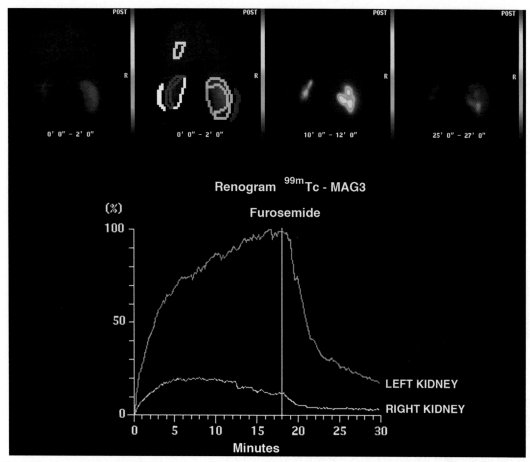

Fig. 2. Renal study with MAG3 in a patient who had suspected obstruction of the right kidney. The upper row of images demonstrates rapid clearance of tracer from a small left kidney but delayed clearance from the normal-sized right kidney. The time-activity curves demonstrate a marked acceleration of clearance after furosemide administration in the left kidney. In contrast, the drug effect is blunted significantly in the right kidney, consistent with partial obstruction.

Other imaging modalities

Renal angiography is the most accurate test for anatomic diagnosis of RAS, but it uses potentially nephrotoxic contrast agents and its associated radiation dose is high compared with other modalities. CT angiography (CTA), magnetic resonance angiography (MRA), and Doppler sonography (DS) are new noninvasive approaches for the diagnosis of renal artery stenosis. DS can be used to monitor recurrent stenosis after corrective therapy and is effective for classifying patients as responders or nonresponders to therapy. Unfortunately, US criteria for RAS based on evaluation of renal peak systolic velocity and renal/aortic ratio are controversial. CTA and MRA provide anatomic information about renal artery stenosis. CTA has higher spatial resolution than MRA and can be used to evaluate the calcium content of atherosclerotic lesions before treatment; however, the associated radiation dose

is high and potentially nephrotoxic contrast agents are required. In contrast, MRA does not expose patients to ionizing radiation or directly nephrotoxic contrast agents. Recently, Eklof and colleagues [92] compared DS, MRA, CTA, DS, and captopril renography for assessing renal artery disease and concluded that MRA and CTA were significantly better than duplex US and captopril renography for detecting hemodynamically significant RAS. A meta-analysis performed by Vasbinder and colleagues [93] supports these findings.

Future prospects

Although captopril renography can play an important role in the evaluation of renovascular hypertension, the use of this test is decreasing. Recently, the clinical use of ACEI renography changed in two ways. First, with the introduction of other new noninvasive imaging techniques, ACEI renography

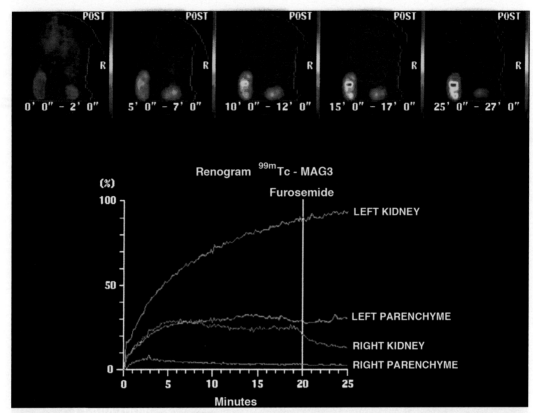

Fig. 3. Renal study with MAG3 in a patient who had suspected renal obstruction. The upper row of images demonstrates significant clearance of tracer from a small right kidney but progressive accumulation of tracer from a normal-sized left kidney. The time-activity curves demonstrate a significant furosemide effect in the right kidney but no effect on the left kidney, consistent with obstruction.

cannot be recommended as the primary imaging procedure for assessing RAS; rather, it usually is used after abnormal results are obtained with MRA and CTA or DS [94]. Secondly, It is more acceptable to use ACEI renography in predicting prognosis of renovascular hypertension and its treatment.

Renography using aspirin or angiotensin II competitors (eg, valsartan) is considered an alternative to captopril renography. These drugs have the advantage of not effecting blood pressure and do not require that treatment with ACEIs be discontinued before imaging. Preliminary studies have suggested that aspirin renography is more sensitive than captopril renography for evaluation of renovascular hypertension [95]. These results are not yet validated in large studies and, therefore, its use is not clinically widespread.

Clinical applications

Renal vascular hypertension

Renal vascular hypertension (RVH) is the most common cause of secondary hypertension. Although it accounts for less than 1% of cases in unselected populations, it is the cause of hypertension in as many as 30% of cases in selected populations [96]. RVH occurs when there is RAS. In older patients, RAS usually is the result of atherosclerosis with increasing luminal narrowing. Fibromuscular dysplasia accounts for approximately 25% of all cases of RVH, and it affects children, young to middle-aged adults, and mostly women under the age of 35 [97]. Other conditions that may be associated with RVH include cholesterol embolic disease, acute arterial thrombosis or embolism, aortic dissection, neurofibromatosis, renal arterial trauma, arterial aneurysm, arteriovenous malformation of the renal artery, and polyarteritis nodosa and other vasculitides.

Pathophysiologically, RVH is a clinical consequence of renin-angiotensin system activation. Ischemia caused by renal artery occlusion results in an elevation of blood pressure by triggering the release of renin, which mediates the conversion of angiotensin I to angiotensin II, which helps maintain physiologic renal perfusion.

RVH can be cured via nephrectomy or vascular repair, and the earlier an arterial stenosis causing RVH

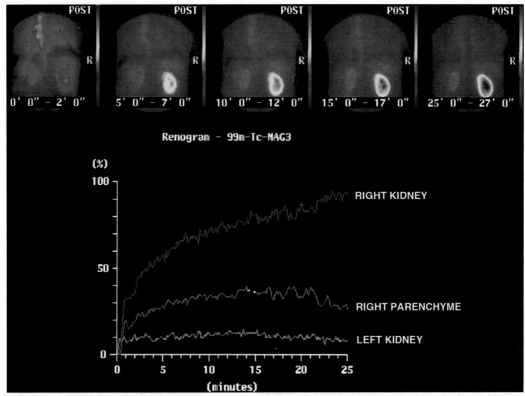

Fig. 4. Renal study with MAG3 in a patient who had hypertension resulting from suspected renal artery stenosis. After captopril administration, the upper row of images demonstrates minimal function of the left kidney but marked retention of tracer on the right. The time-activity curves demonstrate minimal function in the left kidney but progressive retention of tracer on the right. A baseline study (without captopril) demonstrated significant tracer clearance by the right kidney.

is detected the greater the chance for cure. Accordingly, the role of ACEI renography is to exclude RVH in hypertensive populations and, more importantly, to identify the patients who are surgical candidates. The most widely accepted procedure for interpretation of ACEI renography is based on changes in renograms before and after ACE inhibition [98]. In this qualitative grading system, an examination is considered positive if grade decreases on the postcaptopril scan compared with the baseline study. According to a consensus report, ACEI renography can be categorized as low probability, intermediate probability, and high probability for RVH [99]. The sensitivity of the test varies from 83% to 100% and specificity ranges from 62% to 100% [84]. Johansson and colleagues [100] demonstrated that ^{99m}Tc-DTPA captopril renography and duplex US have high specificity and negative predictive values. They suggested that duplex US should be the first-line method when screening for RAS in a hypertensive population. Considering the advantages and limitations of different modalities and the low prevalence of RVH, no method is appropriate as a mass screening produce for the

presence of RVH. It is suggested that a typical diagnostic work-up should first use DS, CTA, or MRA. If this initial evaluation is positive, patients should be studied by ACEI renography.

Maini and colleagues [101] performed aspirin renography in 12 patients who had a clinical suspicion of renovascular hypertension and compared the results with captopril renography using ^{99m}Tc-DTPA. They reported that aspirin renography is superior to captopril renography in the assessment of patients in whom there is suspicion of unilateral and bilateral renovascular hypertension. Despite this success, aspirin renography, like exercise renography and angiotensin receptor blockade renography, requires additional validation [102].

Radionuclide cystography

Radionuclide cystography (RNC) is a method to detect or exclude VUR. There are two different protocols for this test: indirect RNC (IRC) and direct RNC (DRC). IRC does not require bladder catheterization but requires the intravenous injection of the radiopharmaceutical for evaluation of renal function, urine drainage, and detection of VUR. Currently, IRC is not used commonly, because it cannot identify patients who have reflux only during the filling phrase. DRC requires catheterization of the bladder and instillation of radionuclide and fluid for maximum distension of the bladder, allowing imaging during filling and voiding and after voiding. Urinary tract catheterization of children is an important step in this procedure. Dikshit and colleagues [103] reported that the specificity and sensitivity of DRC for detecting VUR are 95.8% and 95%, respectively. Examples of a normal radionuclide voiding cystourethrography (VCUG) and a study in a patient who had significant reflux are illustrated in Fig. 5.

Overall, RNC is an alternative procedure for detecting and excluding VUR with greater sensitivity and specificity compared with VCUG. Radionuclide cystography, however, does not provide the anatomic detail of VCUG. The greatest advantage of RNC is its low radiation exposure, which is of great significance in infants and children.

Indications

According to the Society of Nuclear Medicine, the indications for RNC include initial evaluation of women who have urinary tract infection for reflux, diagnosis of familial reflux, evaluation of VUR after medical management, assessment of the results of antireflux surgery, and serial evaluation of bladder dysfunction (eg, neurogenic bladder) for reflux [104].

Pitfalls and limitations

DRC requires bladder catheterization, which may increase the risk for renal tract infection. In addition, it does not provide anatomic information that is required to classify grade of VUR.

Future prospects

Although RNC is more sensitive than radiographic contrast techniques, it has several limitations, including the necessity of bladder catheterization and the lack of anatomic information. DRC can be used for the diagnosis of VUR as an alternative to VCUG; however, it cannot replace conventional VCUG completely. With continuing improvements in imaging techniques, the disadvantages of RNC may be overcome in the future. Jose and colleagues [105] showed promising results of a study that evaluated radionuclide cystography by direct suprapubic puncture and instillation of the radiotracer

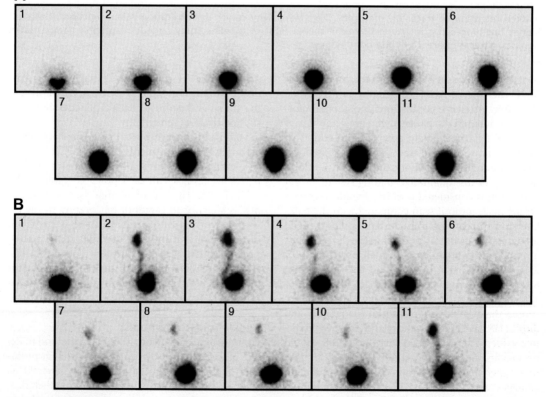

Fig. 5. (A) Radionuclide VCUG in a patient who did not have reflux. (B) Radionuclide VCUG in a patient who had significant reflux.

directly into the bladder, thereby avoiding catheterization [104].

Other imaging modalities

The detection or exclusion of VUR classically is performed by VCUG, which provides detailed anatomic information and can grade the intensity of reflux. High radiation exposure and intermittent imaging are the main disadvantages of VCUG. Currently, echo-enhanced voiding urosonography, indirect voiding urosonography, and magnetic resonance voiding cystography are being investigated for the detection of in children. Ascenti and colleagues [106] reported that contrast-enhanced color voiding DS has high specificity (97%) and sensitivity (81%) and that its diagnostic accuracy is greater than RNC. Magnetic resonance voiding cystography has lower sensitivity for VUR than VCUG but offers the potential of combining an anatomic and functional evaluation of the renal parenchyma and urinary tract and the advantage of investigating VUR without radiation [107].

Clinical applications

Vesicoureteric reflux

VUR occurs when the valve at the ureterovesical junction fails to prevent retrograde flow of urine from the bladder. VUR alone does not result in damage; however, intrarenal reflux of infected urine can result in scarring, hypertension, and chronic renal failure. Almost all children who are diagnosed with VUR are assessed because of febrile urinary tract infection (UTI) or prenatal hydronephrosis; 10% children evaluated for prenatal hydronephrosis are found to have VUR [108]. In addition, VUR is related strongly to genetic factors. The diagnosis of VUR is made most commonly during evaluation of a UTI. Renal parenchymal imaging with ^{99m}Tc-dimercaptosuccinic acid (DMSA) can determine the presence or absence of reflux and measure the postvoiding residue in the bladder. With VUR, radioactivity uptake above the bladder can be seen on the RNC scan. VCUG can be used to diagnose and grade intensity of reflux.

Cortical scintigraphy

UTI may be limited to the bladder (cystitis) or may involve the upper collecting system (pyelitis) or the renal parenchyma (pyelonephritis). The major cause of UTI in children is acute pyelonephritis. Hypertension and high-grade VUR combined with UTI tract infection lead to a high risk for developing renal scarring. More importantly, it is suggested that renal scarring can be prevented or diminished by early diagnosis and treatment of acute pyelonephritis (APN). Therefore, accurate diagnosis is of significant clinical importance.

Renal cortical scintigraphy commonly is performed in infants and children. Although several radiopharmaceuticals are available for this procedure, ^{99m}Tc-DMSA is preferred. Alternative tracers for renal imaging are those with high excretion rate used for renography, such as ^{99m}Tc-MAG3 and ^{123}I-hippuran. These tracers offer the advantage of combining cortical imaging with information about renal excretion; however, they are less useful for the detection of cortical defects. Renal cortical scintigraphy using ^{99m}Tc-DMSA usually is performed to assess the renal sequelae of UTI.

No special preparations are required for cortical scintigraphy; however, it is recommended that children be well hydrated to reduce pelvic retention. The value of single photon emission CT (SPECT) is controversial. Studies by Craig and colleagues and De Sadeleer and colleagues [109,110] concluded that the addition of SPECT imaging increases the risk for false-positive images and interobserver variability. Scintigraphy is performed 2 to 3 hours after tracer injection and should include at least a posterior view, acquired for a minimum of 200,000 counts or 5 minutes using a high-resolution parallel-hole collimator, and both posterior oblique views.

The sensitivity of DMSA for detection of parenchymal defects resulting from infection ranges from 80% to 100% but does not allow differentiation of APN from renal scars [111,112]. The area of highest controversy is the place of cortical scintigraphy in investigations of APN [113].

Indications

Cortical scintigraphy is the most accepted imaging technique for evaluation of chronic renal scars, although it also is performed in the assessment of APN. DMSA scintigraphy also is used in the diagnosis of renal infarctions, horseshoe kidney, multicystic dysplastic kidney, and ectopic kidney. Segmental RAS also may be diagnosed, especially when captopril is administered 1 hour before a radiopharmaceutical.

Pitfalls and limitations

Cortical scintigraphy is accepted as a highly sensitive technique for the detection of focal lesions. It accurately reflects the histologic changes, and interobserver reproducibility is high. Potential technical pitfalls should be recognized, such as normal variants and the difficulty in differentiating acute versus chronic lesions or acquired versus congenital lesions. Although DMSA seems to play a minor role in the traditional approach to UTI, recent studies suggest that this examination might influence the treatment of the acute phase, the indication for chemoprophylaxis and micturating cystography and the duration of follow-up [114,115]. Pitfalls are related mainly to the interpretation of drainage on images and curves. Dilated uropathies represent the main indication of the renography, but the impact of this technique on the management of children is, in many cases, a matter of intense controversy. DRC and IRC are interesting alternatives to the radiographic technique and should be integrated into the diagnosis and follow-up of VUR.

Future prospects

Prospective studies are required to determine whether or not early scintigraphy can influence the type and duration of treatment in cases with a high probability of APN.

Other modalities

Renal DS commonly is used in the evaluation and management of UTI. The advantages of this procedure are its wide availability, low cost, and lack of radiation. Depending on operator dependence, poor interobserver reproducibility, and low sensitivity for the detection of acute inflammatory changes of the renal cortex, however, it can be useful for detecting only severe UTI.

MRU imaging seems a reliable technique for the diagnosis of APN and adds valuable anatomic information for further management. Lonergan and colleagues [116] demonstrated that gadolinium-enhanced inversion-recovery MR imaging enabled detection of more pyelonephritic lesions than did renal cortical scintigraphy and had superior interobserver agreement. Weiser and coworkers [117] demonstrated that MRU has potential for differentiating APN from scar. Disadvantages of MRU imaging include the need for sedation in infants and younger children and the cost of the procedure.

Clinical application: pyelonephritis and renal cortical scarring

APN is a clinical syndrome of chills, fever, and flank pain, which is accompanied by bacteriuria and pyuria. It generally is believed that infants are more susceptible to development of renal scarring after pyelonephritis than children over 5 years of age [114].

APN leads to the development of irreversible renal scarring, which can be avoided by early diagnosis and treatment. Renal scarring resulting from pyelonephritis seems related to VUR but in some cases can be caused by the infection itself [118]. Ajdinovie and colleagues [119] reported that the incidence of DMSA findings is higher in UTI with VUR.

Cortical uptake of DMSA is associated with two factors: renal blood flow and distal tubular cell membrane transport function. An early response to APN is elevated renal vein renin, which results indirectly in ischemia [120]. The pyelonephritic lesions show decreased uptake resulting from regional ischemia [121]. Compared with other imaging modalities, DMSA cortical demography remains the gold standard for the diagnosis of renal cortical scarring and also is useful in accessing sequelae of UTIs [122]. An example of a cortical defected detected by DSMA imaging is illustrated in Fig. 6.

A study by Lavocat and colleagues [123] reported that DMSA imaging should be considered as a reference in the detection and follow-up scarring associated with APN. Other researchers have suggested that acute renography is not necessary because half of the acute lesions are transitory and disappear at follow-up [124,125].

Renal transplant evaluation

Renal transplantation currently is the treatment choice for most patients who have end-stage renal disease. In recent years, recipient survival rate has increased because of advances in histocompatibility testing, surgical techniques, immunosuppressive regimens, and overall care of transplant recipients. The transplanted kidney is subject to many potential complications, which occur at a variety of times after the initial surgery [126,127]. According to the anatomy or treatment, these complications can be classified as prerenal, renal, or postrenal and medical or surgical. Thus, noninvasive methods for

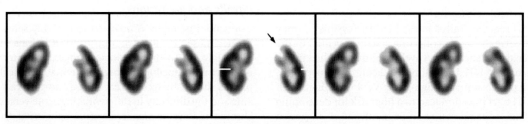

Fig. 6. Selected SPECT images (coronal) of a ^{99m}Tc-DMSA study of a patient who had pyelonephritis. The cortical defect is indicated by the arrow.

monitoring graft function and early detection of major complications are essential. Because of their noninvasive character and repeatability, radionuclide methods are used widely in the evaluation of renal grafts. Perfusion studies (bolus transit or first pass) and renography are the most common procedures for monitoring graft function [128,129].

ATN is an early complication in cadarevic allografts and frequently resolves spontaneously in 1 to 3 weeks [130]. The radionuclide imaging findings associated with this condition are well-preserved perfusion but poor renal function and decreased urine excretion. Persistence of reduced function (without improvement) in vasomotor nephropathy can be superimposed on acute rejection. Examples of radionuclide studies in patients who have ATN and acute rejection are illustrated in Fig. 7.

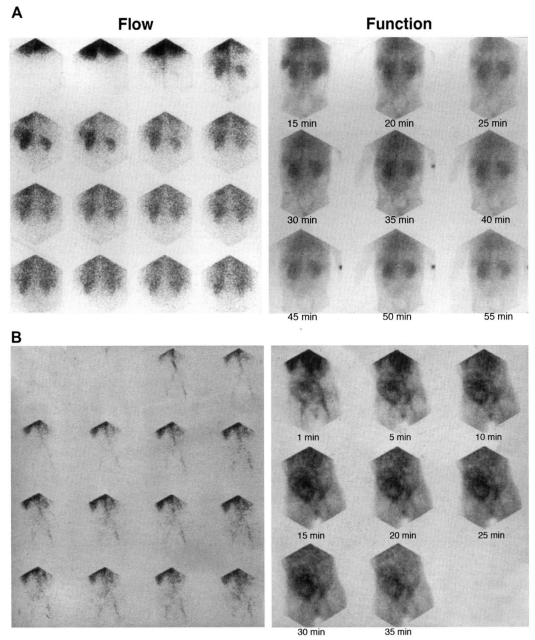

Fig. 7. (*A*) Renal study with ^{99m}Tc-DTPA in a renal transplant patient. The perfusion images demonstrate significant flow to the graft (right sided) with minimal function, consistent with ATN. (*B*) Renal study with ^{99m}Tc-DTPA in a renal transplant patient demonstrating decreased perfusion and function, consistent with graft rejection.

Acute rejection is the most common type of allo-graft rejection, which occurs late in the first postoperative week [131]. The renogram in conjunction with the bolus transit time may be helpful in confirming the diagnosis of acute rejection and can be used to differentiate acute rejection from vasomotor nephropathy. Diminished flow on radionuclide imaging also can be observed in graft thrombosis. A worsening of perfusion and uptake on radionuclide studies within an interval of 2 or 3 days suggests rejection. In addition, quantitative measurements of GFR or effective renal plasma flow are decreased in acute rejection. Doppler US does not demonstrate any specific findings in this condition [132].

Chronic rejection is the major cause of permanent graft failure. The characteristic findings of chronic rejection are cortical thinning and mild hydronephrosis on gray-scale US and radionuclide images [132]. The only unequivocal method, however, for confirming the diagnosis of allograft rejection in transplant patients who have renal dysfunction is early biopsy.

Unfortunately, none of the imaging modalities currently available can be used to specifically determine the cause of allograft rejection. Although over the years, several radiopharmaceutics have been proposed for the diagnosis of transplant rejection, none has been shown adequately specific. Agents tested for this purpose include radiolabeled monoclonal antibodies (^{99m}Tc-labeled OKT3 and ^{111}indium-labeled TNT-1) and autologous platelets labeled with various radionuclides [133,134]. Although these tracers have produced interesting results in preclinical models and preliminary clinical trials, none is deployed in routine clinic practice.

Of all cases of post-transplantation hypertension, 1% to 5% are caused by transplant renal artery stenosis, which may develop early or late in the post-transplantation period [135]. There are many causes of this condition, including suture technique, renal artery trauma during transplantation, torsion of the renal artery, rejection, atherosclerosis in the donor or recipient arteries, and cytomegalovirus infection. In these patients, the findings on captopril scan are similar to those of renovascular hypertension in native kidneys [127]. Compared with other imaging modalities, this procedure has the advantages of being able to exclude transplant hypertension caused by RAS and differentiating functional from nonfunctional RAS noninvasively. Color Doppler flow US is useful for initial screening in transplant RAS. Transplant RAS also can be diagnosed with gadolinium-enhanced MRU and CTA [136]. The CT contrast medium may induce nephropathy,

however, especially when renal insufficiency is present.

The most common cause of ureteral obstruction is ureteral ischemia. The causes may be intrinsic, such as ureteral stricture, blood clots, and calculi, or extrinsic, including fluid collections or masses [137–140]. Because renal allograft rejection has similar presenting features to ureteral obstruction, early diagnosis is difficult. As in native kidneys, diuretic renography may be useful for distinguishing obstructed from nonobstructed kidneys.

CT has limited use in the evaluation of renal transplants as a result of its use of contrast medium and lack of functional information. It can provide detailed anatomic information, however, which cannot be obtained with US because of technical factors, such as bowel loops, surgical sutures, and osseous structures.

MRU is developing rapidly. Despite its disadvantages (discussed previously), it can provide anatomic and functional information of the transplant arterial system, the renal parenchyma, the peritransplant region, and graft GFR. MRI using macrophages labeled with ultrasmall, superparamagnetic, iron-oxide nanoparticles is a new technique used to detect allograft rejection in rats [141]. Although the results are promising, additional studies are required before the technique can be studied in clinical trials.

Summary

Nuclear medicine will continue to have an important and expanding role in the evaluation of patients who have renal disorders. Although currently, research in renal nuclear medicine is not very active, there have been several important contributions for the improvement of clinical care. Technical developments recently applied include tracers that are more specific and appropriate for young children, new types of interventional renography, early injection of furosemide, late postmicturition and gravity-assisted imaging, and, finally, more objective parameters of renal drainage. Standardizations of methodology remain an important issue for renal nuclear medicine.

References

[1] Taplin GV, Meredith OM, Kade H, et al. The radio-isotope renogram. An external test for individual kidney function and upper tract patency. J Lab Clin Med 1956;48:886–8.

[2] McAfree JG, Wanger HN Jr. Visualization of renal parenchyma. Scintiscanning with 203-DHg neohydrin. Radiology 1960;75:820–1.

[3] Raynaud C, Desgrez A, Kellershohn C. Measurement of renal mercury uptake by external

counting. Separate function testing of each kidney. J Urol 1968;99:248–63.

[4] Estorch Cabreram M, Carrio Gasset I. Nephrourology and nuclear medicine today. Arch Esp Urol 2001;54(6):637–48 [in Spanish].

[5] Smith HW. The kidney: structure and function in health and disease. New York: Oxford University Press; 1951. p. 63–66.

[6] Levey AS, Bosch JP, Lewis JB, et al. A more accurate method to estimate glomerular filtration rate from serum creatinine: a new prediction equation. Ann Intern Med 1999;130(6):461–70.

[7] Laterza OF, Prince CP, Mitchell G, et al. An improved estimator of glomerular filtration rate? Clin Chem 2002;48:699–707.

[8] Lin J, Knight EL, Hogan ML, et al. A comparison of prediction equations for estimating glomerular filtration rate in adults without kidney disease Tc-MAG3 scans. J Am Soc Nephrol 2003; 14(10):2573–80.

[9] Eckelman W, Richards P. Instant 99mTc-DTPA. J Nucl Med 1970;11:761.

[10] Klopper JF, Hauser W, Atkins HL. Evaluation of 99mTc-DTPA for the measurement of glomerular filtration rate. J Nucl Med 1972;13:107–10.

[11] Piepsz A, Denis R, Ham HR, et al. A simple method for method for measuring separate glomerular filtration rate using a single injection of 99mTc-DTPA and scintillation camera. J Pediatr 1978;93:430–5.

[12] Tsushima Y, Blomley MJK, Okabe K, et al. Determination of glomerular filtration rate per unit renal volume using computed tomography: correlation with conventional measures of total and divided renal function. J Urol 2001;165:382–5.

[13] Chachati A, Meyers A, Godon JP, et al. Rapid method for the measurement of differential renal function: validation. J Nucl Med 1987;28: 829–36.

[14] Dubovsky EV, Russell CD. Quantitation of renal function with glomerular and tubular agents. Semin Nucl Med 1982;12:308–29.

[15] Gates GF. Glomerular filtration rate: estimation from fractional renal accumulation of (stannous). AJR Am J Roentgenol 1982;138:565–70.

[16] Shore RM, Koff SA, Mentser M. Glomerular filtration rate in children determination from the 99m-Tc-DTPA renogram. Radiology 1984;151: 627–33.

[17] Esteves EP, Halkar RK, Issa MM, et al. Comparison of camera-based 99mTc-MAG3 and 24-hour creatinine clearances for evaluation of kidney function. AJR Am J Roentgenol 2006;187: W316–9.

[18] Waller DG, Christopher MK, Fleming JS, et al. Measurement of glomerular filtration rate with technetium-99m DTPA; comparisons of plasma clearance a techniques. J Nucl Med 1987;28: 372–7.

[19] Gates GF. Filtration fraction and its implication for radionuclide renography using diethylenetriaminepentaacetic acid and mercaptoacetyltriglycine. Clin Nucl Med 2004;29:231–7.

[20] Carlsen O. The gamma camera as an absolute measurement device: determination of glomerular filtration rate in 99mTc-DTPA renography using a dual head gamma camera. Nucl Med Commun 2004;25(10):1021–9.

[21] LaFrance ND, Drew HH, Walser M. Radioisotopic measurement of glomerular filtration rate in severe chronic renal failure. J Nucl Med 1988; 29:1927–30.

[22] Delanaye P, Krzesinski JM. The new Mayo Clinic equation for estimating glomerular filtration rate. Ann Intern Med 2005;142(8):679–80.

[23] Gates GF. Split renal function testing using Tc-99m DTPA; a rapid technique for determining differential glomerular filtration. Clin Nucl Med 1983;8:400–7.

[24] Goates JJ, Morton KA, Whooten WW, et al. Comparison of methods for calculating glomerular filtration rate: technetium-99m DTPA scintigraphic analysis, protein free and whole-plasma clearance of technetium-99m DTPA and iodine-125-iothalamate clearance. J Nucl Med 1990; 31(4):424–9.

[25] Taylor A. Radionuclide renography: a personal approach. Semin Nucl Med 1999;29:102–27.

[26] Thrall James H, Ziessman Harvey A, editors. Nuclear medicine the requisites. 2nd edition. St. Louis (MO): Mosby-Year Book, Inc; 2001. p. 336–50.

[27] Itoh K. Comparison of methods for determination of glomerular filtration rate: Tc-99m-DTPA renography, predicted creatinine clearance method and plasma sample method. Ann Nucl Med 2003;17(7):561–5.

[28] Petersen J, Petersen JR, Talleruphuus U, et al. Glomerulate filtration rate estimated from the uptake phrase of 99mTc-DTPA renography in chronic renal failure. Nephrol Dial Transplant 1999;14:1673–8.

[29] Rehling M, Moller ML, Thamdrup B, et al. Simultaneous measurement of renal clearance and plasma clearance of 99mTc-labelled diethylenetriaminepentaacetate, 51Cr-labelled ethylene-diaminetetra-acetate and inulin in man. Clin Sci 1984;66:613–9.

[30] Piepsz A, Dobbeleir A, Ham HR. Effect of background correction on separate technetium-99m-DTPA renal clearance. J Nucl Med 1990; 31:430–5.

[31] Gruenewald SM, Collins LT, Fawdry RM. Kidney depth measurement and its influence on quantitation of function fromgamma camera renography. Clin Nucl Med 1985;6:398–401.

[32] Itoh K, Tsushima S, Tsukamoto E, et al. Reappraisal camera methods for determination of the glomerular filtration rate with 99mTc-DTPA. Ann Nucl Med 2000;14:143–50.

[33] Prigent A, Cosgriff P, Gates GF, et al. Consensus report on quality control of quantitative measurements of renal function obtained from the

renogram: international consensus committee from the scientific committee of radionuclides in nephrourology. Semin Nucl Med 1999;29: 146–59.

[34] Blaufox MD. Over view of renal nuclear medicine. In: Ell PJ, Gambhir SS, editors. 3rd edition, Nuclear medicine in clinical diagnosis and treatment, vol. 2. Philadelphia: Elsevier Limited; 2004. p. 1497–9.

[35] Piepsz A, Prigeat A, Hall M, et al. At what level of unilateral renal impairment does contralateral functional compensation occur? Pediatr Nephrol 2005;20(11):1593–8.

[36] Sommer FG. Can single-kidney glomerular filtration rate be determinated with contrast-enhanced CT? Radiology 2007;242(2):325–6.

[37] Sommer G, Olcott EW, Chow LC, et al. Measurement of renal extraction fraction with contrast-enhanced CT. Radiology 2005;236(3):1029–33.

[38] Hackstein N, Bauer J, Hauck EW. Measuring single-kidney glomerular filtration rate on single-detector helical CT using a two-point Patlak plot technique in patients with increased interstitial space. AJR Am J Roentgenol 2003;181(1): 147–56.

[39] Daghini E, Juillard L, Haas JA, et al. Comparison of mathematic models for assessment of glomerular filtration rate with electron-beam CT in pigs. Radiology 2007;242(2):417–24.

[40] Lee VS, Rusinek H, Noz ME, et al. Dynamic three-dimensional MR renography for the measurement of single kidney function: initial experience. Radiology 2003;227:289–94.

[41] Krishnamurthi G, Stantz KM, Steinmetz R, et al. Functional imaging in small animals using x-ray computed tomography: study of physiologic measurement reproducibility. IEEE Trans Med Imaging 2005;24(7):832–43.

[42] Hackstein N, Wiegand C, Rau WS, et al. Glomerular filtration rate measured by using triphasic helical CT with a two-point Patlak plot technique. Radiology 2004;230(1):221–6.

[43] O'Dell-Anderson KJ, Twardock R, Grimm JB, et al. Determination of glomerular filtration rate in dogs using contrast-enhanced computed tomography. Vet Radiol Ultrasound 2006; 47(2):127–35.

[44] Baker LRI. Renal disease. In: Warrell DA, Cox TM, Firth JD, editors. Oxford textbook of medicine. 4th edition. Oxford (UK): Oxford University Press; 2003. p. 1024–57.

[45] Brown SCW. Nuclear medicine in the clinical diagnosis and treatment of obstructive uropathy. In: Ell PJ, Gambhir SS, editors. 3rd edition, Nuclear medicine in clinical diagnosis and treatment, vol. 2. Philadelphia: Elsevier Limited; 2004. p. 1581–9.

[46] Begi CA. Role of radionuclide imaging in nephrourology. Med Arh 2006;60(5):328–9.

[47] Rado JP, Bano C, Tako J. Radioisotope renography during furosemide (Lasix) diuresis. Nucl Med Commun 1968;7:212–21.

[48] Thrall JH, Koff SA, Keyes JW Jr. Diuretic radionuclide renography and scintigraphy in the differential diagnosis of hydroureteronephrosis. Semin Nucl Med 1981;11:89–104.

[49] O'Reilly PH. Standardization of diuresis renography techniques. Nucl Med Commun 1998; 19:1–2.

[50] O'Reilly PH, Lawson RS, Shields RA, et al. Idiopathic hydronephrosis: the diuresis renogram—a new non-invasive method of assessing equivocal pelvioureteral junction obstruction. J Urol 1979;121:153–5.

[51] English PJ, Testa HJ, Lawson RS, et al. Modified method of diuresis renography for the assessment of equivocal pelviureteric junction obstruction. Br J Urol 1987;59:10–4.

[52] Imai M. Effect of bumetanide and furosemide on the thick asending limbs of Henle's loop of rabbits and rats perfused in vitro. Eur J Pharmacol 1977;41:409–16.

[53] Turkolmez S, Atasever T, Turkolmez K, et al. Comparison of three different diuretic renal scintigraphy protocols in patients with dilated upper urinary tracts. Clin Nucl Med 2004; 29(3):154–60.

[54] O'Reilly PH. Diuresis renography: recent advances and recommend protocols. Br J Urol 1992;69:113–20.

[55] Upsdell SM, Testa HJ, Lawson RS. The F-15 diuresis renogram in suspected obstruction of the upper urinary tract. Br J Urol 1992;69: 126–31.

[56] Tripathi M, Chandrashekar N, Phom H, et al. Evaluation of dilated upper renal tracts by technetium-99m ethylenedicysteine F+O diuresis renography in infants and children. Ann Nucl Med 2004;18(8):681–7.

[57] Wong DC, Rossleigh MA, Farnsworth RH. F+0 diuresis renography in infants and children. J Nucl Med 1990;40(11):1805–11.

[58] Donoso G, Kuvvenhoven JD, Ham H, et al. 99mTc-MAG3 diuretic renography in children: a comparison between F0 and F+20. Nucl Med Commun 2003;24(11):1189–93.

[59] Liu Y, Ghesani NV, Shurick JH, et al. The F + 0 protocol for diuretic renography results in fewer interrupted studies due to voiding than the F − 15 protocol. J Nucl Med 2005;46(8): 1317–20.

[60] Conway JJ, Maizels M. The "well tempered" diuretic renogram: a standard method to examine the asymptomatic neonate with hydronephrosis or hydroureteronephrosis. A report from combined meetings of The Society for Fetal Urology and members of the pediatric Nuclear Medicine Council—The society of nuclear medicine. J Nucl Med 1992;33:2047–51.

[61] Tremel F, Caravel JP, Siche JP, et al. Diagnostic value of renal scintigraphy with MAG 3 and DTPA in the diagnosis of renal artery stenosis. Arch Mal Coeur Vaiss 1996;89(8): 1035–9.

[62] Upsdell SM, Leeson SM, Brooman PJ, et al. Diuretic-induced urinary flow rates at varing clearance and their relevance to the performance and interpretation of diuresis renography. Br J Urol 1988;61:14–8.

[63] Brown SCW, Upsdell SM, O'Reilly PH. The importance of renal function in the interpretation of diuresis renography. Br J Urol 1992;69:121–5.

[64] Zechmann W. An experimental of approach to explain some misinterpretations of diuresis renography. Nucl Med Commun 1988;9:283–94.

[65] Uero S, Suzuki Y, Murakami T, et al. Quantitative analysis of infantile ureteropelvic junction obstruction by diuretic renography. Ann Nucl Med 2001;15(2):131–6.

[66] Roarke MC, Sandler CM. Provocative imaging. Diuretic renography. [review]. Urol Clin North Am 1998;25(2):227–49.

[67] Oh SJ, Moon DH, Kang W. Supranormal differential renal function is real but may be pathological: assessment by 99m technetium mercaptoacetyltriglycine renal scan of congenital unilateral hydronephrosis. J Urol 2001; 165(6 Pt 2):2300–4.

[68] Garcia EV, Talor A, Manatunga D, et al. A software engine to justify the conclusions of an expert system for detecting renal obstruction on 99mTc-MAG3 scans. J Nucl Med 2007;48(3): 463–70.

[69] Vaidyanathan S, Hughes PL, Soni BM. A comparative study of ultrasound examination of urinary tract performed on spinal cord injury patients with no urinary symptoms and spinal cord injury patients with symptoms related to urinary tract: do findings of ultrasound examination lead to changes in clinical management? ScientificWorldJournal 2006;6:2450–9.

[70] Watkin S, Bowra J, Sharma P, et al. Validation of emergency physician ultrasound in diagnosing hydronephrosis in ureteric colic. Emerg Med Australas 2007;19(3):188–95.

[71] Kemper J, Regier M, Stork A, et al. Improved visualization of the urinary tract in multidetector CT urography (MDCTU): analysis of individual acquisition delay and opacification using furosemide and low-dose test images. J Comput Assist Tomogr 2006;30(5):751–7.

[72] Nolte-Ernsting C, Staatz G, Wildberger J, et al. MR-urography and CT-urography: princles, examination techniques, applications. Rofo 2003;175(2):211–22.

[73] Riccabona M. Pediatric MRU-its potensial and its role in the diagnostic work-up of upper urinary tract dilatation in infants and children. World J Urol 2004;22(2):79–87.

[74] Woodward M, Frank D. Postnatal management of antenatal hydronephrosis. BJU Int 2002;89: 149–56.

[75] Eskild-Jensen A, Gordon I, Piepsz A, et al. Congential unilateral hydronephrosis: a review of the impact of diuretic renography on clinical treatment. J Urol 2005;173:1471–6.

[76] Shokeir AA, El-Diasty T, Eassa W, et al. Diagnosis of noncalcareous hydronephrosis; role of magnetic resonance urography and noncontrast computed tomography. Urology 2004;63: 225–9.

[77] Chu WC, Lam WW, Chan KW, et al. Dynamic gadolinium-enhanced magnetic resonance urography for assessing drainage in dilated pelvicalyceal system with moderate renal function: preliminary results and comparison with diuresis renography. BJU Int 2004;93(6): 830–4.

[78] Sfakianakis GN, Cohen DJ, Braunstein RH, et al. MAG3-F0 scintigraphy in decision making for emergy intervation in renal colic after helical CT positive for a urolith. J Nucl Med 2000; 41:1813–22.

[79] Fommei E, Ghione S, Palla L, et al. Renal scintigraphic captopril test in the diagnosis of renal vascular hypertension. Hypertension 1987;10: 212–20.

[80] Majd M, Potter BM, Guzzetta PC, et al. Effect of captopril on efficacy of renal scintigraphy in detection of renal artery stenosis. [abstract]. J Nucl Med 1983;24(Suppl 5):23.

[81] Fine EJ, Blaufox MD. The Einstein/Cornell collaborative protocol to assess efficacy and methodology in captopril scintigraphy: early results in patients with essential hypertension. Report of the Einstein/Cornell Collaborative Hypertension Group. Am J Hypertens 1991;4(12 Pt 2): 716s–20s.

[82] Claveau-Tremblay R, Turpin S, De Brackeleer M, et al. False-positive captopril renography in patients taking calcium antagonists. J Nucl Med 1998;39:1621–6.

[83] Kopecky RT, Thomas FD, McAfee JG. Furosemide augments the effects of captopril on nuclear studies in renovascular stenosis. Hypertension 1987;10:181–8.

[84] Prigent A, Taylor A. The role of ACE inhibitor renography in the diagnosis of renovascular hypertension. In: Robert E Henkin, Davide Bova, Stephen M Karesh, et-al, editors. Nuclear medicine. Philadelphia: Elsevier Limited; 2006. p. 1051–75.

[85] Lagomarsino E, Orellana P, Munoz J, et al. Captopril scintigraphy in the study of arterial hypertension in pediatrics. Pediatr Nephrol 2004;19(1):66–70.

[86] Nally JV Jr, Black HR. State-of-the-art review: captopril renography—pathophysiological considerations and clinical observations. [review]. Semin Nucl Med 1992;22(2):85–97.

[87] Dondi M, Fanti S, De Fabritiis A, et al. Prognostic value of captopril renal scintigraphy in renovascular hypertension. J Nucl Med 1992;33(11): 2040–4.

[88] Bujenovic LS. Renovascular hypertension: a noninvasive screening approach using captopril renography. J Am Board Fam Pract 1995; 8(4):295–9.

[89] Nally JV, Barton DP. Contemporary approach to diagnosis and evaluation of renovascular hypertension [review]. Urol Clin North Am 2001; 28(4):781–91.

[90] Koyanagi T, Nonomura K, Takeuchi I. Surgery for renovascular disease: a single-center experience in revascularizing renal artery stenosis and aneurysm. Urol Int 2002;68:24–31.

[91] Blaufox MD, Fine EJ, Heller S, et al. Prospective study of simultaneous orthoiodohippurate and diethylenetriaminepentaacetic acid captopril renography. The Einstein/Cornell Collaborative Hypertension Group. J Nucl Med 1998;39: 522–8.

[92] Eklof H, Ahlstrom A, Magnusson A, et al. A prospective comparison of duplex ultrasonography, captopril renography, MRA, and CTA in assessing renal artery stenosis. Acta Radiol 2006;47(8):764–74.

[93] Vasbinder GB, Nelemans PJ, Kessels AG, et al. Diagnostic tests for renal artery stenosis in patients suspected of having renovascular hypertension: a meta-analysis. Ann Intern Med 2001;14(16):724–33.

[94] Boubaker A, Prior JO, Meuwly JY, et al. Radionuclide investigations of the urinary tract in the era of multimodality imaging. J Nucl Med 2006;47:1819–36.

[95] Karanikas G, Becherer A, Wiesner K, et al. ACE inhibition is superior to angiotensin receptor blockade for renography in rena artery stenosis. Eur J Nucl Med 2002;29(3):312–8.

[96] Fields LF, Burt VL, Jeffery A, et al. The burden of adult hypertension in the United States 1999 to 2000. A rising tide. Hypertension 2004;44: 398–404.

[97] Helin KH, Lepantalo M, Edgren J. Predicting the outcome of invasive treatment of renal artery disease. J Intern Med 2000;247(1): 105–10.

[98] Nally JV Jr, Chen C, Fine E, et al. Diagnostic critirior of renovascular hypertension with captopril renography. A consensus statement. Am J Hypertens 1991;4:749S–53S.

[99] Talor A, Nally J, Aurell M, et al. Consensus report on ACE inhibitor renography for detecting-renovascular hypertension. J Nucl Med 1996; 37:1876–82.

[100] Johansson M, Jensen G, Aurell M, et al. Evaluation of duplex ultrasound and captopril renography for detection of renovascular hypertension. Kidney Int 2000;58(2):774–82.

[101] Maini A, Gambhir S, Singhal M, et al. Aspirin renography in the diagnosis of renovascular hypertension: a comparative study with captopril renography. Nucl Med Commun 2000;21: 325–31.

[102] Mudun A, Falay O, Eryilmaz A, et al. Can exercise renography be an alternative to ACE inhibitor renography in hypertensive patients who are suspicious for renal artery stenosis? Clin Nucl Med 2004;29(1):27–34.

[103] Dikshit MP, Acharya VN, Shikare S, et al. Comparison of direct radionuclide cystography with micturating cystourethrography for the diagnosis of vesicoureteric reflux, and its correlation with cystoscopic appearances of the ureteric. Nephrol Dial Transplant 1993;8:600–2.

[104] Klassen PS, Svetkey LP. Diagnosis and management of renovascular hrpertension. Cardiol Rev 2000;8(1):17–29.

[105] Jose TE, Mohiudheen H, Patel C, et al. Direct radionuclide cystography by supra-pubic puncture: comparison with conventional voiding cystourethrography. Nucl Med Commun 2004; 25(4):383–5.

[106] Ascenti G, Zimbaro G, Mazziotti S, et al. Vesicoureteral reflux: comparison between urosonography and radionuclide cystography. Pediatr Nephrol 2003;18(8):768–71.

[107] Lee SK, Chang Y, Park NH, et al. Magnetic resonance voiding cystography in the diagnosis of vesicoureteral reflux: comparative study with voiding cystourethrography. J Magn Reson Imaging 2005;21(4):406–14.

[108] Swerkersson S, Jodal U, Six R, et al. Relationship among vesicoureteral reflux, urinary tract infection and renal damage in children. J Urol 2007;178(2):647–51.

[109] Craig JC, Irwig L, Ford M, et al. Reliability of DMSA for the diagnosis of renal parenchymal abnormality in children. Eur J Nucl Med 2000;27:1610–6.

[110] De Sadeleer C, Bossuyt A, Goes E, et al. Renal technetium-99m DMSA SPECT in normal volunteers. J Nucl Med 1996;37(8):1346–9.

[111] Piepsz A, Ham HR. Pediatric application of renal nuclear medicine. Semin Nucl Med 2006; 36:16–35.

[112] Kovanlikaya A, Okkay N, Cakmakci H, et al. Comparison of MRI and renal scintigraphy findings in childhood acute pyelonephritis: preliminary experience. Eur J Radiol 2004;49: 76–80.

[113] Piepsz A. Cortical scintigraphy and urinary tract infection in children. Nephrol Dial Transplant 2002;17:560–2.

[114] Benador D, Benador N, Slosman D, et al. Are younger children at higher risk of renal sequelae after pyelonephritis? Lancet 1997; 349(9044):17–9.

[115] Sukamoto E, Itoh K, Morita K, et al. Reappraisal of Tc-99m DMSA scintigraphy for follow up in children with vesicoureteral reflux. Ann Nucl Med 1999;13(6):401–6.

[116] Lonergan GL, Pennington DJ, Morrison JC, et al. Children pyelonephritis: comparison of gadolinium-enhanced MR imaging and renal cortical scintigraphy for diagnosis. Radiology 1998;207:377–84.

[117] Weiser AC, Amukele SA, Leonidas JC, et al. The role of gadolinium enhanced magnetic resonance imaging for children with suspected acute pyelonephritis. J Urol 2003;169:2308–11.

[118] Taskinen S, Ronnholm K. Post-pyelonephritic renal scars are not associated with vesicoureteral reflux in children. J Urol 2005;173(4):1345–8.

[119] Ajdinovic B, Jaukovic L, Krstic Z, et al. Technetium-99m-dimercaptosuccinic acid renal scintigraphy in children with urinary tract infection. Hell J Nucl Med 2006;9(1):27–30.

[120] Kaack MB, Dowling KJ, Patterson GM, et al. Immunology of pyelonephritis. VIII. E coli cause granuocytic aggregation and renal ischemia. J Urol 1986;136:1117–22.

[121] Rushton HG, Majd M. Dimercaptosuccinic acid renal scintigraphy for the evaluation of pyelonephritis and scarring: a review of experimental and clinical studies. J Urol 1993;148(pt2):1726–32.

[122] Lavocat MP, Granjon D, Allard D, et al. Imaging of prelonephritis. Pediatr Radiol 1997;27:159–65.

[123] Lavocat MP, Granjon D, Guimpied Y, et al. The importance of 99Tcm-DMSA renal scintigraphy in the follow-up of acute pyelonephritis in children: comparison with urographic data. Nucl Med Commun 1998;19(7):703–10.

[124] Agras K, Ortapamuk H, Naldoken S, et al. Resolution of cortical lesions on serial renal scans in children with acute pyelonephritis. Pediatr Radiol 2007;37(2):153–8.

[125] Zaki M, Badawi M, AlMutari G, et al. Acute pyelonephritis and renal scarring in Kuwaiti children: a follow-up study using 99mTc DMSA renal scintigraphy. Pediatr Nephrol 2005;20(8):1116–9 [epub 2005 Jun 23].

[126] Diethelm AG, Dubovsky EV, Whelchel JD, et al. Diagnosis of impaired renal function after kidney transplantation using renal scintigraphy, renal plasma flow and urinary excretion of hippurate. Ann Surg 1981;191:604–16.

[127] Dubovsky EV, Russel CD, Erbas B. Radionuclide evaluation of renal transplants. Semin Nucl Med 1995;25:49–59.

[128] Ozgen Kiratti P, Gordon I. DMSA findings in the evaluation of pediatric renal allograft. Turk J Pediatr 2006;48(4):328–33.

[129] Aktas A, Haberal M. Indicators of acute rejection on Tc-99m DTPA renal scintigraphy. Transplant Proc 2006;38(2):443–8.

[130] Thrall JH, Ziessman HA, editors. Nuclear medicine—the requisites. 2nd edition. St. Louis (MO): Mosby-Year Book, Inc; 1995. p. 349–69.

[131] Frokiaer J, Thomsen HS. Renal transplant evaluation. In: Ell PJ, Gambhir SS, editors. 3rd edition, Nuclear medicine in clinical diagnosis and treatment, vol. 2. Philadelphia: Elsevier Limited; 2004. p. 1652–9.

[132] Brown ED, Chen MY, Wolfman NT, et al. Complications of renal transplantation: evaluation with US and radionuclide imaging. Radiographics 2000;20:607–22.

[133] Martins FP, Souza SA, Goncalves RT. Preliminary results of 99mTc-OKT3 scintigraphy to evaluate acute rejection in renal transplants. Transplant Proc 2004;36(9):2664–7.

[134] Chen F, Wisner JR, Omachi H, et al. Localisation of monoclonal antibody TNT-1 in experimental kidney infarction of the mouse. FASEB J 1990;4:3033–9.

[135] Luke RG, Curtus J. Biology and treatment of transplant hypertension. In: Laragh JH, Brenner BM, editors. Hypertension: pathophysiology, diagnosis, and management. 2nd edition. New York: Raven; 1995. p. 2471–83.

[136] van Helvoort-Postulart D, Dirksen CD, Nelemans PJ, et al. Renal artery stenosis cost effectiveness of diagnosis and treatment. Radiology 2007;244(2):505–13.

[137] Huang AJ, Lee VS, RusineK H. Functional renal MR imaging. [review]. Magn Reson Imaging Clin N Am 2004;12(3):469–86 vi.

[138] Sandhu C, Patel U. Renal transplantation dysfunction: the role of interventional radiology. Clin Radiol 2002;57:772–83.

[139] Orons PD, Zajko AB. Angiography and interventional aspects of renal transplantation. Radiol Clin North Am 1995;33:461–71.

[140] Bhagat VJ, Gordon RL, Osorio RW, et al. Ureteral obstructions and leaks after renal transplantation: outcome of percutaneous antegrade ureteral stent placement in44 patients. Radiology 1998;209:159–67.

[141] Ye Q, Yang D, Williams M, et al. In vivo detection of acute rat renal allograft rejection by MRI with USPIO particles. Kidney Int 2002;61(3):1124–35.

RADIOLOGIC
CLINICS
OF NORTH AMERICA

Radiol Clin N Am 46 (2008) 45–64

ELSEVIER
SAUNDERS

Interventional Uroradiology

Raul N. Uppot, MD*, Debra A. Gervais, MD, Peter R. Mueller, MD

- Imaging modalities
  Ultrasound
  Fluoroscopy
  Angiography
  Computed tomography
  Interventional MR imaging
- Preprocedure planning
  Conscious sedation
- Interventional urologic procedures
  Biopsy
  Nonfocal renal biopsy
  Focal renal biopsy
  Renal cyst aspiration biopsy
  Adrenal biopsy
  Prostate biopsy
  Transvaginal biopsy

- Image-guided percutaneous drainage
  and aspiration
  Percutaneous nephrostomy
  Suprapubic tube insertion
  Stone management
  Percutaneous ureteral lithotripsy
  Ureteral stents
  Ureteral embolization
- Renal vascular interventions
  Management of renal artery stenosis
  Renal embolization
- Ablation
  Radiofrequency or cryoablation
  Renal ablation
  Adrenal ablation
- Summary
- References

Percutaneous urologic interventions comprise a wide range of techniques, including biopsies, drainages, stone management, ureteral stenting, renal vascular interventions, and tumor ablations. With advances in imaging capabilities and percutaneous instruments, many urologic diseases that were once managed surgically are now managed with minimally invasive image-guided techniques, using only conscious sedation.

Interventional uroradiology has evolved from simple renal biopsies for diagnostic confirmation, to percutaneous management of stones, to ablation of renal and adrenal tumors. Central to this evolution is the close cooperation with the urologist and nephrologist, each of whom provides specific skill sets and knowledge that can be used to

successfully manage the patient. The purpose of this article is to detail the wide range of image-guided interventional techniques, including a discussion of indications, methods, success rates, and complications.

Imaging modalities

Advances in imaging capabilities have spurred the evolution of minimally invasive techniques. Compared with open surgery, image guidance allows one to target the pathology of interest while avoiding injury to adjacent normal tissue. Modalities used in interventional uroradiology include ultrasound, fluoroscopy, angiography, CT, and MR imaging.

Division of Abdominal Imaging and Interventional Radiology, Department of Radiology, Massachusetts General Hospital, 55 Fruit Street; White #270, Boston, MA 02114, USA
* Corresponding author.
E-mail address: ruppot@partners.org (R.N. Uppot).

doi:10.1016/j.rcl.2008.01.010

Ultrasound

Typically, a 2-mHz to 4-mHz transducer is used for most urologic procedures. Ultrasound is an excellent modality at distinguishing cysts versus solid masses. The contrast between solid renal parenchyma and fluid filled calyces makes ultrasound a useful tool for imaging the kidneys (Fig. 1). Real time targeting using ultrasound allows one to more easily approach the kidneys, which move with patient respiration. The advantages of ultrasound include no radiation and real time visualization. The disadvantages include potential for poor penetration and poor visualization of the kidneys or renal pathology because of overlying bowel gas or patient body habitus.

Ultrasound is useful for biopsies, cysts aspiration, nephrostomy, suprapubic tube placement, and may even be used for tumor ablations. Typically, to approach the kidneys, patients are placed prone, prone oblique, or in an ipsilateral side down decubitus position.

Fluoroscopy

Fluoroscopy is used in interventional urology to evaluate and access the collecting system. Real time visualization of the collecting system with contrast allows visualization of the entire collecting system, from the calyces to the bladder (Fig. 2). Pathology within the collecting system can be accessed and treated.

The advantages of fluoroscopy include real time visualization and good contrast between the collecting system and the renal parenchyma. The disadvantages include radiation to the patient and nonvisualization of adjacent solid organs. Allergy to intravenous contrast does not necessarily mean that iodine cannot be used in the collecting system. Iodine-based agents may still be carefully injected

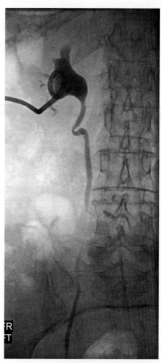

Fig. 2. Fluoroscopic coronal spot image of the left renal collecting system, including renal pelvis and ureter, after injection of an existing nephrostomy tube.

into the collecting system as long as the patient does not have a history of anaphylaxis.

Fluoroscopy is used for percutaneous nephrostomy, ureteral stent, and suprapubic tube placement. Typically, to approach the collecting system patients are placed prone or prone oblique.

Angiography

Although magnetic resonance angiography has replaced the need for many diagnostic renal angiograms, angiography is still used in the treatment of renal vascular disorders. Similar to fluoroscopy, angiography allows real time visualization of the renal vasculature with injection of contrast via femoral vessel access (Fig. 3).

The advantages of angiography include real time visualization and good contrast between renal vasculature and the remaining organs. The disadvantages include radiation, nonvisualization of adjacent solid organs, potential for an allergic reaction to iodine-based contrast, and risk for contrast-induced renal insufficiency or failure. Potential allergic reaction may be addressed with either pretreatment with steroids and antihistamines or by using gadolinium or carbon dioxide as substitute contrast agents. Contrast-induced renal insufficiency may also be addressed using the same

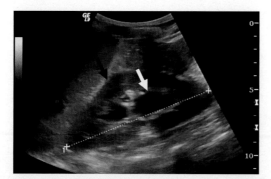

Fig. 1. Sagittal ultrasound image of the kidneys shows clear distinction between the renal parenchyma (*black arrow*) and the dilated renal collecting system (*white arrow*). Ultrasound is useful in interventional urology to target the collecting system.

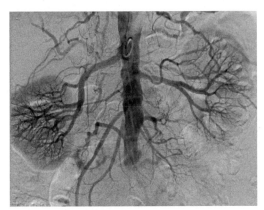

Fig. 3. Spot angiographic image after contrast injection into the descending aorta opacifying both renal arteries and renal vasculature.

substitute contrast agents and pre treatment with N-acetylcysteine and vigorous hydration.

Angiography is used for balloon dilation, stenting, and for embolization in the management of tumors or renal trauma. To access the renal vasculature, patients are typically placed supine for access to the femoral vessels.

Computed tomography

CT allows clear visualization of all the components of the urologic system, including renal parenchyma, collecting system, and vasculature (Fig. 4). Advances in multidetector CT (MDCT) now allows reformatting in any plane, which allows for improved targeting during interventional procedures.

The advantage of MDCT includes clear visualization of all organs structures, improved spatial resolution, and improved instrument visibility. The disadvantages include increased cost and increased

ionizing radiation exposure. In addition, standard CT does not typically allow for real-time visualization. However, CT fluoroscopy is an option that does allow real time visualization. CT fluoroscopy however, increases radiation exposure to the radiologist, when the radiologist reaches into the gantry to advance interventional instruments.

Interventional MR imaging

Interventional MR imaging is a new modality that may be used for urologic treatments. Currently, its primary use in interventional uroradiology is for cryoablation of renal tumors.

The advantages of interventional MR include no radiation and excellent tissue contrast. MR imaging allows visualization, in real time, of the growth of the ice ball in cryoablation and allows for very specific targeting of the tumor and its margins. The disadvantages of interventional MR include limitations in patients who cannot undergo an MR imaging study because of pacemaker, need for cardiac monitoring, or other metallic implants. Also, all instruments used in interventional procedures must be MR imaging compatible.

Preprocedure planning

Before any interventional urologic procedure, proper planning is essential. It is important to review pre procedure imaging to assess the pathology and plan for choice of modality, patient positioning, and access to the lesion. The patient's clinical history and laboratory data are reviewed. Assessment of whether the patient can receive conscious sedation, lie prone or supine for extended periods, and whether they can fit on available imaging equipment is made.

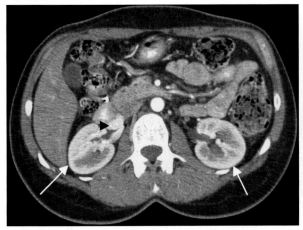
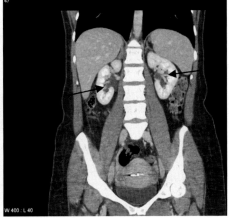

Fig. 4. Axial and coronal contrast enhanced MDCT of the kidneys showing renal parenchyma (*white arrows*), collecting system (*black arrows*), and vasculature (*black arrowhead right kidney*).

Laboratory data are reviewed: particularly the blood urea nitrogen, creatinine, prothrombin, thromboplastin time, international normalized ratio (INR), and platelets. Ideally, laboratory data should be recent (less than 3 months old). Abnormalities in INR must be corrected by withholding anticoagulation mediations (ie, heparin), giving vitamin K, or correcting the coagulation abnormality with fresh frozen plasma. Platelets should also be administered prior to or during the procedure for patients with low platelet counts. Ideally, INR should be less than or equal to 1.5 and platelets less than or equal to 50,000 th/cmm.

Conscious sedation

The majority of interventional urologic procedures are performed using both local and conscious sedation. A few nonfocal renal biopsies may be performed using only local anesthetic. Prolonged and extensive ablation cases or patients at high risk for conscious sedation because of prior myocardial infarction, stroke, and respiratory disease may need to undergo sedation by an anesthesiologist.

Conscious sedation used at the authors' institution includes midazolam and fentanyl. Locally, lidocaine is administered at a maximum dosage of 300 mg (30 cc of 1% lidocaine). Midazolam dose is weight based at 0.5 mg/kg to 1 mg/kg, and fentanyl dose is 1 mcg/kg to 3 mcg/kg. Before any procedure requiring conscious sedation, patients will need to be fasting to avoid the risk of aspiration during conscious sedation.

Interventional urologic procedures

Biopsy

Indications for biopsy include: to establish a diagnosis of benign or malignant, to stage a known malignancy, and to establish a diagnosis of malignancy in diffuse disease.

Interventional urologic biopsies include: nonfocal renal biopsies, focal renal biopsies, renal cyst aspiration, adrenal biopsy, ureteral biopsy, percutaneous bladder biopsies, and transrectal or transgluteal prostate biopsies [1–7]. The remainder of this section will review the indications, methods, success rate, and potential complications of these biopsies.

Nonfocal renal biopsy

Indications

Indications for nonfocal renal biopsy include assessing for cause of renal failure (nephropathies) or for cause for renal transplant rejection.

Methods

Nonfocal renal biopsies may occasionally be performed using only local anesthetic. For biopsies of the native kidney, the patient is placed prone or contralateral side down under ultrasound guidance. After the skin is prepped in a sterile manner and draped, a 15-gauge needle is advanced, using real-time ultrasound guidance, into the renal cortex. One or two core biopsy samples are obtained. The biopsy needle is subsequently removed and pressure applied to the area. Biopsy of a renal transplant is performed in a similar fashion; however, patients are typically placed in a supine position and the transplanted kidney, typically in the anterior pelvis, is targeted using ultrasound (Fig. 5).

Focal renal biopsy

Indications

The incidence of renal cell carcinoma has been increasing. In the United States it is estimated that there were 38,890 new cases and 129,000 deaths from renal cell carcinoma in 2006 [8]. Imaging has improved in the detection of smaller renal masses and percutaneous focal renal biopsy is now more imperative to establish a diagnosis before operative nephrectomy or ablation.

Methods

Focal renal biopsies may be performed with either ultrasound or CT guidance, with the decision based on ability to visualize and target the lesion using ultrasound. The majority of the authors' renal biopsies are performed under CT guidance using a 17-gauge coaxial needle allowing 18-gauge core biopsies (Fig. 6). Patients are typically placed prone or in the ipsilateral side down decubitus position to decrease respiratory motion of the kidney (Fig. 7A). After the patient is positioned and conscious sedation achieved, the skin entrance site, identified

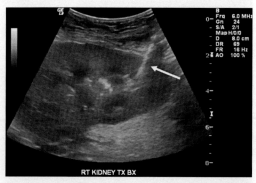

Fig. 5. Sagittal ultrasound image shows biopsy needle (*arrow*) entering lower pole cortex of a transplanted right lower pelvic kidney. Procedure is performed to evaluate for evidence of renal transplant rejection.

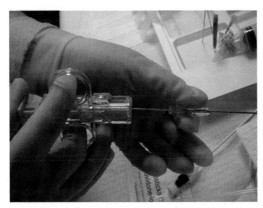

Fig. 6. Photograph showing insertion of 18-gauge biopsy gun into 17-gauge coaxial needle. The majority of the authors' focal biopsies are performed using this coaxial system, which allows one to obtain multiple samples through the coaxial needle while only passing the renal capsule just once with the 17-gauge needle.

using a radiopaque grid, is prepped using sterile technique and draped. Under sterile conditions, the 17-gauge coaxial needle is advanced into the lesion and its position is confirmed on CT (Fig. 7B).

If the lesion cannot be visualized on the unenhanced images, the initial diagnostic contrast-enhanced CT is used as a reference to target the lesion on the unenhanced preliminary interventional CT image. After the lesion is targeted with the coaxial needle using internal landmarks, intravenous contrast may be administered to identify the lesion

and the relative position of the coaxial needle (Fig. 8). If the initially placed coaxial needle does not target the lesion, its position can be used as a reference marker for placement of a second coaxial needle to target the lesion.

Once the coaxial needle is positioned within the lesion, multiple 22-gauge fine needle aspirates are obtained. Subsequently, multiple 18-gauge core biopsy samples are obtained and sent in saline to pathology. The coaxial needle is then removed and a dressing applied to the area. A final postprocedure ultrasound or CT image is obtained to assess the amount of perinephric hemorrhage and to exclude injury to adjacent organs or lung.

From a procedural standpoint, the most difficult focal renal biopsies are small exophytic lesions. These small exophytic lesions are difficult to target because of poor visualization on ultrasound and extensive motion on CT. Occasionally, multiple tandem coaxial needles are inserted to attempt to trap and target a small lesion.

Renal cyst aspiration biopsy

Indications
Renal cyst aspiration biopsies are performed to establish a diagnosis of benign or malignant cystic renal cell in a suspicious cystic lesion.

Methods
Similar to a focal renal biopsy, renal cyst aspiration is targeted with ultrasound or CT guidance after

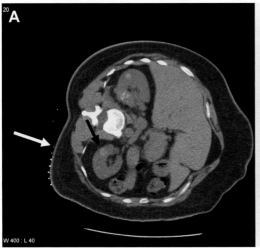

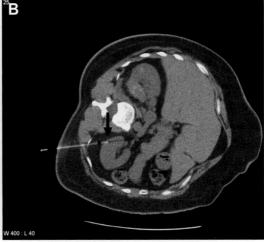

Fig. 7. (*A*) Axial CT image of a focal renal biopsy with the ipsilateral side of the kidney down to splint the kidney's motion, which occurs with normal patient respiration. A grid placed at the entrance site localized the site of entry (*white arrow*). The lesion to be biopsied is visualized as minimally hyperdense on this noncontrast CT image (*black arrow*). (*B*) Axial CT of a focal renal biopsy shows coaxial needle inserted through the subcutaneous tissue targeting the renal lesion (*arrow*).

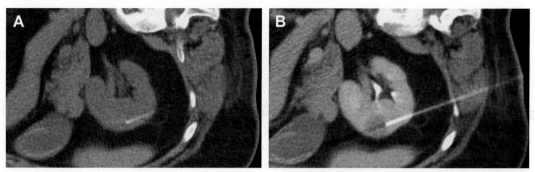

Fig. 8. Axial CT images of a focal renal biopsy. (*A*) Axial CT showing biopsy needle positioned in the presumed location of the focal renal lesion, based on the location of the renal vessels and the configuration of the renal calyces. (*B*) Subsequently, after needle placement, contrast was administered and the lesion became visible. The needle location proved to be adequate for proper biopsy.

conscious sedation, prepping, and draping of the patient. In contradistinction to focal solid renal mass biopsy, for a renal cyst aspiration, a coaxial needle is used to access the cyst. The contents of the cyst are then partially aspirated and sent to pathology. Subsequently, air or contrast is injected into the cyst to opacify any solid nodules or areas of wall thickening. This area is then targeted for biopsy using 22-gauge fine needle aspirates and 18-gauge core biopsies (Fig. 9).

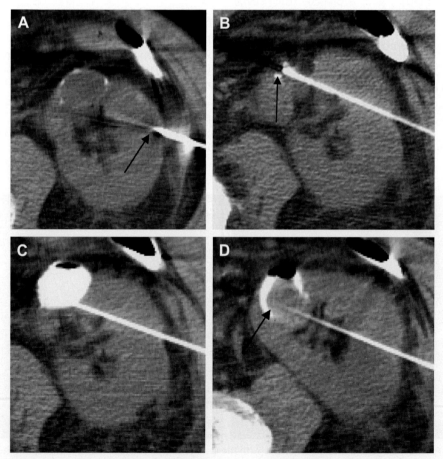

Fig. 9. Renal cyst aspiration and biopsy. (*A*) Axial CT image shows needle entering renal parenchyma extending toward renal cyst (*arrow*). (*B*) Axial CT image shows needle aspirating all the fluid from the cyst (*arrow*). (*C*) Axial CT shows cyst injected with 1:20 dilute contrast. (*D*) Axial CT shows visible solid component of the cyst targeted for biopsy (*arrow*).

Success rate

The overall sensitivity of all renal biopsies is 70% to 100% and the specificity is 100% [4–7,9–15]. There is no significant difference in success between ultrasound versus CT-guided biopsies [9].

Complications

Complications include bleeding (Fig. 10), infection, and injury to adjacent organs, including the colon, the liver, spleen, and lungs (Fig. 11). The overall mortality rate is 0.031% [16].

Bleeding can occur because of injury to renal vessels, bleeding from a vascular tumor or, in cases of persistent bleeding, from arterio-venous fistulas. With every biopsy, there is mild perinephirc bleeding recently reported to be up to 44% [9]. However, this bleeding is usually self-limiting, and clinically significant bleeding is unusual. The risk of needle tract seeding is low (0.017%) and only six cases have been reported in the literature [17–22].

Adrenal biopsy

Indication

Adrenal biopsies are performed to establish a diagnosis of malignancy [23–30]. Typical scenarios for adrenal biopsy include indeterminate adrenal mass per CT or MR imaging or a fluoro-2-deoxy-D-glucose positron emission tomography positive adrenal mass.

Methods

Adrenal biopsies are typically performed under CT guidance. Patients are placed in an ipsilateral decubitus position and the adrenal mass is targeted using the grid. Adrenal biopsies are sometimes blocked by the adjacent lung. In addition, the

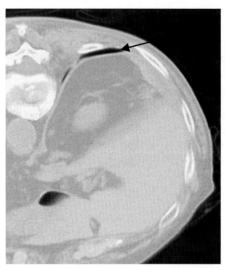

Fig. 11. Axial prone CT after biopsy of a focal renal mass shows a tiny pneumothorax (*arrow*). Patient was asymptomatic and after follow-up chest radiograph 4 hours later did not show any pneumothorax, the patient was discharged.

kidney or vertebral body may prevent access to the mass. Access to the adrenal may be obtained via a transrenal or transhepatic approach, if necessary. Twenty-two gauge fine needle aspirates and 18-gauge cores are obtained and sent to pathology.

Success rate

With CT-guided biopsies, sufficient biopsy material for diagnosis is obtained in 80% to 95% of patients [31–34]. In a prospective multicenter study of 220 consecutive adrenal biopsies, the overall sensitivity for malignancy was 94.6% and specificity 95.3%, if adequate tissue was obtained [34]. The negative predictive value of a biopsy is dependent upon several factors, including lesion size, morphology, biopsy needle size, and the oncologic history of the patient. In patients without a known oncology history, the negative predictive value is 91%, and even in patients with a history of lung cancer, the negative predictive value was 92% [35].

Complications

As with any biopsy, risks include bleeding and infection. In addition, there is risk of a pneumothorax from a transpleural approach. There is also a risk of a hypertensive crisis [36,37].

Prostate biopsy

Indications

Prostate biopsies are typically performed for elevation of prostate specific antigen or for follow-up of a patient with known prostate cancer [38].

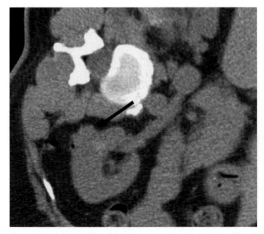

Fig. 10. Axial CT after biopsy, in same patient as **Fig. 8,** shows minimal post biopsy perinephric hemorrhage (*arrow*).

Methods

Prostate biopsies are typically performed via transrectal ultrasound guidance. The patient is placed in a left lateral decubitus position. Patients typically take a course of pre and postprocedure antibiotics. In addition, intramuscular 80-mg gentamicin is administered at the time of the procedure. After a rectal examination is performed, a transrectal ultrasound probe is inserted and preliminary images of the prostate are obtained. Lidocaine is then administered in the nerve plexus adjacent to the seminal vesicles for both lobes of the prostate (Fig. 12A). Subsequently, using the probe guide, a 19-gauge needle is inserted and five biopsy samples from the peripheral zone (apex to base) and one biopsy sample from the central zone of each gland of the prostate are obtained (Fig. 12B). Care must be taken during the biopsy to avoid any peripheral vessels or the central urethra. Any focal hypodensities visualized within the peripheral zone must also be targeted for biopsy. After the biopsy, the transrectal probe is removed and digital rectal pressure is placed to tamponade any bleeding. Patients are advised that they may see small blood in their stool, urine, or semen for up to 10 days after the biopsy.

If a patient does not have a rectum because of abdomino-perineal resection, the prostate can be biopsied via a transgluteal approach under CT guidance.

Success rate

In a review that combined 87 studies with a total of 20,698 subjects, it was found that increasing the number of core biopsy samples was significantly associated with increased cancer yield. Obtaining 12 laterally directed cores, compared with the sextant scheme, detected 31% more cancer and did not increase the complication rate. Obtaining 18 to 24 cores did not detect significantly more cancers and potentially increased the adverse events [39].

Complications

Hematuria and hematospermia are seen in up to greater than 80% of patients who undergo a prostate biopsy [40]. Almost all patients will also experience some level of pain or discomfort, depending on their pain threshold and the type of sedation or local anesthesia used [41]. The pain can be significant, and up to 19% of patients may decline a future biopsy [42].

Other complications include perirectal bleeding (up to 37%) [40], infection, vasovagal reaction [43], urinary retention [44], epididymitis [45], periprostatic hematoma [46], and a single reported case of disseminated intravascular coagulation [47].

Transvaginal biopsy

Indications

Biopsy of pelvic masses that are not accessible via the transcutaneous approach may be achieved via the transvaginal approach.

Methods

Transvaginal biopsies may be very painful and require conscious sedation. Patients are placed a dorsolithotomy position. Similar to a transrectal biopsy, a transvaginal probe is loaded with a plastic needle guide. After the transvaginal examination is performed, a speculum is inserted and the vaginal vault is prepped. The transvaginal probe is then inserted. When the lesion is identified, the needle is inserted through the guide and punctures through the vaginal wall to biopsy the lesion under real-time visualization with ultrasound (Fig. 13).

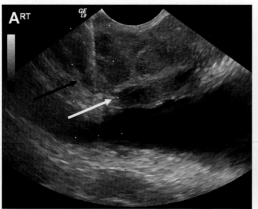 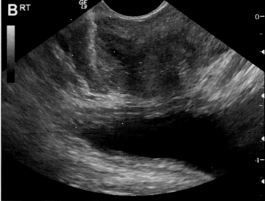

Fig. 12. (A) Transrectal ultrasound image from a prostate biopsy shows administration of anesthetic into prostatic nerve plexus located at the junction between the seminal vesicle (*white arrow*) and the base of the prostate (*black arrow*). (B) Transrectal prostate ultrasound shows targeting of the peripheral zone of the prostate.

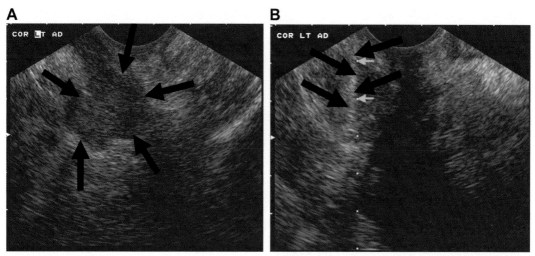

Fig. 13. (A) Transvaginal ultrasound showing lobulated hypoechoic right adnexal mass (*arrows*). (B) Transvaginal biopsy is performed (*arrows*).

Success rate

In a study of 61 subjects who underwent transvaginal ultrasound-guided biopsy or fine needle aspiration, the sensitivity was 82% [48].

Complications

Complication rate is reported to be low [49,50] and include bleeding, infection, and vaginal, ovarian, or bladder injury.

Image-guided percutaneous drainage and aspiration

Drainages or aspirations are performed for three reasons: to diagnose and manage an infected collection; to relieve an area of obstruction; and to decompress a fluid-filled cavity causing pain. Urologic drainage procedures include nephrostomy tubes, nephroureteral stents, and perinephric abscess drainages.

Once the catheter is placed, postprocedure care of the catheter must be performed, including frequent saline flushes to maintain the patency of the tube. In addition, follow-up ultrasound or CT studies and tube injection studies are performed to confirm resolution of the collection and clearing of the obstruction before tube removal.

Percutaneous nephrostomy

Indications

Percutaneous nephrostomy is performed to relieve urinary obstruction or divert the urinary stream away from the ureter or bladder. Percutaneous nephrostomies can be emergent cases because of risk of pyuria and sepsis from a stagnant urine collection.

Methods

Patients are given preprocedure antibiotics. The procedure is performed using both ultrasound and fluoroscopy under conscious sedation. Patients are placed on the fluoroscopy table in a prone oblique position to access the renal collecting system via the avascular plane. If the dilated calyces are visualized under ultrasound, ultrasound guidance may be used to access the renal collecting system. The urine is then aspirated and sent for microbiologic analysis. Subsequently, an equivalent or lesser amount of contrast may be carefully injected to opacify the collecting system. Ideal access to the collecting system would be through the avascular plane of the kidney via a peripheral calyx. If the initial access is not ideal, fluoroscopy may be used to guide an 18-gauge sheathed needle into the appropriate calyx. Once access is obtained, a soft tip wire is inserted to access the collecting system and is replaced with a stiff wire. Ultimately, the tract is serially dilated to an 8 French hole and a percutaneous nephrostomy pigtail catheter is placed into the renal pelvis (Fig. 14). The catheter is secured to the patient.

Occasionally, the calices are not dilated or not well visualized. Access to the renal collecting system can then be performed either using landmarks, such as an internal radiopaque calculus, or by administering intravenous contrast and waiting for the delayed phase excretion of the contrast into the renal collecting system.

Success rate

The success rate approaches 100% for dilated systems and approximately 80% for nondilated systems [51].

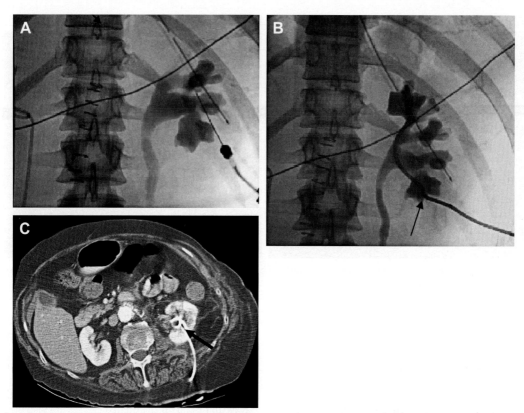

Fig. 14. Ultrasound guidance was used to gain access to dilated renal collecting system using a 22-gauge needle (*not shown*). (*A*) After urine is aspirated, an equivalent amount of contrast is injected under fluoroscopy to opacify the renal collecting system. A more suitable access site is chosen in the lower pole calyx of the right kidney and this calyx was accessed under fluoroscopy using an 18-gauge ring needle and exchanged for an Amplatz wire. (*B*) An 8 French nephrostomy tube is advanced into the right renal collecting system and decompresses the system via the lower pole access (*arrow*). (*C*) Axial CT in a different patient shows a left nephrostomy tube in position (*arrow*).

Complications

Complications include bleeding, infection, and injury to adjacent organs, kidney, and ureter. There is also a risk of injury to the renal vasculature.

Suprapubic tube insertion

Indications

Indications for a suprapubic tube insertion include relieving bladder outlet obstruction, draining a nonfunctioning, neurogenic bladder, keeping a perforated bladder decompressed, and diverting urine from a urethral injury [52].

Methods

A suprapubic tube can be placed via two methods: either by using ultrasound and fluoroscopy or just using fluoroscopy. For each approach, a urethral Foley catheter is necessary. The bladder is first filled with water soluble iodinated contrast material. The skin is then prepped and draped. Preprocedure imaging may be used to confirm location of the sigmoid colon in relation to the bladder. Under ultrasound guidance, a 12 French Foley loaded on a trocar may be used to gain access to the bladder (Fig. 15). The Foley is then released from its trocar, and the foley is advanced into the bladder over the inner core stiffener. The Foley balloon is then inflated. Urine is emptied from the bladder and contrast is instilled into the bladder under fluoroscopy, confirming position of the Foley catheter and confirming no contrast leak. Minimal contrast leak is occasionally seen and is secondary to minimal leaking that occurs during placement of the catheter into the bladder.

If using only fluoroscopy, a sheathed needle may be used to access the bladder under fluoroscopy (Fig. 16). Once urine is aspirated through the sheathed needle, a 3J-wire is inserted into the bladder under fluoroscopy. Using an angled guiding catheter, the 3J-wire is exchanged for an Amplatz

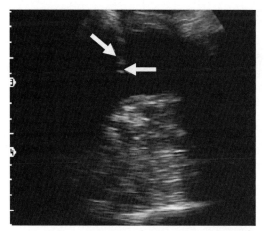

Fig. 15. Ultrasound guidance was used to obtain access to a filled bladder using a Foley catheter loaded onto a trocar.

and serial dilatation of the tract is performed over the Amplatz. Finally, an 8 to 12 French suprapubic Foley catheter is inserted over the Amplatz wire into the bladder.

Success rate
Success rate for suprapubic tube insertion has been reported to approach 100% and is comparable to surgical insertion [53,54].

Complications
Complications include bleeding, infection, and bladder or bowel perforation.

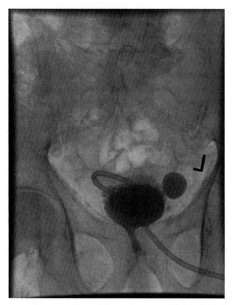

Fig. 16. Fluoroscopy with a contrast-distended bladder may also be used to place a suprapubic tube.

Stone management
Management of stone disease, including renal, ureteral, and bladder stones requires close cooperation between the urologist and interventional radiologist. Percutaneous management of stone disease is possible because of availability of sonographic lithotripsy, performed by the urologist. However, before performing a lithotripsy, percutaneous access of the renal collecting system is necessary.

Indications
Most renal or ureteral calculi are able to pass on their own without intervention. Typically, ureteral calculi less than 5 mm are able to pass on their own. Larger, distal ureteral calculi may be managed by the urologist by basket retrieval via a transurethral approach. Large proximal calculi or large renal calculi will require percutaneous intervention, including a nephrostomy tube to relieve the obstruction, and placement of percutaneous wire through the renal collecting system in ureter and to the bladder for lithotripsy access.

Percutaneous ureteral lithotripsy
Indications
Percutaneous ureteral lithotripsy is indicated for management of large renal stones with lithotripsy [53]. Percutaneous access to the kidney is obtained so that the urologist may use the wires as a guide for lithotripsy.

Methods
The patient is placed prone on the fluoroscopy table. After antibiotics are given and conscious sedation is obtained, the kidneys are accessed either using ultrasound, if there is a dilated collecting system, or fluoroscopy, if there is a radiopaque stone. The most ideal access for the urologist is a calyx that bears the stone. Once access is obtained, either a 3J-wire or occasionally, an angled glidewire is used to cross the obstructing stone and gain access to the ureter. Two wires can then be advanced to the bladder to provide a "working wire" and a "safety wire" (Fig. 17). The urologist can then gain access to the wires in the bladder and perform the lithotripsy.

Success rate
Success of lithotripsy is 98.3% for targeted renal stones and 88.2% for ureteral stones [55].

Complications
Complications include bleeding, infection, renal injury, ureteral perforation, dissection, and bladder injury.

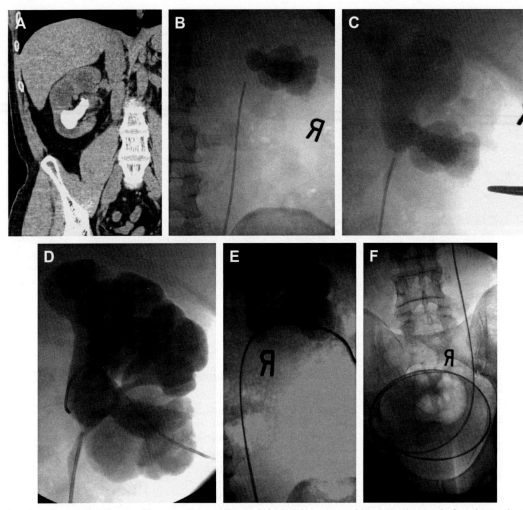

Fig. 17. In the management of large collecting system calculi (*A*), access to kidney is obtained after the urologist places a retrograde stent (*B*). The skin site is localized (*C*) and accessed with a wire and a Kumpe catheter (*D*). Two Amplatz percutaneous wires are placed extending from the skin through the renal collecting system (*E*) to the bladder (*F*).

Ureteral stents

Indications
Ureteral stents are placed to bypass an obstructing stone or to stent across of an area of stricture or ureteral laceration. Stents may be placed by the urologist via a transurethral approach or by the interventional radiologist via a percutaneous approach [56]. The decision as to method of stent placement is based upon the location and accessibility of the ureteral pathology.

Methods
After informed consent is obtained, the patient is placed prone on the fluoroscopy table. After antibiotics and conscious sedation are administered, the renal collecting system is accessed either via previously placed nephrostomy tube or via a primary access (see method above) to opacify the entire renal collecting system from the renal calices to the bladder. The area of ureteral pathology (stone, stricture, extravasation) is then identified. A soft tip wire is then advanced across the ureteral pathology into the bladder and then exchanged for a stiff wire. A 10 French sheath is then placed into the renal collecting system. Subsequently, over the stiff wire, a double pigtail ureteral stent is advanced with the distal portion in the bladder. The inner stiffener of the ureteral stent is then slowly retracted, activating the distal pigtail. Subsequently, the inner stiffener and Amplatz wire are removed and the proximal pigtail is deployed within the renal pelvis. A safety wire attached to the proximal portion of the ureteral stent allows minor adjustments to the stent (Fig. 18). Using the sheath, a stiff wire is inserted and a safety nephrostomy tube is placed into the

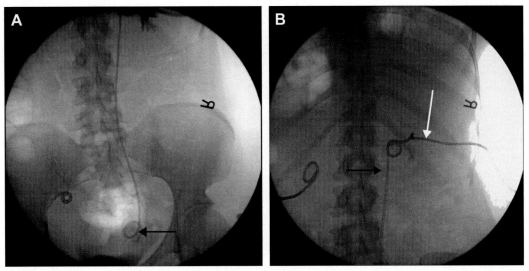

Fig. 18. Fluoroscopic image showing (*A*) distal (*arrow*) and (*B*) proximal (*black arrow*) placement of an internal ureteral stent. A safety nephrostomy wire is often left in place in the immediate 48 hours after stent placement (*white arrow*).

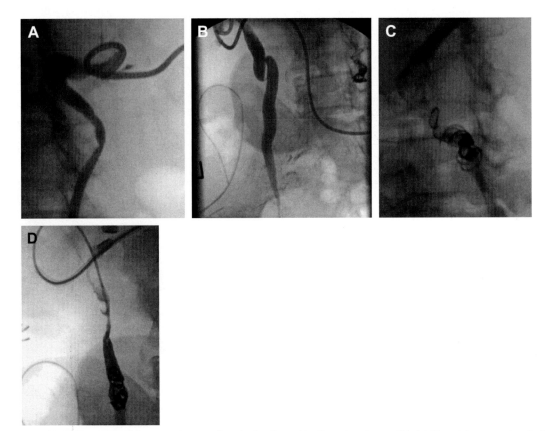

Fig. 19. (*A–D*) Fluoroscopic images shows coil embolization of both ureters in a patient with pelvic cancer treated with permanent urinary diversion. (*A, B*) Both renal collecting systems are accessed via indwelling nephrostomy tubes. (*C, D*) An angled guiding catheter delivers 10/8 tornado coils and gelfoam to obstruct the flow within the ureter. Complete obstruction to flow may take weeks while the ureter strictures.

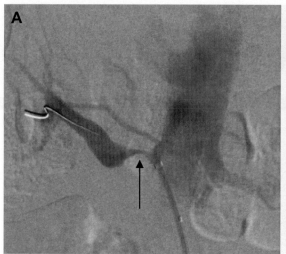
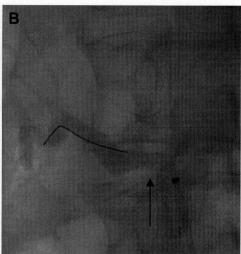

Fig. 20. Renal angiography and stenting. (*A*) Stenotic renal artery is selected via femoral artery approach (*arrow*). (*B*) The stenosis is balloon dilated and a stent is placed across it (*arrow*).

renal collecting system. The safety nephrostomy is left in for 24 to 48 hours to ensure that blood clots and stones created and dislodged during the procedure do not obstruct the stent. The safety nephrostomy tube is subsequently removed under fluoroscopy.

Success rate

Using a midpole access and a peel-away sheath, technical success for antegrade stent placement approaches 100% [53,56]. The 3-month patency rate is reported to be 95% and drops to 54% at 6 months [53,56].

Complications

Complications include bleeding, infection, ureteral or renal injury, deployment of the stent too distally, and deployment of the proximal portion of the stent outside the renal collecting system in the renal parenchyma or outside the kidney [57].

Ureteral embolization

Indications

Ureteral embolization is occasionally performed as an option of last resort in patients with unresectable tumors of the pelvis. Typically patients will have long-standing nephrostomy tubes and will require ureteral embolization to treat distal urine leaks refractory to other treatments.

Methods

After informed consent is obtained, the patient is placed prone on the fluoroscopy table. After antibiotics and conscious sedation are administered, the renal collecting system is accessed via the previously

placed nephrostomy tube. Contrast injection can opacify the renal collecting system and ureter and provide a road map for ureteral embolization. The nephrostomy tube is exchanged for a stiff wire, which is advanced to the distal most portion of the ureter. Over the stiff wire, a small catheter is positioned in the distal ureter. Via the small catheter, multiple coils are then deployed into the ureter until contrast injection confirms slow flow within the ureter (Fig. 19). Gelfoam can also be injected into the ureter. Typically, embolization of the ureter will not immediately occlude the ureter. Coils placed will require time to cause an inflammatory reaction within the ureter for obstruction to

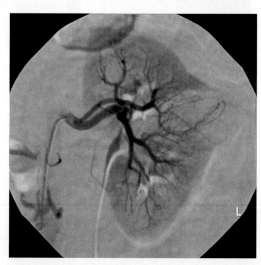

Fig. 21. Renal angiography and subselective embolization to decrease vascularity of hypervascular renal tumor. After the tumor vascularity is identified, gelfoam and coils are injected.

occur; therefore, effectiveness is assessed with follow-up contrast injection studies.

Success rate

In a study of 34 patients who underwent ureteral embolization for ureteral fistulas and incontinence, the procedure was technically successful in 100% of the patients [58]. Complications included coil migration into the renal pelvis in 2 patients and nephrostomy tube occlusion requiring replacement in 3 patients [58].

Complications

Complications include bleeding, infection, ureteral or renal injury, and deployment of the coils within the renal pelvis.

Renal vascular interventions

Renal vascular interventions include angiography, ballooning and stenting of the renal artery, and embolization of renal pseudoaneurysms.

Management of renal artery stenosis

Indications

Renal artery stenosis is managed in patients who have a clinically significant and hemodynamically significant stenosis. Typically, patients have uncontrollable hypertension and imaging showing greater than 50% narrowing of the renal artery. Hemodynamically significant stenosis is defined as a gradient of greater than 20 mm Hg. Renal artery

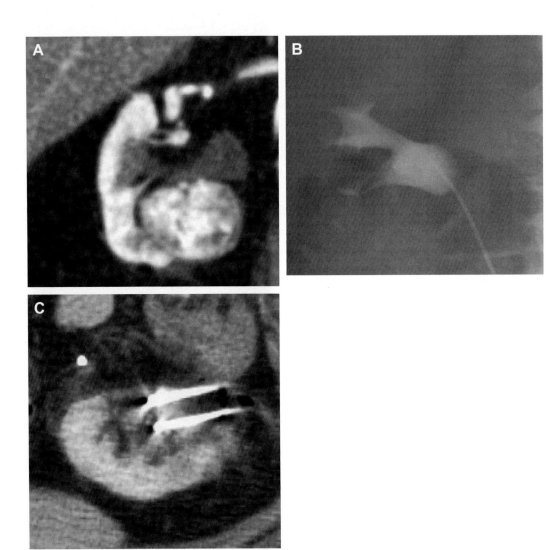

Fig. 22. (*A*) Axial CT shows central renal tumor close to the proximal ureter. (*B*) Using a cystoscope in the interventional suite, the urologist inserts a ureteral stent and its position is confirmed on fluoroscopy. (*C*) The ureteral stent is infused with cold 5% dextrose solution and ablation of the central tumor is performed.

stenosis is managed with balloon dilatation or stenting.

Methods
After informed consent is obtained, the patient is placed supine on the angiography table. The renal artery is accessed via the femoral artery. Contrast injection confirms the anatomy and shows the area of stenosis. The stenosis is then crossed using a wire and balloon dilation is performed. Subsequently, a stent is placed across the stenosis (Fig. 20).

Success rate
Technical success of renal angioplasty is dependent on the original pathology and location: artherosclerosis (ostial) 40%, artherosclerosis (proximal) 85%, fibromuscular dysplasia 90%, Takayasu's arteritis 85%. Stenting increases success rate to 95% [53].

Complications
Complications include bleeding, infection, contrast allergy, and renal artery or renal injury.

Renal embolization

Indications
Renal embolization is performed for the management of persistent renal hemorrhage from trauma, biopsy, or bleeding angiomyolipoma.

Methods
The renal artery is accessed as described above. Contrast is injected to identify the site of extravasation or pseudoaneurysm. Subselective catheter is used to gain access to the vessel proximal to the extravasation or pseudoaneurysm (Fig. 21). If there is extravasation, gelfoam is injected to embolize the hemorrhage. If there is a pseudoaneurysm, coils are used to embolize the proximal feeding and distal emptying vessels.

Success rate
In the largest series of renal embolizations performed for a variety of indications, embolization was successful on the first attempt in 87% of the patients [59].

Complications
Complications include bleeding, infection, renal artery injury, renal infarction, post embolization syndrome, and allergic reaction.

Ablation

Ablation using either heat (radiofrequency ablation) or freezing (cryoblation) is now used as an alternative to surgery in the management of renal or adrenal tumors in patients who are poor operative candidates [60–65]. Ablations are performed using either ultrasound, CT, or interventional MR imaging guidance [65].

Radiofrequency or cryoablation ablation
Radiofrequency ablation (RFA) is the management of tumors using heat. Multiple manufacturers have designed equipment for radiofrequency ablation that relies on heat based cytotoxicity to destroy

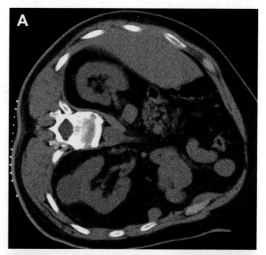

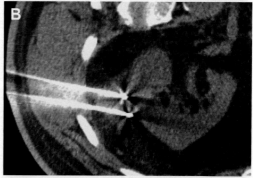

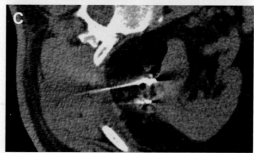

Fig. 23. Axial CT images of a radiofrequency ablation of a left renal tumor. Multiple overlapping treatments are performed to cover the entire extent of the tumor.

the tumor. Cytotoxicity is achieved by attaining temperatures greater than 50° to 60° centigrade. The size of the ablation is dependent upon the type of electrode used and the number of overlapping treatments performed.

Cryoablation is the management of tumors using freezing techniques. Cytotoxicity is achieved by alternatively freezing and thawing tumor tissue.

Renal ablation

Although ablation can be performed on tumors of any size, success is most likely for tumors less than or equal to 4 cm [60]. Tumors may be classified into three areas: exophytic, parenchymal, or central. Central tumors are more challenging because of the proximity of central renal vessels and the renal collecting system and ureter. Proximity of the tumor to the vessels may result in direct vessel injury from the inserted probes or inadequate tumor margin treatment because of heat sink affect preventing adequate treatment of the tumor margin adjacent to the vessel. The ureter can also be injured with radiofrequency or cryoablation, resulting in stricture or laceration. A useful mechanism to reduce ureteric injury is to insert a ureteral stent and flush it with cold 5% dextrose solution to serve as a heat sink, and thus protect the ureter (Fig. 22).

Methods

Under imaging guidance, probes are inserted into the tumor. Multiple overlapping ablations are performed covering the entire volume of the tumor

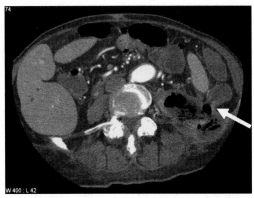

Fig. 25. Axial CT showing delayed colon injury (*arrow*) s/p RFA, likely because of a ruptured diverticulum.

(Fig. 23). If using radiofrequency ablation, images may be acquired after each treatment to confirm treatment success. If using cryoablation, the zone of ablation may be identified with the growing ice ball using either CT or MR imaging.

Success rate

Complete necrosis can be achieved in 90% of cases performed if treated lesion sizes are limited to 4 cm or less. Increasing the lesion size cutoff to 5.8 cm will include 99% of patients who could achieve complete necrosis; however, the rate of necrosis drops to 63% [60].

Complications

Complications include bleeding, infection, vascular, ureteral injury (Fig. 24), injury to adjacent organs (Fig. 25), and inadequate treatment resulting in residual or recurrent tumor (Fig. 26).

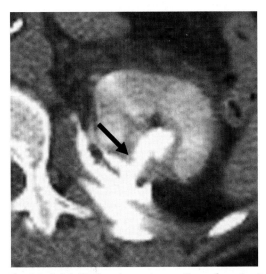

Fig. 24. Axial CT showing extravasation of contrast from lower pole calyx after RFA (*arrow*). These cases are managed with percutaneous nephrostomy and urinoma drainage.

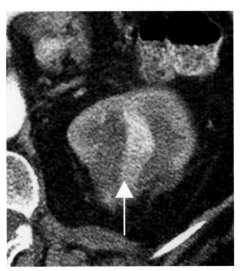

Fig. 26. Axial contrast enhanced CT shows area of enhancement after RFA, suspicious for residual tumor (*arrow*).

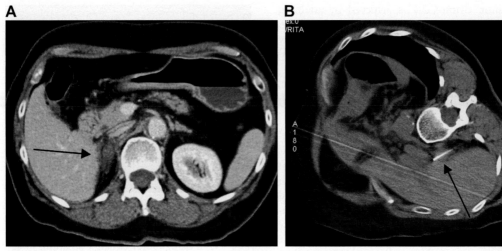

A

B

Fig. 27. (A) Axial contrast enhanced CT shows right adrenal mass (*arrow*). (B) This mass was treated with radio-frequency ablation (*arrow*).

Adrenal ablation

Indications
Adrenal ablations are performed in patients with a metastatic or primary adrenal neoplasm who are poor surgical candidates [66,67].

Methods
Because of the risk of a hypertensive crisis during ablation of the adrenal, cases are typically performed with preparations for a hypertensive crisis. Patients are placed in an ipsilateral decubitus or prone position. Under CT, ultrasound, or MR imaging guidance, ablation probes are inserted into the tumor. Ablations are then performed covering the entire extent of the tumor (Fig. 27). The authors' experience has shown that there may be variations in blood pressure during the treatment sessions.

Success rate
Success rate for adrenal radiofrequency ablation has been reported to be 15.3% for lesions measuring 3.9 cm and followed for a mean of 11.2 months [66].

Complications
Complications include bleeding, infection, hypertensive crisis, and injury to adjacent organs including kidney, lungs, pancreas.

Summary

Interventional urologic procedures have dramatically altered the clinical management of many urologic diseases. Advances in imaging capabilities and percutaneous instruments allow management of urologic diseases as outpatient procedures with

minimal morbidity and mortality. Continued developments in imaging capabilities and instrument designs will continue to advance the field of interventional uroradiology.

References

[1] Wood BJ, Khan MA, McGovern F, et al. Imaging guided biopsy of renal masses: indications, accuracy and impact on clinical management. J Urol 1999;161:1470.
[2] Wunderlich H, Hindermann W, Al Mustafa AM, et al. The accuracy of 250 fine needle biopsies of renal tumors. J Urol 2005;174:44–6.
[3] Brierly RD, Thomas PJ, Harrison NW, et al. Evaluation of fine-needle aspiration cytology for renal masses. BJU Int 2000;85:14–8.
[4] Richter F, Kasabian NG, Irwin RJ Jr, et al. Accuracy of diagnosis by guided biopsy of renal mass lesions classified indeterminate by imaging studies. Urology 2000;55:348–52.
[5] Hara I, Miyake H, Hara S, et al. Role of percutaneous image-guided biopsy in the evaluation of renal masses. Urol Int 2001;67:199–202.
[6] Eshed I, Elias S, Sidi AA. Diagnostic value of CT-guided biopsy of indeterminate renal masses. Clin Radiol 2004;59:262–7.
[7] Lechevallier E, Andre M, Barriol D, et al. Fine-needle percutaneous biopsy of renal masses with helical CT guidance. Radiology 2000;216:506–10.
[8] Jemal A, Siegel R, Ward E, et al. Cancer statistics, 2006. CA Cancer J Clin 2006;56:106–30.
[9] Lechevallier E, Andre M, Barriol D, et al. Fine-needle percutaneous biopsy of renal masses with helical CT guidance. Radiology 2000;216:506–10.
[10] Neuzillet Y, Lechevallier E, Andre M, et al. Accuracy and clinical role of fine needle percutaneous biopsy with computerized tomography guidance

of small (less than 4.0 cm) renal masses. J Urol 2004;171:1802–5.

[11] Herts BR, Baker ME. The current role of percutaneous biopsy in the evaluation of renal masses. Semin Urol Oncol 1995;13:254–61.

[12] Caoili EM, Bude RO, Higgins EJ, et al. Evaluation of sonographically guided percutaneous core biopsy of renal masses. AJR Am J Roentgenol 2002; 179:373–8.

[13] Rybicki FJ, Shu KM, Cibas ES, et al. Percutaneous biopsy of renal masses: sensitivity and negative predictive value stratified by clinical setting and size of masses. AJR 2003;180:1281–7.

[14] Dechet CB, Zincke H, Sebo TJ, et al. Prospective analysis of computerized tomography and needle biopsy with permanent sectioning to determine the nature of solid renal masses in adults. J Urol 2003;169:71–4.

[15] Shah RB, Bakshi N, Hafez KS, et al. Image-guided biopsy in the evaluation of renal mass lesions in contemporary urological practice: indications, adequacy, clinical impact, and limitations of the pathological diagnosis. Hum Pathol 2005;36:1309–15.

[16] Smith ED. Complications of percutaneous abdominal fine-needle biopsy. Radiology 1991; 178:253–8.

[17] Gibbons RP, Bush WH Jr, Burnett LL. Needle tract seeding following aspiration of renal cell carcinoma. J Urol 1977;118:865–7.

[18] Kiser GC, Totonchy M, Barry JM. Needle tract seeding after percutaneous renal adenocarcinoma aspiration. J Urol 1986;136:1292–3.

[19] Shenoy PD, Lakhkar BN, Ghosh MK, et al. Cutaneous seeding of renal carcinoma by Chiba needle aspiration biopsy: Case report. Acta Radiol 1991;32:50–2.

[20] Wehle MJ, Grabstald H. Contraindications to needle aspiration of a solid renal mass: tumor dissemination by renal needle aspiration. J Urol 1986;136:446–8.

[21] Auvert J, Abbou CC, Lavarenne V. Needle tract seeding following puncture of renal oncocytoma. Prog Clin Biol Res 1982;100:597–8.

[22] Abe M, Saitoh M. Selective renal tumour biopsy under ultrasonic guidance. Br J Urol 1992;70:7–11.

[23] Hussain S. Gantry angulation in CT-guided percutaneous adrenal biopsy. AJR 1996;166(3):537–9.

[24] Mesurolle B, Ariche-Cohen M, Tardivon A, et al. Retrospective analysis of 44 adrenal puncture biopsies under x-ray computed tomographic guidance. J Radiol 1996;77(1):17–21.

[25] Karampekios S, Hatjidakis AA, Drositis J, et al. Artificial paravertebral widening for percutaneous CT-guided adrenal biopsy. J Comput Assist Tomogr 1998;22(2):308–10.

[26] Choyke PL. From needles to numbers: can non-invasive imaging distinguish benign and malignant adrenal lesions? World J Urol 1998;16(1): 29–34, UI: 9542012.

[27] Arellano RS, Boland GW, Mueller PR. Adrenal biopsy in a patient with lung cancer: imaging algorithm and biopsy indications, technique, and complications. AJR 2000;175(6):1613–7.

[28] Mignon F, Mesurolle B. CT guided adrenal biopsies: remaining indications? J Radiol 2002; 83(4 Pt 1):419–28.

[29] Harisinghani MG, Maher MM, Hahn PF, et al. Predictive value of benign percutaneous adrenal biopsies in oncology patients. Clin Radiol 2002; 57(10):898–901.

[30] Konig CW, Pereira PL, Trubenbach J, et al. MR imaging-guided adrenal biopsy using an open low-field-strength scanner and MR fluoroscopy. AJR 2003;180(6):1567–70.

[31] Saeger W, Fassnacht M, Chita R, et al. High diagnostic accuracy of adrenal core biopsy: results of the German and Austrian adrenal network multicenter trial in 220 consecutive patients. Hum Pathol 2003;34(2):180–6.

[32] Silverman SG, Mueller PR, Pinkney LP, et al. Predictive value of image-guided adrenal biopsy: analysis of results of 101 biopsies. Radiology 1993;187:715–8.

[33] Welch TJ, Sheedy PF II, Johnson CM, et al. CT-guided biopsy: prospective analysis of 1,000 procedures. Radiology 1989;171:493–6.

[34] Moore TP, Moulton JS. Coaxial percutaneous biopsy technique with automated biopsy devices: value in improving accuracy and negative predictive value. Radiology 1993;186: 515–22.

[35] Phillips MD, Silverman SG, Cibas ES, et al. Negative predictive value of imaging-guided abdominal biopsy results: cytologic classification and implications for patient management. AJR 1998;171:693–6.

[36] Atwell TD, Wass CT, Charboneau W, et al. Malignant hypertension during cyroablation of an adrenal gland tumor. J Vasc Interv Radiol 2006;17: 573–5.

[37] Chini EN, Brown MJ, Farrell MA, et al. Hypertensive crisis in a patient undergoing percutaneous radiofrequency ablation of an adrenal mass under general anesthesia. Anesth Analg 2004;99: 1867–9.

[38] Raja J, Ramachandran N, Munneke G, et al. Current status of transrectal ultrasound-guided prostate biopsy in the diagnosis of prostate cancer. Clin Radiol 2006;61(2):142–53.

[39] Eichler K, Hempel S, Wilby J, et al. Diagnostic value of systematic biopsy methods in the investigation of prostate cancer: a systematic review. J Urol 2006;175(5):1605–12.

[40] Ghani KR, Dundas D, Patel U. Bleeding after transrectal ultrasonography-guided prostate biopsy: a study of 7-day morbidity after a six-, eight- and 12-core biopsy protocol. BJU Int 2004;94:1014–20.

[41] Irani J, Fournier F, Bon D, et al. Patient tolerance of transrectal ultrasound-guided biopsy of the prostate. Br J Urol 1997;79:608–10.

[42] Seymour H, Perry MJ, Lee-Elliot C, et al. Pain after transrectal ultrasonography-guided prostate

biopsy: the advantages of periprostatic local anaesthesia. BJU Int 2001;88:540–4.

[43] Rodriguez LV, Terris MK. Risks and complications of transrectal ultrasound guided prostate needle biopsy: a prospective study and review of the literature. J Urol 1998;160:2115–20.

[44] Borboroglu PG, Comer SW, Riffenburgh RH, et al. Extensive repeat transrectal ultrasound guided prostate biopsy in patients with previous benign sextant biopsies. J Urol 2000;163:158–62.

[45] Donzella JG, Merrick GS, Lindert DJ, et al. Epididymitis after transrectal ultrasound-guided needle biopsy of prostate gland. Urology 2004; 63:306–8.

[46] Saad A, Hanbury DC, McNicholas TA, et al. Acute periprostatic haematoma following a transrectal ultrasound-guided needle biopsy of the prostate. Prostate Cancer Prostatic Dis 2002;5:63–4.

[47] Al-Otaibi MF, Al-Taweel W, Bin-Saleh S, et al. Disseminated intravascular coagulation following transrectal ultrasound guided prostate biopsy. J Urol 2004;171:346.

[48] Faulkner RL, Mohiyiddeen L, McVey R, et al. Transvaginal biopsy in the diagnosis of ovarian cancer. BJOG 2005;112(7):991–3.

[49] Bret PM, Guibaud L, Atri M, et al. Transvaginal US-guided aspiration of ovarian cysts and solid pelvic masses. Radiology 1992;185(2):377–80.

[50] Ylagan LR, Mutch DG, Davila RM. Transvaginal fine needle aspiration biopsy. Acta Cytol 2001; 45(6):927–30.

[51] Maher MM, Fotheringham T, Lee MJ. Percutaneous nephrostomy. Semin Interv Radiol 2000;17: 329–39.

[52] Pender SM, Lee MJ. Percutaneous suprapubic cystostomy for long term bladder drainage. Semin Interv Radiol 1996;13(2):93–9.

[53] Lee MJ. Percutaneous genitourinary interventions. In: Kaufman JA, Lee MJ, editors. The requisites: vascular & interventional radiology. 1st edition. St. Louis (MO): Mosby; 2004.

[54] Lee MJ, Papanicolaou N, Nocks BN, et al. Fluoroscopically guided percutaneous suprapubic cystostomy for long-term bladder drainage: an alternative to surgical cystostomy. Radiology 1993;188:787–9.

[55] Segura JW, Patterson DE, LeRoy A, et al. Percutaneous removal of kidney stones: review of 1000 cases. J Urol 1985;134:1077–81.

[56] Lu DS, Papanicolaou N, Girard M, et al. Percutaneous internal ureteral stent placement: review of technical issues and solutions in 50 consecutive cases. Clin Radiol 1994;49:256–61.

[57] Lee WJ, Smith AD, Cubelli V, et al. Complications of percutaneous nephrolithotomy. AJR 1987;148:177–80.

[58] Farrell TA, Wallace M, Hicks ME. Long-term results of transrenal ureteral occlusion with use of Gianturco coils and gelatin sponge pledgets. J Vasc Interv Radiol 1997;8:449–52.

[59] Jacobson AI, Amukele SA, Marcovich R, et al. Efficacy and morbidity of therapeutic renal embolization in the spectrum of urologic disease. Journal of Endourology 2003;17(6):385–91.

[60] Gervais DA, McGovern FJ, Arellano RA, et al. Radiofrequency ablation of renal cell carcinoma: Part I, Indications, Results, and Role in Patient Management over a 6-Year Period and Ablation of 100 tumors. AJR 2005;185:64–71.

[61] Gervais DA, Arellano RA, McGovern FJ, et al. Radiofrequency ablation of renal cell carcinoma: part 2, Lessons learned with ablaltion of 100 tumors. Am J Roentgenol 2005;185:72–80.

[62] Desai MM, Gill IS. Current status of cryoablation and radiofrequency ablation in the management of renal tumors. Curr Opin Urol 2002;12(5): 387–93.

[63] Lee DI, Clayman RV. Percutaneous approaches to renal cryoablation. J Endourol 2004;18(7): 643–6.

[64] Tuncali K, Morrison PR, Tatli S, et al. MRI-guided percutaneous cryoablation of renal tumors: use of external manual displacement of adjacent bowel loops. Eur J Radiol 2006;59(2): 198–202.

[65] Silverman SG, Tuncali K, van Sonnenberg E, et al. Renal tumors: MR imaging-guided percutaneous cryotherapy–initial experience in 23 patients. Radiology 2005;236(2):716–24.

[66] Mayo-Smith WW, Dupuy DE. Adrenal neoplasms: CT-guided radiofrequency ablation—preliminary results. Radiology 2004;231: 225–30.

[67] Lo WK, van Sonnenberg E, Shankar S, et al. Percutaneous CT-guided radiofrequency ablation of symptomatic bilateral adrenal metastases in a single session. J Vasc Interv Radiol 2006; 17(1):175–9.

ELSEVIER
SAUNDERS

RADIOLOGIC
CLINICS
OF NORTH AMERICA

Radiol Clin N Am 46 (2008) 65–78

Imaging Techniques for Adrenal Lesion Characterization

Michael A. Blake, MRCPI, FFR(RCSI), FRCR[a,b,*],
Nagaraj-Setty Holalkere, MD[a,b], Giles W. Boland, MD[a,b]

- Prevalence and causes of adrenal lesions
- Principles of adrenal imaging
- Morphologic imaging—CT and MR imaging
- Lipid-sensitive imaging techniques—CT and MR imaging
- CT techniques

- MR imaging techniques
- CT washouts of the adrenals
- Positron emission tomography and positron emission tomography/CT
- Adrenal biopsy
- Summary
- References

Radiology plays a critical role in the characterization of adrenal lesions. This review discusses the major adrenal imaging techniques currently available, including newly developed promising techniques, and outlines their underlying anatomic and physiologic imaging principles. It focuses primarily on the incidental adrenal lesion (IALs), or incidentalomas, which are adrenal nodules or masses discovered during imaging performed for indications other than adrenal disease [1]. With the burgeoning use of imaging, IALs are encountered more frequently, seen in approximately 4% to 6% of the imaged population [2–4]. The majority of IALs prove benign in patients who do not have a known history of cancer [4–9]. Alternatively, once patients have a known diagnosis of an extraadrenal malignancy, the chance that an incidentally detected adrenal mass is malignant increases significantly [1]. Characterization of an adrenal lesion in these patients is essential to predict the prognosis of the primary disease and assess staging and direct therapy. The review finishes by discussing the role of adrenal biopsy briefly, indicated less frequently because of the noninvasive imaging advances designed to characterize adrenal lesions.

Prevalence and causes of adrenal lesions

IALs are detected in approximately 0.2% of CT scans performed on patients ages 20 to 29 years and increases to 7% to 10% of scans in older patients [1,3,6,7]. Adrenal masses are common in the general population, with a mean prevalence determined from several large autopsy studies of 2.3% [8]. Categories of adrenal lesions include functioning or nonfunctioning masses, primary or metastatic, and benign or malignant. The large majority of IALs are nonfunctioning cortical adenomas and 6% are functioning autonomous cortisol-secreting (5%) and sex-hormone– or aldosterone-producing tumors (1%) [1–3]. Other benign lesions making up approximately 1% to 2%

[a] Harvard Medical School, Boston, MA, USA
[b] Department of Radiology, Division of Abdominal Imaging and Intervention, Massachusetts General Hospital, 55 Fruit Street, Boston, MA 02114, USA
* Corresponding author. Department of Radiology, Division of Abdominal Imaging and Intervention, Massachusetts General Hospital, Harvard Medical School, 55 Fruit Street, Boston, MA 02114.
E-mail address: mblake2@partners.org (M.A. Blake).

0033-8389/08/$ – see front matter © 2008 Elsevier Inc. All rights reserved.
radiologic.theclinics.com

doi:10.1016/j.rcl.2008.01.003

combined of all adrenal lesions include myelolipoma (reported up to 9% of detected lesions), adrenal cysts, hemorrhage, hemangioma, ganglioneuroma, neuroblastoma, and granulomatous disease [1–4].

Malignant IALs account for approximately 2% to 3% of all detected lesions, increasing in number and proportion with patient age [1]. Investigators who are oncology based state this figure as much higher, however, up to 30% [3]. In most clinical practices, adrenal carcinomas and pheochromocytomas are uncommon tumors, probably accounting for less than 5% combined of all detected IALs [10]. Other rare adrenal malignancies include primary lymphoma of the adrenal, hemangiosarcoma, and neuroblastoma [11].

Nonetheless, the chance of an IAL being malignant depends greatly on whether or not patients have an underlying extra adrenal malignancy. Up to 27% of oncologic patients are reported to have microscopic adrenal metastases and approximately 50% of incidentally detected adrenal lesions in such patients represent metastatic disease [1,3,8,12]. Given this propensity for and the clinical importance of adrenal metastatic involvement, accurate diagnosis of adrenal masses is of critical importance in oncologic patients, in particular. Fortunately, as discussed later, noninvasive adrenal imaging techniques usually determine if a mass is benign or likely malignant.

Principles of adrenal imaging

The characterization of a detected IAL depends on if it is functioning or nonfunctioning and then benign or malignant. Functioning cortical adenomas and pheochromocytomas are characterized best by clinical assessment and appropriate biochemical analyses.

For a nonhyperfunctioning mass, the imaging and clinical challenge is to determine if the mass detected is benign or malignant. Accurate adrenal lesion characterization is critical for appropriate patient management and adrenal-imaging tests must be as specific as possible [13]. An adrenal characterization test, to be clinically useful, also should be reasonably sensitive, but it is far more sensible to accept that some lesions are indeterminate rather than risk missing a malignancy.

Morphologic features alone, although sometimes helpful, often are limited by poor test specificity. Other imaging techniques, however, have been developed that do satisfy the test requirements. These tests, using CT, MR imaging, and positron emission tomography (PET) and PET/CT, take advantage of three key physiologic principles: the intracellular lipid concentration of a mass, intravenous (IV) contrast washout behavior of a mass, and the metabolic activity of a mass. Each of these major adrenal imaging methods is examined in this review and useful adrenal morphologic features and new adrenal imaging developments are highlighted.

Morphologic imaging—CT and MR imaging

An important but sometimes overlooked principle is that IAL characterization often is made by comparison with any relevant prior imaging tests (Fig. 1). In general, long-term stability is consistent with a benign lesion but any adrenal lesion that increases significantly in size on interval imaging, usually 6 months, can be considered malignant. Some benign lesions (adenomas and myelolipomas), however, rarely increase in size very slightly over time and adrenal hemorrhage will cause abrupt adrenal enlargement [14]. In general, however, a significant increase in size during 6 months

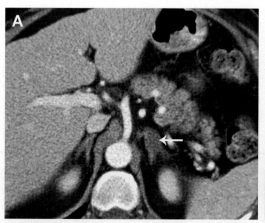
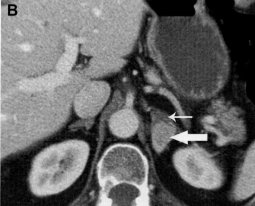

Fig. 1. Value of comparing with prior examinations. (*A*) CT scan demonstrating a low-density benign adenoma (*arrow*). (*B*) CT scan 6 months later shows development of a new enhancing mass (*large arrow*) displacing the former adenoma (*small arrow*) (collision tumor).

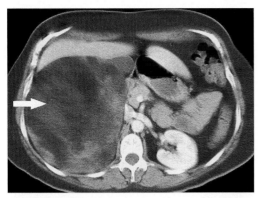

Fig. 2. Adrenal myelolipoma. Contrast-enhanced CT scan showing fat-containing mass (*arrow*) in right adrenal consistent with a myelolipoma.

is considered indicative of malignancy until proved otherwise.

Large size of an adrenal lesion, in general, is a suspicious feature for malignancy [1]. An IAL greater than 4 cm is reported to have an increased chance of malignancy of approximately 70% (and 85% if larger than 6 cm) [1,3]. Some investigators dispute these high figures, but it is unusual in clinical practice to see benign lesions greater than 4 cm other than these exceptions: (1) benign myelolipomas, but these usually are recognized confidently by the presence of macroscopic fat (Fig. 2) [1,4,14] and (2) benign pheochromocytomas, but they often are diagnosed biochemically and, furthermore, are removed given their malignant systemic circulation effects [15]. If patients have no other history of malignancy and a unilateral lesion larger than 4 to 5 cm, adrenal adenocarcinoma should be strongly suspected [16]. Adrenocortical carcinomas also have a propensity to involve the adrenal veins and inferior vena cava (IVC), and the tumor thrombus

can be well displayed by contrast-enhanced CT or MR imaging (Fig. 3).

Lesion characterization usually depends on imaging principles other than morphologic features, although some such features can be helpful if used with care and in an informed manner. Most lesions, however, regardless of type, are small (<3 cm) when discovered and smooth and uniform in shape. Adrenal lesions, benign and, especially, malignant, may appear heterogeneous, particularly after the administration of IV contrast media. The finding of large necrotic areas within a mass usually represents malignancy. Metastases, however, when first detected, often are homogeneous and appear similar to adenomas, especially when small. Most adrenal cysts, because of their lack of enhancement and uniform nature, can be characterized morphologically (Fig. 4), although some are complex and difficult to distinguish from necrotic adrenal carcinomas [4,8,17].

The shape or margins of an adrenal lesion sometimes can assist in characterization, as large lesions with irregular borders usually are malignant (see Fig. 3). Adenomas sometimes demonstrate irregular margins, however, and even in patients who have a known extra-adrenal malignancy, multinodularity of the adrenals with preservation of adreniform shape usually is associated with benignity [18]. Adrenal shape and borders also can be assessed with multiplanar reformations and volume renderings, which readily are available with multidetector CT (see Fig. 4).

Lipid-sensitive imaging techniques—CT and MR imaging

CT and MR imaging lipid techniques can take advantage of up to 70% of adrenal adenomas

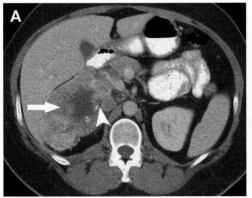
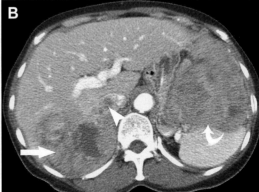

Fig. 3. Adrenal carcinoma. (*A*) Large irregularly enhancing adrenal mass (*arrow*) on contrast-enhanced CT with evidence of invasion of the IVC (*arrowhead*) and demonstrated delayed retention of contrast consistent with an adrenal carcinoma. (*B*) Large irregularly enhancing adrenal mass (*arrow*) on contrast-enhanced CT with evidence of invasion of the IVC (*arrowhead*) and left upper-quadrant, large soft tissue mass (*curved arrow*) representing metastatic disease.

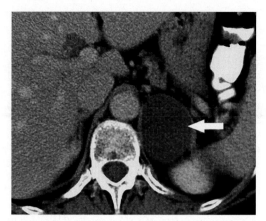

Fig. 4. Left adrenal cyst. CT showing nonenhancing 2.5-cm left adrenal lesion (*arrow*) displacing normal adrenal parenchyma consistent with a cyst.

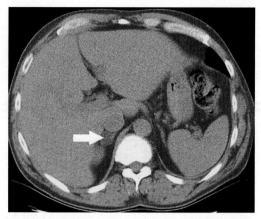

Fig. 5. Low-density adenoma. Right adrenal mass (*arrow*) measuring 6 HU on noncontrast CT representing a pathologically proved adenoma.

containing abundant intracellular fat, in contrast to almost all malignant lesions [19–24]. The presence of substantial amounts of intracellular fat is critical in making the specific diagnosis of adenoma with unenhanced CT or MR imaging.

CT techniques

Lee and colleagues were the first to report, in a seminal paper in 1991, that unenhanced CT attenuation could differentiate effectively many adrenal adenomas from nonadenomatous disease [22]. In their study, they demonstrated that the mean attenuation of adrenal adenomas (−2.2 Hounsfield units [HU]) was significantly lower than that of nonadenomas (28.9 HU). By choosing an attenuation threshold of 0 HU, these lesions could be differentiated with a sensitivity/specificity of 47%/100%. Korobkin and colleagues [19] then demonstrated an inverse linear relationship between fat concentration and the unenhanced CT attenuation value (Fig. 5). In contrast, almost all nonadenomatous lesions have a paucity of intracellular fat, and thus, higher CT attenuation values.

The attenuation measuring technique involves placing a region of interest (ROI) over the adrenal gland, avoiding hemorrhagic, necrotic, or calcified areas [4,19,23]. The ROI should be placed over one half to two thirds of the lesion area to decrease noise artifact and to avoid partial voluming effects from neighboring fat [4,19,23,24].

Boland and colleagues [13], using a meta-analysis study, demonstrated that if the CT attenuation threshold was 10 HU, then the test sensitivity increased (71%) while preserving high specificity (98%). The 10-HU threshold now is the standard by which radiologists differentiate lipid-rich adenomas from most other adrenal lesions on

unenhanced CT. Up to 30% of adenomas, however, do not have abundant intracellular fat and, thus, show attenuation values greater than 10 HU on unenhanced CT, as do almost all malignant lesions [4,8,22–28]. Lesions above 10 HU on an unenhanced CT are considered indeterminate and other tests generally are required to characterize them. Furthermore, most CT scans that include the adrenals are performed after administration of IV contrast media so unenhanced attenuation measurements cannot be made. In addition, there is too much overlap between the attenuation values of adenomas and nonadenomas on dynamic enhanced CT to enable these entities to be distinguished [23–29].

Bae and colleagues [30], however, have reported a CT histogram analysis method that is more sensitive than the 10-HU threshold method for the diagnosis of adrenal adenoma on unenhanced and enhanced CT. The technique presumes that most adenomas (either lipid rich or lipid poor) contain sufficient intracytoplasmic fat for lesion characterization. The histogram analysis technique again involves placing an ROI (as previously discussed) and then processing with a histogram analysis tool, available on most current CT viewing workstations [30]. This gives the number and range of pixel attenuation measurements, which then can be visualized graphically (Fig. 6). The histogram is a graphic plot of pixel attenuation (CT numbers) along the X axis versus the frequency of pixels at each attenuation value along the Y axis. It allows estimation, therefore, of tissue attenuation distribution in a lesion rather than calculation of an overall mean attenuation in a ROI as with conventional CT densitometry. The technique also allows the measurement of mean attenuation, number of pixels, and range of pixel attenuation for all pixels in the ROI. The

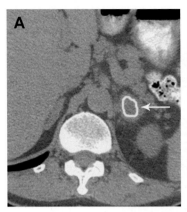
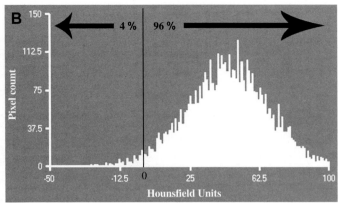

Fig. 6. Histogram analysis of adrenal mass. (*A*) CT scan showing left adrenal lesion with ROI placed within it. (*B*) Graphic display of distribution of HU values in the mass.

investigators proposed that lesions should be considered benign only if the negative pixel count is greater than 10%, as some nonadenomatous lesions sometimes contain negative pixels. Other investigators, however, have found the test sensitivity too low (71% and 12% for unenhanced and contrast-enhanced CT, respectively) for use in standard clinical practice [31,32]. Although volumetric analysis may improve its performance, the practical value of the histogram analysis method remains uncertain [32].

Dual-energy CT is a well-established technique for determining bone mineral density, is used for differentiating fatty liver from low-density masses in the liver, and can be applied to detecting fat in adrenal lesions [33,34]. The technique is based on the principle that differences in X-ray attenuation diminish with increasing energy of X rays used. This phenomenon can be exploited to quantify fat in the adrenal glands by measuring the difference in CT attenuation acquired at 140- and 80-kg voltage peaks (kV[p]). If the difference of attenuation between the two kV(p) images is greater than 6 HU, then it is suggestive of fat-containing lesions [33,34]. This technique could be applied in the adrenal to identify lesions, such as adenomas or myelolipomas. There are as yet no published papers discussing this technique for adrenal lesion characterization; however, a recent abstract presented by Li and colleagues [35] contains promising results. The technique is simple and can be performed on any scanner using routine software available on picture archiving and communication systems for analysis. The main weaknesses of this technique are the minimal increase in radiation dose and increased noise that results from the additional 80-kV(p) images. Further studies are necessary to understand its role in characterization of adrenal, particularly lipid poor, adenomas in comparison to the other well-established imaging techniques.

MR imaging techniques

Chemical-shift MR imaging (CSI) also characterizes adenomas by detecting their intracellular fat content but by exploiting the different resonant frequencies of fat and water protons rather than by attenuation differences as with CT [4,8,33–36]. Water protons precess at a higher frequency than fat protons so that the MR signals of water and lipid protons within a voxel can cancel each other out during out-of-phase (OOP) gradient-echo imaging [33–37]. This leads to signal loss relative to the in-phase (IP) images when, in contrast, the signals combine. Similar to his CT findings, Korobkin demonstrated there was an inverse linear relationship up to equal voxel concentrations of fat and water protons between the percentage of lipid-rich cells and the relative change in magnetic resonance (MR) signal intensity on CSI [19]. There needs to be a balance of fat and water protons (as seen with many lipid-rich adenomas) for signal loss on OOP CSI to occur (Fig. 7). Pure fat voxels (as seen in myelolipomas) show little or no signal loss on OOP imaging, as there are few, if any, water protons to cancel out the fat signal [8,38].

This CSI signal loss can be measured quantitatively, as the adrenal-to-spleen chemical-shift ratio, by dividing the lesion-to-spleen signal intensity ratios on the IP images by the OOP images. A CSI ratio of less than 0.71 indicates a lipid-rich adenoma [37]. The alternative adrenal signal intensity index is calculated as [(IP signal intensity−OOP signal intensity)/(IP signal intensity)] × 100%; using this formula, a measurement of greater than 16.5% is consistent with a lipid-rich adenoma [39]. In clinical practice, however, most radiologists evaluate chemical-shift change visually or qualitatively using muscle or spleen as the internal reference organ, which is more convenient and as effective as

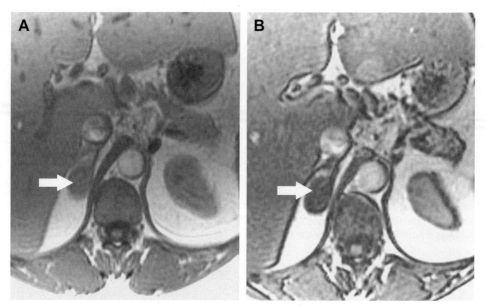

Fig. 7. CSI adenoma. MR image showing left adrenal masses (*arrows*) showing signal intensity drop between IP (*A*) and OOP (*B*) images consistent with adenoma. Notice how the liver also drops in signal on OOP imaging due to fatty liver, a behavior that makes it unsuitable as an internal standard reference organ.

quantitative methods [40,41]. The liver should not be used as the internal reference organ, as it also can show loss of OOP signal with fatty liver (see Fig. 7) [8,40].

The sensitivity and specificity of CSI for the differentiation of adrenal lesions are reported at 78% to 100% and 87% to 100%, respectively [35]. Studies suggest that there is no significant difference between the CT and CSI tests for characterizing lipid-rich adenomas but that CSI might be superior when evaluating lipid poor adenomas, up to an attenuation of 30 HU [42,43]. CT contrast washout tests, however (discussed later), have proved the most accurate diagnostic imaging tool with which to differentiate adrenal lesions [4,5,23,26,28,29,44,45].

An important MR advance that can be applied to adrenal imaging is parallel MR imaging, which, by taking advantage of an array of coils' inherent ability to encode multiple lines of MR data simultaneously, can be used to reduce scan time or increase spatial resolution. A MR advance that also may be applied to adrenal imaging is MR diffusion and MR spectroscopy (MRS), and initial preliminary reports are promising [46–48].

Diffusion-weighted imaging (DWI) can provide insight into water composition within a tumor [46]. Diffusion is thermally induced motion of water molecules in biologic tissues, called Brownian motion. Changes in tissue structure, such as cell membranes, vascular structures, and viscosity of the media, can limit or restrict the amount

of diffusion. Benign tumors tend to have a balanced increase of cells and intercellular space whereas malignant tumors usually have a disproportionate increase of cells (mitotic activity) as compared with interstitial tissue. These properties of malignancies result in selective restriction of diffusion of water molecules that may provide strong evidence for malignancy in an adrenal lesion (Fig. 8).

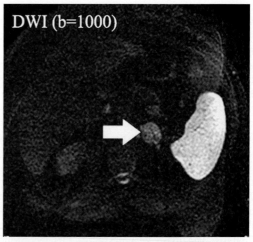

Fig. 8. Diffusion MR image of metastasis. MR image of a 52-year-old man who had a history of renal cell cancer that demonstrates a hyperintense adrenal lesion (*arrow*) on left side on a high b-value DWI consistent with restricted diffusion, which typically is seen in malignant lesions. The lesion proved to be a renal cell cancer metastasis on histopathology.

Alternatively, the lack of restricted diffusion may correlate with a benign lesion [46,47]. The diffusion data can be presented as signal intensity or as an image map of the apparent diffusion coefficient (ADC). Calculation of the ADC requires two or more acquisitions with different diffusion weightings. As yet, there are no published studies on the usefulness of DWI and ADC maps in characterization of adrenal lesions. Uhl and colleagues [47], however, have demonstrated restricted diffusion in 7 of 7 (100%) neuroblastomas, including two in adrenal glands. Based on this and the authors' early experience with this technique, the authors believe that the DWI and ADC maps may increase the accuracy of detection of malignancy in the adrenal gland. The lack of radiation and IV contrast requirements represent major advantages of DWI whereas the lack of experience with the technique and lack of published data remain the main current limitations.

MRS is useful in quantification of liver fat and is useful in identifying fat in benign adrenal lesions [48]. In vivo nuclear MRS is advancing because of the development of effective MR instrumentation and increasing availability of whole-body MR imaging systems. Absolute quantification of metabolite concentrations is useful, as a lipid peak at 1.3 ppm on the MR spectra in an adrenal lesion could characterize adrenal lesions confidently as benign. Quantification of choline-containing compounds at 3 to 3.3 ppm also is of great interest, as such compounds are increased in malignancy [48]. Researchers actively are investigating adrenal lesion characterization as a practical application of MRS. MRS has the potential to emerge as a promising tool in adrenal imaging with the continuing developments in MR scanners and postprocessing techniques.

Perfusion imaging is well established for brain tumors and has proved valuable in other abdominal tumors, such as hepatocellular carcinoma and rectal cancer [49]. Similar to these tumors, malignant adrenal tumors are likely to demonstrate higher permeability surface as a result of the presence of disorganized neovasculature and increased blood flow in contrast to benign adenomatous lesions, where the vascular organization is preserved [50]. Thus, CT or MR perfusion (dynamic or functional) imaging also may prove useful in the characterization of indeterminate adrenal lesions. Currently, CT and MR perfusion imaging are being evaluated for various organs in the body and their application in adrenal lesion evaluation not yet is evaluated fully. From the authors' experience with a few selected patients, however, perfusion imaging is another potential tool for adrenal lesion characterization but further study is needed.

CT washouts of the adrenals

After the successful noncontrast CT attenuation results for characterization of lipid-rich lesions, other investigators reported that the CT densitometry could characterize some adrenal lesions by performing attenuation measurements after different scan delays up to 1 hour [24,26,27]. They noticed that after administering IV contrast, adenomas tended to de-enhance faster than nonadenomatous lesions [5]. Malignancies have abnormal vasculature with a high microvascular density leading to slow blood flow and abnormally high vascular endothelial permeability [51]. Because of these vascular abnormalities, administered IV contrast agents more likely accumulate, and are retained for a longer period, in malignant tissues. These differences explain why contrast agent washout rates are significantly faster from benign adenomas compared with malignant masses [24,26,27].

An absolute attenuation measurement on a delayed scan has not been found practical as it depends on the type, total dose, and injection rate of IV contrast material and patient cardiac output [4,5,23,28]. The ratio of the washout-delayed attenuation, however, when compared with the dynamic enhanced attenuation, can help characterize adrenal lesions with great accuracy [5,27]. This phenomenon first was noticed by MR imaging investigators but considered too variable for use in routine MR clinical practice [50]. Korobkin and colleagues described a corresponding CT washout value with sensitivities and specificities for the diagnosis of adrenal adenoma. The percentage washout represents the percentage of the dynamic enhancement that is washed out at delayed scanning [4,5,26]. If the unenhanced attenuation value is available, an absolute percentage washout (APW) can be calculated. If no unenhanced scan is available, it is as useful to calculate the relative percentage washout (RPW). Many reports have corroborated the accuracy of using APW or RPW, and these measures now are used commonly in standard clinical practice. The RPW and APW are calculated as follows:

$$RPW = \frac{100 \times (\text{enhanced HU} - \text{delayed HU})}{\text{enhanced HU}}$$

$$APW = \frac{100 \times (\text{enhanced HU} - \text{delayed HU})}{\text{enhanced HU} - \text{noncontrast HU}}$$

The only difference between the respective formulae is that RPW gives a 0 value to the noncontrast HU field, whereas APW incorporates the true noncontrast attenuation value. Many investigators use a 40% threshold on a 15-minute delayed scan for RPW (or 60% for APW). Any adrenal lesion that demonstrates greater than 40% RPW (or >60% APW) at 15 minutes indicates an adenoma, with almost perfect sensitivity/specificity. Lesions that demonstrate RPW washouts less than 40% (or <60% APW) on a 15-minute delayed scan almost always are malignant (Fig. 9) [23,28,29,44,46]. Some investigators choose a 10-minute delay scan as more time efficient for CT scheduling and find the RPW 40% threshold (38% in the authors' series) as effective on a 10-minute delayed study [46,48]. There are some caveats to this technique: a noncontrast attenuation less than 0 H supercedes the washout profile in the evaluation of an adrenal mass; all noncalcified and nonhemorrhagic adrenal lesions measuring over 43 HU precontrast should be considered malignant, whatever the washout values. These data-driven caveats are intuitive as few

malignant lesions are expected to measure less than HU and few adenomas expected to measure greater than 43 HU. Furthermore, the inconsistent behavior by pheochromocytomas in terms of fat content and contrast washout also should be remembered when assessing an adrenal mass, especially in the correct clinical setting [15,45]. While bearing in mind these caveats, the APW value should be calculated when available, as it is a truer measure of de-enhancement. For 10-minute delay scans, the optimal APW threshold was 52% compared with 60% on the 15-minute delay scans. The lower threshold values on 10-minute delay postcontrast scans compared with 15 minutes delayed scans are to be expected, as the 10-minute delay gives 5 minutes less time for lesions to de-enhance. Importantly, most lipid poor adenomas also can be characterized using this technique leading to a much higher sensitivity for differentiating adrenal lesions using RPW than using unenhanced CT alone (Fig. 10) [23,28,29,44,45].

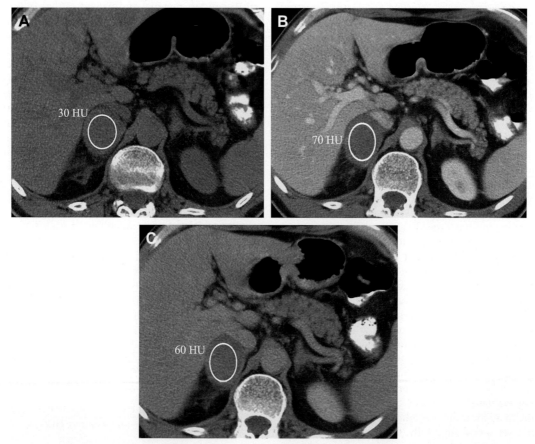

Fig. 9. Adrenal metastasis from lung cancer on washout analysis. Right adrenal mass giving ROI measurements of 30 HU precontrast (*A*), 70 HU on dynamic imaging (*B*), and 60 HU on delayed 10-minute images (*C*). The lesion is indeterminate by noncontrast criteria greater than 10 HU but as the RPW = 50% and APW = 66.6%, it is consistent with an indeterminate lesion (suspicious for malignancy).

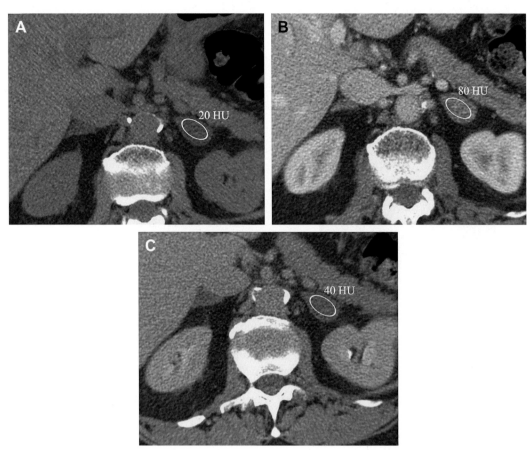

Fig. 10. Lipid-poor adrenal adenoma on washout analysis. Right adrenal mass giving ROI measurements of 20 HU precontrast (*A*), 80 HU on dynamic imaging (*B*), and 40 HU on delayed 10-minute images (*C*). The lesion is indeterminate by noncontrast criteria greater than 10 HU, but as the RPW = 50% and APW = 66.6%, it is consistent with a lipid-poor adenoma.

Positron emission tomography and positron emission tomography/CT

Several radioisotopes are used to help characterize adrenal lesions, including NP-59 iodomethylnorcholesterol, metaiodobenzylguanidine (MIBG), and 18F-fluorodeoxyglucose PET (FDG-PET) [51–69]. Although NP-59 iodomethylnorcholesterol has a high positive predictive value for the detection of adenoma, it is not used effectively in clinical practice. MIBG may be helpful in the evaluation of some pheochromocytomas, particularly if ectopic or metastatic [54,62,64]. Most pheochromocytomas show increased FDG uptake but more impressive results are reported with fluorodopamine PET and 11C-hydroxyephedrine PET, both of which having greater specificity for characterizing pheochromocytoma [69–72].

In practice, an increasing number of adrenal lesions are detected and characterized with FDG-PET or, in particular, FDG-PET/CT. In general, malignant masses usually show increased FDG uptake

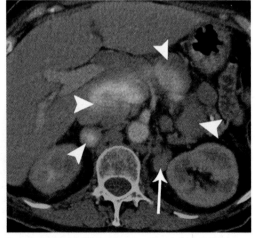

Fig. 11. PET CT of lymphoma. Overlaid PET/CT image demonstrating a left adrenal mass (*arrow*) and multiple upper-abdominal lymph nodes (*arrowheads*), all showing increased FDG activity resulting from involvement with lymphoma.

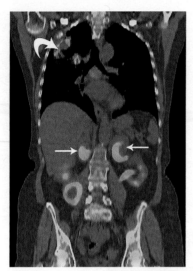

Fig. 12. Adrenal metastases from lung cancer on PET/CT. Axial and coronal PET/CT images demonstrating intense FDG uptake in the primary left upper lobe lung carcinoma (*curved arrow*) and in the adrenal metastases (*arrows*).

due to increased glucose metabolism (Figs. 11 and 12), whereas benign noninflammatory masses, in general, do not show significantly increased uptake [51,54]. Many studies have demonstrated that FDG-PET imaging can help differentiate benign from malignant adrenal disease [45,51–53,55–61,63, 64,67,68]. Early metastatic disease sometimes can be detected using this technique.

Sensitivity/specificity results reported for PET or PET/CT imaging range from 93%/80%, respectively, to 100%/100% [45,67,68], although most investigators believe that specificity is closer to 95% [57,67]. Some adrenal adenomas (5%) and inflammatory and infectious lesions demonstrate slight increased radiotracer uptake compared with the liver (the internal reference organ for normal uptake). Occasionally necrotic or hemorrhagic malignant adrenal lesions may cause false-negative findings showing poor FDG uptake [67]. PET imaging is not reliable for lesions less than 1 cm in size, as metastatic lesions of this size may demonstrate less radiotracer uptake than normal liver [67].

The use of PET/CT offers clear advantages over PET alone, as lesion morphology on CT can be coregistered with the metabolic activity from PET, allowing for accurate anatomic localization of any FDG abnormalities (Fig. 13). Furthermore, CT densitometry and washout measurements (if a contrast-enhanced CT and delays also are performed) can be incorporated into the analysis. Thus, three of the most effective tests used to characterize adrenal lesions may be combined in one scan. Under these circumstances, it has been demonstrated that sensitivity/specificity lesion characterization in a report with 41 masses was 100%/100%, although further studies with larger patient numbers are required to corroborate these findings [44]. Results in practice likely are less perfect as there is some clustering of benign and malignant lesions around the adrenal/liver threshold ratio on PET and the washout

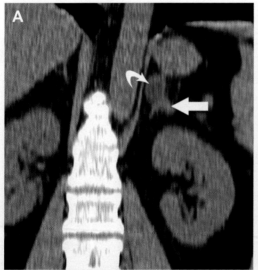
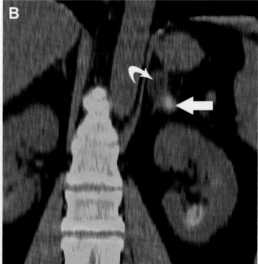

Fig. 13. Collision tumors. Coronal reconstruction of contrast-enhanced CT scan (*A*) shows low-density left adrenal lesion (*curved arrow*) stable compared with previous scans consistent with an adenoma in a patient who had breast cancer. CT scan, however, also shows a new enhancing mass (*arrow*) in left adrenal. Overlaid PET/CT image (*B*) demonstrating that the new lesion shows increased FDG uptake, consistent with breast cancer metastasis, displacing the low-density, non–FDG-avid adenoma (collision tumors).

thresholds on CT [45]. Most patients who have known adrenal lesions likely are referred for characterization with PET or PET/CT only if CT densitometry or washout analyses are inconclusive on a separate CT study. PET/CT is becoming the oncology imaging test of choice for many tumors, so greater numbers of adrenal lesions will be encountered and diagnosed on PET/CT in the future.

Adrenal biopsy

The number of requested adrenal biopsies has been reduced significantly by the improved accuracy of current adrenal imaging techniques [73]. Biopsy still is required in some cases, however, particularly if patients have an underlying extra-adrenal malignancy. Sometimes imaging findings with conventional adrenal imaging tests are indeterminate, there is suspicion that the lesion still could be malignant, or there are discordant imaging results. The frequency and necessity for adrenal biopsy depend to a certain extent on a department's familiarity with adrenal imaging and biopsy techniques.

CT-guided percutaneous needle aspiration biopsy (PNAB) is a well-established technique and the method of choice for sampling adrenal lesions. The procedure usually is performed with patients in the decubitus position, with the adrenal mass ipsilateral side down to reduce the risk for pneumothorax (Fig. 14). Rarely, it may be necessary to use a transhepatic approach. Adrenal biopsy procedures have a good safety record with a low complication rate (most commonly adrenal hemorrhage or pneumothorax) and good accuracy rates (83%–96% diagnostic accuracy) [74,75]. It should be

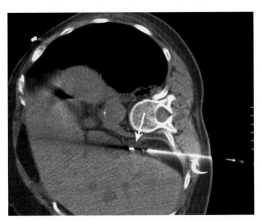

Fig. 14. Adrenal biopsy. CT image from CT guided biopsy of an indeterminate right adrenal lesion (*arrow*) with the needle in place. The patient has been placed in a right side down decubitus to reduce the risk for a biopsy-induced pneumothorax by decreasing the amount of visualized lung on this side at the percutaneous access level.

remembered, however, that sampling error sometimes leads to false-negative PNAB results. Collision tumors affecting the adrenal gland (see Fig. 13) (when two different tumors coexist in the adrenal) occasionally occur and PET/CT helps identify and direct appropriate biopsy in such circumstances [76]. Biopsy generally is not indicated for patients who have suspected pheochromocytoma because of the risk for precipitating a hypertensive crisis, although these tumors sometimes are biopsied inadvertently without untoward clinical complications [74,75]. If biopsy absolutely is required in a suspected case of pheochromocytoma, then appropriate prophylaxis blockade with endocrine and anesthesiology consultation should be sought.

Summary

Adrenal imaging techniques have undergone significant advances in recent years, allowing characterization of most adrenal lesions discovered at imaging. CT, MR imaging, PET, and PET/CT all are clinically useful in differentiating benign from malignant adrenal lesions although all use fundamentally different principles to make their adrenal diagnoses. Recently developed applications of dual-energy CT and histogram analysis may offer additional information. The new functional imaging techniques, such as perfusion, DWI, and MRS, may play a role in lesion characterization in the near future. Image-guided adrenal biopsy occasionally should be considered for treatment planning or for the uncommon lesions that remain indeterminate by imaging. The overall goal of adrenal imaging is to detect and achieve accurate characterization of most adrenal lesions and to direct patient management correctly.

References

[1] Young WF Jr. The incidentally discovered adrenal mass. N Engl J Med 2007;356:601–10.

[2] Bovio S, Cataldi A, Reimondo G, et al. Prevalence of adrenal incidentaloma in a contemporary computerized tomography series. J Endocrinol Invest 2006;29:298–302.

[3] Mansmann G, Lau J, Blak E, et al. The clinically inapparent adrenal mass. Update in diagnosis and treatment. Endocr Rev 2004;25(2):309–40.

[4] Dunnick NR, Korobkin M. Imaging of adrenal incidentalmomas. AJR Am J Roentgenol 2002; 179:559–68.

[5] Korobkin M. CT characterization of adrenal masses: the time has come. Radiology 2000; 217:629–32.

[6] Kloos RT, Gross MD, Francis IR, et al. Incidentally discovered adrenal masses. Endocr Rev 1995;16:460–84.

[7] Young WF Jr. Management approaches to adrenal incidentalomas: a view from Rochester, Minnesota. Endocrinol Metab Clin North Am 2000; 29:159–85.

[8] Barzon L, Sonino N, Fallo F, et al. Prevalence and natural history of adrenal incidentalomas. Eur J Endocrinol 2003;149:273–85.

[9] Song JH, Chaudhry FS, Mayo-Smith WW. The incidental indeterminate adrenal mass on CT (>10HU) in patients without cancer. Is further imaging necessary? Follow-up of 321 consecutive indeterminate adrenal masses. AJR Am J Roentgenol 2007;189:1119–23.

[10] Slattery JM, Blake MA, Kalra MK, et al. Adrenocortical carcinoma: contrast washout characteristics on CT. AJR Am J Roentgenol 2006;187: W21–4.

[11] Angeli A, Osella G, Ali A, et al. Adrenal incidentaloma: an overview of clinical and epidemiological data from the National Italian Study Group. Horm Res 1997;47:279–83.

[12] Abrams HL, Spiro R, Goldstein N. Metastases in carcinoma: analysis of 1000 autopsied cases. Cancer 1950;3:74–85.

[13] Boland GW, Lee MJ, Gazelle GS, et al. Characterization of adrenal masses using unenhanced CT: an analysis of the CT literature. AJR Am J Roentgenol 1998;171:201–4.

[14] Russell C, Goodacre BW, vanSonnenberg E, et al. Spontaneous rupture of adrenal myelolipoma: spiral CT appearance. Abdom Imaging 2000;25: 431–4.

[15] Blake MA, Kalra MK, Maher MM, et al. Pheochromocytoma: an imaging chameleon. Radiographics 2004;24:S87–9.

[16] Szolar DH, Melvyn Korobkin M, Reittner P, et al. Adrenocortical carcinomas and adrenal pheochromocytomas: mass and enhancement loss evaluation at delayed contrast-enhanced CT. Radiology 2005;234:479–85.

[17] Rozenblit A, Morehouse HT, Amis SE Jr. Cystic adrenal lesions: CT features. Radiology 1996; 201:541–8.

[18] Benitah N, Yeh BM, Qayyum A. Minor morphologic abnormalities of adrenal glands at CT: prognostic importance in patients with lung cancer. Radiology 2005;235:517–22.

[19] Korobkin M, Giordano TJ, Brodeur FJ, et al. Adrenal adenomas: relationship between histologic lipid and CT and MR findings. Radiology 1996; 200:743–7.

[20] Anderson JB, Gray GF. Adrenal pathology. In: Vaughan ED, Carey RM, editors. Adrenal disorders. New York: Thieme Medical; 1989. p. 18–9.

[21] Carney JA. Adrenal gland. In: Sternberg SS, editor. Histology for pathologists. New York: Raven; 1992. p. 150–4.

[22] Lee MJ, Hahn PF, Papanicolau N, et al. Benign and malignant adrenal masses: CT distinction with attenuation coefficients, size, and observer analysis. Radiology 1991;179:415–8.

[23] Caoili EM, Korobkin M, Francis IR, et al. Adrenal masses: characterization with combined unenhanced and delayed enhanced CT. Radiology 2002;222:629–33.

[24] Boland GW, Hahn PF, Pena C, et al. Adrenal masses: characterization with delayed contrast-enhanced CT. Radiology 1997;202:693–6.

[25] Korobkin M, Brodeur FJ, Yutzy GG, et al. Differentiation of adrenal adenomas from nonadenomas using CT attenuation values. AJR Am J Roentgenol 1996;166:531–6.

[26] Korobkin M, Brodeur FJ, Francis IR, et al. CT time-attenuation washout curves of adrenal adenomas and nonadenomas. AJR Am J Roentgenol 1998;170:747–52.

[27] Szolar DH, Kammerhuber FH. Adrenal adenomas and nonadenomas: assessment of washout at delayed contrast-enhanced CT. Radiology 1998;207:369–75.

[28] Pena CS, Boland GW, Hahn PF, et al. Characterization of indeterminate (lipid-poor) adrenal masses: use of washout characteristics at contrast-enhanced CT. Radiology 2000;217: 798–802.

[29] Caoili EM, Korobkin M, Francis IR, et al. Delayed enhanced CT of lipid-poor adrenal adenomas. AJR Am J Roentgenol 2000;175:1411–5.

[30] Bae KT, Fuangtharnthip P, Prasad SR, et al. Adrenal masses: CT characterization with histogram analysis method. Radiology 2003;228:735–42.

[31] Jhaveri KS, Wong F, Ghai S, et al. Comparison of CT histogram analysis and chemical shift MRI in the characterization of indeterminate adrenal nodules. Am J Roentgenol 2006;187:1303–8.

[32] Remer EM, Motta-Ramirez GA, Shepardson LB, et al. CT histogram analysis in pathologically proven adrenal masses. Am J Roentgenol 2006; 187:191–6.

[33] Wang B, Gao Z, Zou Q, et al. Quantitative diagnosis of fatty liver with dual-energy CT. An experimental study in rabbits. Acta Radiol 2003; 44(1):92–7.

[34] Raptopoulos V, Karellas A, Bernstein J, et al. Value of dual-energy CT in differentiating focal fatty infiltration of the liver from low-density masses. AJR Am J Roentgenol 1991;157(4): 721–5.

[35] Li J, Kalra MK, Small WC. Adrenal mass: differentiation by attenuation characteristics using dual-energy MDCT. Am J Roentgenol 2007;188(Suppl 5):A59–62.

[36] Korobkin M, Lombardi TJ, Aisen AM, et al. Characterization of adrenal masses with chemical shift and gadolinium-enhanced MR imaging. Radiology 1995;197:411–8.

[37] Outwater EK, Siegelman ES, Huang AB, et al. Adrenal masses: correlation between CT attenuation value and chemical shift ratio at MR imaging with in-phase and opposed-phase sequences. Radiology 1996;200:749–52.

[38] Fujiyoshi F, Nakajo M, Kukukura Y, et al. Characterization of adrenal tumors by chemical shift

fast-low angle shot MR imaging: comparison of four methods of quantitative evaluation. Am J Roentgenol 2003;180:1649–57.

[39] Mayo-Smith WW, Lee M, McNicholas MM, et al. Characterization of adrenal masses (<5 cm) by use of chemical shift MR imaging: observer performance versus quantitative measures. Am J Roentgenol 1995;165:91–5.

[40] McNicholas MM, Lee MJ, Mayo-Smith WW, et al. An imaging algorithm for the differential diagnosis of adrenal adenomas and metastases. Am J Roentgenol 1995;165:1453–9.

[41] Israel GM, Korobkin M, Wang C, et al. Comparison of unenhanced CT and chemical shift MRI in evaluating lipid-rich adrenal adenomas. AJR Am J Roentgenol 2004;183:215–9.

[42] Haider MA, Ghai S, Jhaveri K, et al. Chemical shift MR imaging of hyperattenuating (>10 HU) adrenal masses: does it still have a role? Radiology 2004;231:711–6.

[43] Park BK, Kim CK, Kim B, et al. Comparison of delayed enhanced CT and chemical shift MR for evaluating hyperattenuating incidental adrenal masses. Radiology 2007;243: 760–5.

[44] Blake MA, Slattery JM, Kalra MK, et al. Adrenal lesions: characterization with fused PET/CT image in patients with proved or suspected malignancy—initial experience. Radiology 2006;238: 970–7.

[45] Blake MA, Kalra MK, Sweeney AT, et al. Distinguishing benign from malignant adrenal masses: multi–detector row CT protocol with 10-minute delay. Radiology 2005;238:578–85.

[46] Luypaert R, Boujraf S, Sourbron S, et al. Diffusion and perfusion MRI: basic physics. Eur J Radiol 2001;38(1):19–27.

[47] Uhl M, Altehoefer C, Kontny U, et al. MRI-diffusion imaging of neuroblastomas: first results and correlation to histology. Eur Radiol 2002;12(9): 2335–8.

[48] Faria JF, Goldman SM, Szejnfeld J, et al. Adrenal masses: characterization with in vivo proton MR spectroscopy—initial experience. Radiology 2007;245:788–97.

[49] Sahani DV, Holalkere NS, Mueller PR, et al. Advanced hepatocellular carcinoma: CT perfusion of liver and tumor tissue—initial experience. Radiology 2007;243(3):736–43.

[50] Jain RK, Munn LL, Fukumura D. Dissecting tumour pathophysiology using intravital microscopy. Nat Rev Cancer 2002;2:266–76.

[51] Krestin GP, Steinbrich W, Friedmann G. Adrenal masses: evaluation with fast gradient-echo MR imaging and Gd-DTPA-enhanced dynamic studies. Radiology 1989;171:675–80.

[52] Murea S, Mainolfi C, Bazzicalupo I, et al. Imaging of adrenal tumors using FDG-PET: comparison of benign and malignant lesions. AJR Am J Roentgenol 1999;173:25–9.

[53] Boland GW, Goldberg MA, Lee MJ, et al. Indeterminate adrenal mass in patients with cancer: evaluation at PET with 2-[F-18]-fluoro-2-deoxy-D-glucose. Radiology 1995;194:131–4.

[54] Erasmus JJ, Patz EF Jr, McAdams HP, et al. Evaluation of adrenal masses in patients with bronchogenic carcinoma using 18F-fluorodeoxyglucose positron emission tomography. AJR Am J Roentgenol 1997;168:1357–60.

[55] Maurea S, Klain M, Mainolfi C, et al. The diagnostic role of radionuclide imaging in evaluation of patients with nonhypersecreting adrenal masses. J Nucl Med 2001;42:884–92.

[56] Gupta NC, Graeber GM, Tamim WJ, et al. Clinical utility of PET-FDG imaging in differentiation of benign from malignant adrenal masses in lung cancer. Clin Lung Cancer 2001;3: 59–64.

[57] Rohren EM, Turkington TG, Coleman RE. Clinical applications of PET in oncology. Radiology 2004;231:305–32.

[58] Elaini AB, Shetty SK, Chapman VM, et al. Improved detection and characterization of adrenal disease with PET-CT. Radiographics 2007;27: 755–67.

[59] Metser U, Miller E, Lerman H, et al. 18F-FDG PET/CT in the evaluation of adrenal masses. J Nucl Med 2006;47:32–7.

[60] Rao SK, Caride VJ, Ponn R, et al. F-18 fluorodeoxyglucose positron emission tomography-positive benign adrenal cortical adenoma: imaging features and pathologic correlation. Clin Nucl Med 2004;29:300–2.

[61] Bagheri B, Maurer AH, Cone L, et al. Characterization of the normal adrenal gland with 18F-FDG PET/CT. J Nucl Med 2004;45:1340–3.

[62] Francis IR, Smid A, Gross MD, et al. Adrenal masses in oncologic patients: functional and morphologic evaluation. Radiology 1988;166: 353–9.

[63] Francis IR, Glazer GM, Shapiro B, et al. Complementary roles of CT and 131I-MIBG scintigraphy in diagnosing pheochromocytoma. AJR Am J Roentgenol 1983;141:719–25.

[64] Shulkin BL, Koeppe RA, Francis IR, et al. Pheochromocytomas that do not accumulate metaiodobenzylguanidine: localization with PET and administration of FDG. Radiology 1993;186: 711–5.

[65] Shapiro B, Copp JE, Sisson JC, et al. Iodine-131 metaiodobenzylguanidine for the locating of suspected pheochromocytoma: experience in 400 cases. J Nucl Med 1985;26:576–85.

[66] Maurea S, Cuocolo A, Reynolds JC, et al. Iodine-131-metaiodobenzylguanidine scintigraphy in preoperative and postoperative evaluation of paragangliomas: comparison with CT and MRI. J Nucl Med 1993;34:173–9.

[67] Freitas JE. Adrenal cortical and medullary imaging. Semin Nucl Med 1995;25:235–50.

[68] Chong S, Lee KS, Kim AH. Integrated PET-CT for the characterization of adrenal lesions in cancer patients: diagnostic efficacy and interpretation pitfalls. Radiographics 2006;26:1811–26.

[69] Yun M, Kim W, Alnafisi N, et al. 18F-FDG PET in characterizing adrenal lesions detected on CT or MRI. J Nucl Med 2001;42:1795–9.

[70] Shulkin Bl, Thompson NW, Shapiro B, et al. Pheochromocytomas: imaging with 2-[fluorine -18]fluoro-2-deoxy-D-glucose PET. Radiology 1999;212:35–41.

[71] Ilias I, Yu J, Carrasquillo JA, et al. Superiority of 6-[18F]-fluorodopamine positron emission tomography versus [131I] metaiodobenzylguanidine scintigraphy in the localization of metastatic pheochromocytoma. J Clin Endocrinol Metab 2003;88:4083–7.

[72] Trampal C, Engler H, Juhlin C, et al. Pheochromocytomas: detection with 11C hydroxyephedrine PET. Radiology 2004;230:423–8.

[73] Paulsen SD, Nghiem HV, Korobkin M, et al. Changing role of imaging-guided percutaneous biopsy of adrenal masses: evaluation of 50 adrenal biopsies. AJR Am J Roentgenol 2004;182: 1033–103.

[74] Welch TJ, Sheedy PF II, Stephens DH, et al. Percutaneous adrenal biopsy: review of a 10-year experience. Radiology 1994;193: 341–4.

[75] Silverman SG, Mueller PR, Pinkney LP, et al. Predictive value of image-guided adrenal biopsy: analysis of results of 101 biopsies. Radiology 1993;187:715–8.

[76] Blake MA, Sweeney AT, Kalra MK, et al. Collision adrenal tumors on PET/CT. Am J Roentgenol 2004;183(3):864–5.

RADIOLOGIC CLINICS OF NORTH AMERICA

Radiol Clin N Am 46 (2008) 79–93

ELSEVIER
SAUNDERS

Imaging of the Renal Donor and Transplant Recipient

Anand K. Singh, MD[a,b], Dushyant V. Sahani, MD[a,b],*

- Renal donor evaluation
  Surgical considerations for donor nephrectomy
  Imaging in donors
  Multidetector CT versus MR imaging for evaluation of renal donors
  Multidetector CT technique
  MR imaging in evaluation of renal donors
  Role of image postprocessing

- Renal transplant recipient evaluation
  Surgical considerations in recipients
  Role of ultrasound and Doppler
  Complications and imaging considerations in recipients
- Summary
- References

Renal transplant remains the mainstay of the treatment of end-stage renal disease. With improvement in management strategies and the diverse imaging options, the yearly survival of recipients with functional kidneys has improved significantly. This improved survival is attributed to factors such as immunosuppressive therapy planning in recipients, human leukocyte antigen matching, surgeon experience, and recipient's age. Transplantation offers the closest thing to a normal state if the transplanted kidney can replace the failed kidneys. Living-donor kidney transplants are playing a vital role in bridging the gap between decreased supply of, and increased demand for, kidneys for transplant. Early detection and characterization of complications in the recipient are of immense clinical relevance, allowing timely intervention to prevent graft failure.

With the advances in several imaging options like multidetector CT (MDCT), MR imaging, and ultrasound, along with recent technical upgrades in

image postprocessing, meticulous donor selection and early detection of transplant complication are now possible [1,2].

Renal donor evaluation

Surgical considerations for donor nephrectomy

It is important that the healthy kidney be left in the donor and the other harvested for the recipient. After confirmation of normal size, location, and function of donor kidneys, a precise delineation of the donor kidney's vascular and collecting system anatomy is a vital prerequisite for presurgical planning. Although the kidney with the less complex vascular anatomy is preferred for harvesting, it is equally important to ensure that the single donor kidney to be left out is free of pathologies such as stones, cysts, and so forth. Such details would also help the surgeon decide if the preferred and less invasive

a Department of Radiology, Division of Abdominal Imaging and Intervention, Massachusetts General Hospital, White-2-270, 55 Fruit Street, Boston, MA 02114, USA
b Harvard Medical School, Boston, MA, USA
* Corresponding author. Department of Radiology, Division of Abdominal Imaging and Intervention, Massachusetts General Hospital, White 2-270, 55 Fruit Street, Boston, MA 02114.
E-mail address: dsahani@partners.org (D.V. Sahani).

0033-8389/08/$ – see front matter © 2008 Elsevier Inc. All rights reserved.
radiologic.theclinics.com
doi:10.1016/j.rcl.2008.01.009

laparoscopic approach to donor nephrectomy is possible or whether an open approach should be adopted [3]. In view of this, the presence of a tiny single calculus (<5 mm diameter) or a cyst of same size in one of the donor kidneys is not a contraindication for its retrieval for a recipient, irrespective of the complexities in its vascular variants. If both donor kidneys are normal, then the kidney with the less complex vascular anatomy is preferred, making a less invasive laparoscopic approach for nephrectomy feasible. The left kidney is usually preferred for a recipient because it provides a longer segment of the renal vein, which joins the inferior vena cava (IVC), and thus provides more maneuverability to the surgeon to suture the donor vessel patch to the recipient's iliac vein.

In addition to defining the vascular anatomy and variants, imaging should clearly depict pathologic conditions like renal artery atherosclerosis, fibromuscular dysplasia, aneurysm, and thrombosis. Accessory renal arteries are seen in up to 30% of cases, and they usually originate from the aorta. Occasionally, these arteries may arise from the iliac arteries and rarely, from the mesenteric and lumbar arteries [4]. Delineation and clear outlining of small accessory arteries, which can be as small as 1 to 2mm in diameter, are important imaging prerequisites from a surgical standpoint. Furthermore, a clear differentiation between two separate accessory arteries from prehilar branching (renal artery branching within 20 mm of renal artery origin) is extremely helpful and can sometimes help avoid torrential bleeding complications [5].

Similarly, multiple renal veins are seen in up to 30% of patients. An important presurgical imaging communication is confirmation of the presence or absence of venous variants such as the circumaortic renal vein (a single renal vein that is split or two renal veins encircling the aorta before joining the IVC), an isolated retroaortic left renal vein, and abnormalities such as venous thrombosis and varices [4].

Recently, the assessing of kidney volume before transplant has also gained importance, because transplant of the larger donor kidney has a more favorable posttransplant outcome rate.

Imaging in donors

With the advent of MDCT and advances in the MR scanner, current donor evaluation protocols are improving rapidly. Both these imaging modalities have proven promising in detecting vascular and collecting system variants with an established increase in readers' confidence [6]. With this development, the use of catheter angiography for mapping renal vasculature has virtually faded. Furthermore, the value of image postprocessing has added to increased acceptability of the CT and MR images to

referring physicians because postprocessed images provide a close simulation to the operative findings during surgery [7]. The high–resolution, thin-slice acquisitions provided by the newer CT and MR imaging scanners make it now possible to detect thin accessory renal arteries (**Fig. 1**) [8]. CT and MR urography also provide a clear delineation of the pyeloureteral anatomy, with added benefits provided by three-dimensional (3D) postprocessing.

Multidetector CT versus MR imaging for evaluation of renal donors

The better spatial resolution, faster speed, and greater cost effectiveness of CT have led to a wide acceptance of CT over MR imaging in most centers. Although CT and MR angiography have demonstrated substantial agreement in the preoperative evaluation of renal donors [9], more published research data on the integrity of CT technique, contrast volume, and injection rates, and various revolutionary CT protocol techniques, have definitely tilted the balance toward MDCT, leading to its widespread acceptance for imaging renal donors. The interobserver disagreement in the interpretation of CT and MR angiography is related to overreading and underreading of small vessels (1–2 mm in diameter) (**Fig. 2**) [10,11]. With the similarity of CT and MR imaging accuracies, the potential advantages and disadvantages associated with each modality have been widely discussed recently.

MR angiography is a safe and noninvasive technique for comprehensive evaluation of renal donors. It is radiation free and particularly advantageous in patients who are prone to allergic reaction from iodinated contrast media. The limitations of

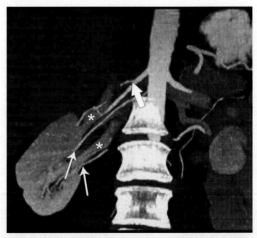

Fig. 1. A console-generated coronal maximum intensity projection in a 56-year-old female donor showing three arteries (*thin arrows*) supplying the right kidney, branching of the right main renal artery (*thick arrow*), and two renal veins (*asterisks*).

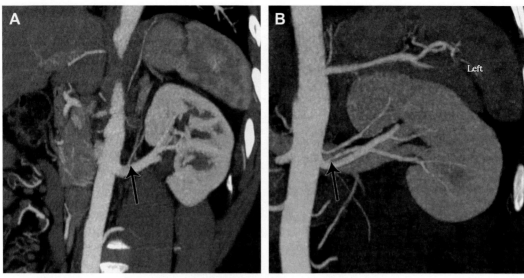

Fig. 2. MDCT coronal maximum intensity projection images in a 48-year-old female donor (*A*) and a 54-year-old male donor (*B*), showing early branching (*arrows*) of the main left renal arteries.

MR imaging include decreased spatial resolution and restrictions in slab length, which can lead to failure to image large volumes [10]. These limitations can lead to misinterpretations, especially in cases where the accessory artery arises from the iliac vessel or where the lower ureter has a tiny stone [11]. Such considerations have led to increased acceptance of CT angiography for the preoperative evaluation of renal donors.

Multidetector CT technique

Earlier four-phase CT acquisition for donor evaluation usually used precontrast, arterial, venous, and 4- to 10-minute delayed phases. However, because of concerns about radiation dose, particularly in healthy renal donors, various studies have suggested a reduction in phase acquisitions and an alteration in scan parameters. From these, it is now generally accepted that the use of a dedicated venous phase acquisition can be avoided by increasing the delay time for the arterial phase, which produces contrast opacification of renal veins and the adjoining IVC, along with the renal arteries and aorta. For arterial phase acquisitions, most authorities have recommended an empiric delay time of 25 seconds [12]. However, use of automated bolus tracking software is favored because accuracy in the timing of image acquisition is so important. Accurate depiction of lumbar and adrenal veins may necessitate a dedicated venous phase acquisition at 55 to 65 seconds delay. However, in the authors' experience, obtaining a delayed arterial phase acquisition with 25 to 30 seconds' delay and using postprocessing algorithms on these CT datasets of delayed arterial phase axial sections, differentiation

among lumbar vessels and accessory renal arteries and identification of adrenal and gonadal veins can easily be achieved. Acquisitions with such delays should be thin (1–2 mm) to ensure good quality of postprocessed images for detection of arterial and venous variants (Fig. 3).

Some groups have also gone to the extent of omitting the excretory phase, believing that the localizer radiograph or CT excretory phase scout images are sufficient to outline the pyeloureteral anatomy (Figs. 4 and 5) [13]. However, because of the possibility of overlooking some rare urothelial neoplasms, this proposal has still not become universally accepted.

Excretory phase acquisition is usually acquired after 4 to 8 minutes' delay time of contrast injection. In the authors' institution, they usually obtain an 80-kilovolt (peak) (kV[p]) excretory phase scout image before the excretory phase acquisition because such a kilovoltage value provides closer approximation to the k-edge value of iodinated contrast in the collecting system and enhances the visibility and delineation on scout images [14]. In view of dose savings for renal donors, the excretory phase acquisitions should be thicker (eg, 10 mm thickness obtained at 10 mm intervals) so that the proximal two thirds of the pelvicalyceal system is covered by the scan, with exclusion of the pelvic portion. Although some authorities still use excretory phase acquisitions of lesser thickness covering the entire pelvicalyceal system up to the pelvis, the authors feel that knowledge of the proximal two thirds of the collecting system, which can easily be revealed by scout images, is generally sufficient. Thicker 10 mm CT acquisitions of the restricted

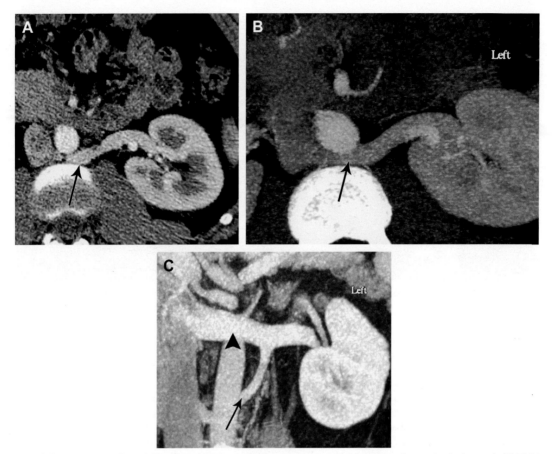

Fig. 3. (*A*) CT angiography axial image of a 45-year-old male donor with a retroaortic renal vein (*arrow*). (*B*) Thick axial MDCT volume maximum intensity projection showing a retroaortic renal vein in a 47-year-old female donor. (*C*) Thick coronal MDCT volume maximum intensity projection showing a circumaortic renal vein in a 51-year-old male donor. Anterior (*arrowhead*) and retroaortic (*arrow*) portions of left renal vein are seen.

portion can also assess for distal urothelial pathologies, which can lead to a significant reduction in radiation dose for these healthy subjects.

Recent papers have advocated omitting the precontrast phase for the CT evaluation of these healthy subjects and have pointed out the efficacy of contrast-enhanced arterial phase images for detection of small calculus up to 8 mm [15,16]. However, because of the prevalence of some false-positive detections, further validation of this work is needed.

Given these considerations, the protocol at the authors' institution is tailored to include a precontrast phase, an arterial phase (25-second delay) of thin section acquisition, and thicker (10 mm) excretory phase acquisition of the upper two thirds of the collecting system, in addition to the delayed-phase CT scout images (Table 1). A further increase in dose savings and cost effectiveness can be achieved by using a higher concentration of contrast media in smaller volumes with higher injection rates and by optimizing scan parameters, such as tube current (milliamperes) and tube voltage (kilovolts).

Some believe that before scanning the patient, it is advisable to obtain good distension of the pelvicalyceal system by ensuring adequate intake of oral contrast. However, fluid-distended bowel loops may interfere with the quality of postprocessed images; as a result, most discourage the use of oral contrast in their CT angiography protocols.

The administration of intravenous contrast media should be designed so that it coincides with and complements the speed of phase acquisition. In the authors' institution, nonionic contrast (300 or 370 mg iodine/mL concentration) is administered at a rate of 4 to 5 mL/s. The contrast media dose is based on the patient's body weight (550–600 mg iodine/kg weight). The maximum permissible limit with respect to injectable volume of contrast is 120 mL of 300 mg iodine and 100 mL of 370 mg Iodine.

MR imaging in evaluation of renal donors

Certain MR imaging sequences pertinent to preoperative evaluation of renal donors are illustrated

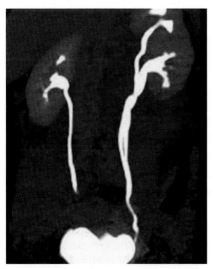

Fig. 4. Incomplete duplication of the left collecting system seen in thick-volume coronal maximum intensity projection image generated from the delayed-phase MDCT acquisitions in a 44-year-male donor.

in Table 2. The postcontrast sequence after a timing bolus is usually a 3D fast-gradient echo sequence (repetition time 5.00 ms, echo time 2.3 ms, flip angle 30°) using 25 to 30 mL intravenous gadolinium with immediate postinjection acquisition followed by three scan series acquisitions per breath hold. Lastly, coronal 3D fast-gradient echo with fat suppression is obtained immediately after the dynamic series of delayed contrast-enhanced images. Coronal T2-weighted images can serve as a localizer sequence, whereas characterization of fluid-filled

lesions like cysts and abscesses can be better appreciated on the axial T2-weighted fat-suppressed sequence. In- and out-of-phase sequences are useful for confirmation of small amounts of fat, whereas the postcontrast gradient-echo fat-suppressed sequence can be useful for delineating renal venous anatomy and detecting thrombus.

In imaging of renal donors, a special emphasis needs to be placed on sequences that optimally delineate the vascular anatomy. Use of a larger flip angle (up to 45°) can be applied to the MR arteriography sequence to reduce the background noise around the bright-appearing contrast-enhanced renal arteries [17]. The venous acquisition should be acquired immediately after the arterial and it is advisable to use a lower flip angle (15–25°) to better visualize the renal veins, which contain less contrast volume than renal arteries because of the nephrographic phase washout [17]. The acquired data can then be sent for postprocessing, where two-dimensional and 3D volume maximum intensity projections (MIPs) and volume-rendered (VR) images are created at dedicated workstations.

With the advent of 3-tesla and higher-generation MR scanners, a better signal-to-noise ratio is now achievable, with shorter sequence acquisition times, which greatly adds to the resolution of the images and enhances the quality of postprocessed images. However, the full potential and advantages of these scanners are still under evaluation.

Role of image postprocessing

These recent advances in CT and MR imaging have emphasized the benefits and quality of the

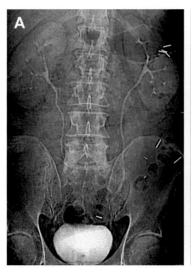
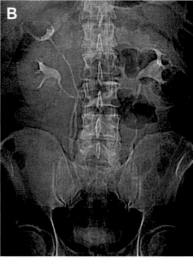

Fig. 5. (*A*) Low-dose (80 kilovolt [peak]) CT scout (localizer) images obtained 6 minutes after contrast injection in 47-year-old male donor showing normal collecting system. Surgical staples from prior surgery are seen in the left abdomen. (*B*) Low-dose CT scout shows presence of incomplete duplication of right collecting system with normal left collecting system anatomy in a 54-year-old female donor.

Table 1:   **Sixteen- and 64-slice multidetector CT protocol for renal donors**

Phase	Scan range	Slice thickness (mm)	Interval (mm)
Precontrast	Dome of diaphragm to iliac crest	10	10
Automated bolus triggering used to obtain a delay of 25 seconds after contrast injection			
Arterial phase	Dome of diaphragm to iliac crest	1.250 (16-slice MDCT) 0.625 (64-slice MDCT)	0.625
6 minute delayed scout images of the abdomen and pelvis: 80 kV(p), 10 mA (anteroposterior scout)			
6 minute delayed phase	Dome of diaphragm to iliac crest	10	10

Contrast injection: up to 120 mL of 370 mg iodine/mL or up to 150 mL of 300 mg iodine/mL at 4 mL/s; 40 mL saline chase. Noise index is 10–5, depending on body weight.

postprocessed 3D images (Figs. 6, 7). Image postprocessing provides not only a simplified display of information of entire MDCT or MR data sets but also a close simulation of the operative field of view to the surgeon. A stack of MIP reformats obtained in a plane parallel to the renal vessel axis outlines the renal vascular anatomy better (Fig. 8) [7]. VR and MIP screen-capture images in various desired angles such as the coronal or oblique coronal planes are becoming increasingly popular with surgeons for preoperative mapping of donor kidney anatomy [7,18,19]. From recent study results and experience, it is now believed that 3D images obtained at various desired angles alone can provide all the useful information to the readers, and independent viewing of axial images is essential only for increasing diagnostic confidence in the visualization of smaller accessory arteries or the differentiation of two thin accessory arteries from an early arterial branching [7]. Furthermore, because of increased clinical acceptability of the 3D images, image postprocessing has evolved to become an integral part of donor imaging. MDCT image postprocessing protocol is given in Table 3.

An enhanced realization of postprocessing benefits is particularly evident in renal donor imaging with the ready availability of donor kidney volumes because the larger kidney is usually preferred from the donor, provided the other kidney is functionally normal and free of pathologies.

Renal transplant recipient evaluation

Assessment for graft dysfunction immediately after surgery is imperative because it can channel the medical management appropriately in cases with complications. Ultrasound, Doppler, and nuclear medicine are the main imaging modalities used for immediate assessment of transplanted kidneys. Ultrasound plays a crucial role in the imaging of recipients immediately after surgery and has proven useful for follow-up in such patients [20,21]. Moreover, ultrasound has emerged as a simple-to-use and a cost-effective modality. An added vital advantage is its usefulness in image-guided percutaneous interventions, whereas Doppler ultrasound remains the mainstay for detecting most vascular complications.

Radionuclide imaging is a good tool to demonstrate graft function [22] and is usually used in cases where rejection is suspected. For the evaluation of a renal transplant recipient, MDCT and MR imaging

Table 2:   **MR protocol for imaging renal donors**

MR sequence	Repetition time (ms)	Echo time (ms)	Fat suppression (±)	Breath hold (±)
Axial T2W FSE	2500	90	+	+
Axial T1W GE (in-phase and out-of-phase)	170	4.7/2.3	–	+
Coronal T2W FSE	1500	105	–	–
Postcontrast 3D axial fat-saturated (bolus timing +20 –30 mL intravenous gadolinium)[a]	5.0	2.3	–	+

Abbreviations: FSE, fast spin-echo; GE, gradient echo; T1W, T1-weighted; T2W, T2-weighted.
[a] Immediate acquisition after injection followed by acquisitions at 30, 70, and 120 seconds.

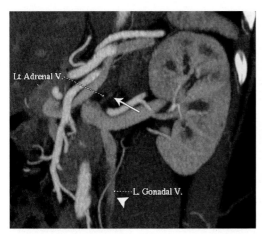

Fig. 6. The left adrenal vein (*arrow*) and left gonadal vein (*arrowhead*) on a coronal MDCT reformat of a 49-year-old male donor.

are usually used as adjunct modalities either to confirm the findings of the ultrasound or to image large patients because of unsatisfactory ultrasound images. Catheter angiography still retains its gold standard value in the diagnosis and treatment of postsurgery vascular complications in a recipient, but its use has diminished greatly because of the popularity gained by MR imaging in the delineation of vascular pathologies such as renal artery stenosis (RAS) and renal vein thrombosis.

Surgical considerations in recipients

Renal allografts are usually placed in the iliac fossa, extraperitoneally. The cadaver kidneys are harvested with an intact main renal artery and an adjoining cut portion of the aorta. The aortic portion is then trimmed in such a way that it can be exactly sutured to the recipient's external iliac artery (end to side

anastomosis) (Fig. 9) [23,24]. However, in some cases, the internal iliac artery is preferred. In a case with multiple arteries, if the origin is present on a single aortic patch, the above procedure is followed. However, in a case of arteries with a distant origin or polar arteries, anastomosis to the main renal artery is usually done.

Similarly, the renal vein is harvested with the adjoining portion of the IVC and is anastomosed to the external iliac vein. The left renal vein is longer than the right, which usually makes the left kidney preferable for harvesting in donors, and allows direct suturing of the left renal vein on the native iliacs. However, in cases where the right kidney is harvested because of the vascular complexities of the left kidney, a large segment of the donor's IVC is usually retrieved, making the anastomotic procedure in the recipient more cumbersome.

Ureteral anastomosis is the most difficult part of the surgery, which involves implantation of the cut ureteral end from the donor, directly into the recipient's bladder muscle [23]. The double ureter can be transplanted separately or each one partially anastomosed to the other beforehand and then transplanted as a single unit [25].

Usually, the venous anastomosis is performed first, followed by arterial anastomosis, and finally, the ureteral anastomosis. In the case of iliac artery atherosclerosis in the recipient, the less affected side is usually chosen for a transplant.

Role of ultrasound and Doppler

Ultrasound still remains the most preferred and economic modality for imaging recipients after transplant. It is noninvasive, can be easily done at the bedside, and is conveniently repeatable to assess response or monitor treatment in such patients.

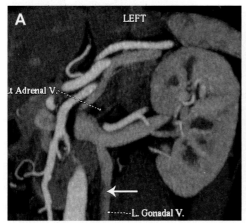
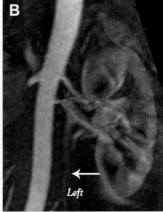

Fig. 7. Delineation of left gonadal vein (*arrow*) in a 44-year-old male donor is better appreciated on a coronal MDCT reformat (*A*) than a coronal postcontrast T1-weighted MR (*B*) because of improved resolution provided from MDCT.

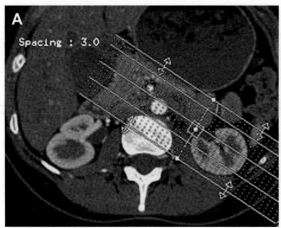
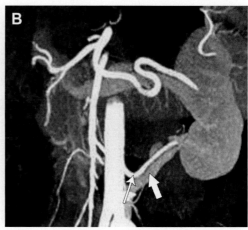

Fig. 8. CT angiography images of left kidney in a 32-year-old female donor. (*A*) Reconstruction design used at the workstation for generation of 6-mm oblique coronal MIPs planned parallel to the obliquity of renal vasculature. (*B*) Oblique coronal MIP showing accessory artery (*thin arrow*) and vein (*thick arrow*) at the lower pole. Accessory venous origin is from the left common iliac vein.

A transplant kidney can easily be visualized in either iliac fossa and is usually placed a few centimeters below the skin surface. However, certain factors may alter the image resolution, including postoperative edema in the skin and soft tissue, the patient's build, and the distance of the kidney below the skin surface.

A transplant kidney usually appears morphologically similar to a native kidney, except for some subtle differences. Usually, the peripheral parenchyma is well defined and hypoechoic, compared with the bright appearance of the echogenic renal sinus. Also, in the transplant kidney, the pyramids are usually well delineated and easily differentiated from the adjacent parenchyma (Fig. 10). They usually appear more hypoechoic, compared with the remaining parenchyma. A transplanted kidney

may also display a mild degree of hydronephrosis, which is usually due to edema at the site where the transplanted ureter is anastomosed to the native's bladder. This hydronephrosis usually resolves in time and may act as a baseline for subsequent ultrasounds of the recipient.

Color Doppler provides a satisfactory and immediate assessment of the blood perfusion in the transplanted kidney. However, spectral Doppler is always used for quantification. Usually, the flow in the interlobar artery of the transplant kidney should demonstrate a waveform similar to the

Table 3: Postprocessing protocol for generation of maximum intensity projections using multidetector CT data sets at workstations			
View	Algorithm used	Slice thickness (mm)	Overlap (mm)
Axial	MIP	6	3.0
Coronal	MIP	6	3.0
Oblique coronals[a]	MIP	—	3.0
Delayed (single) coronal oblique[b]	MIP	7	3.5

[a] Obtained for both kidneys.
[b] Including both kidneys.

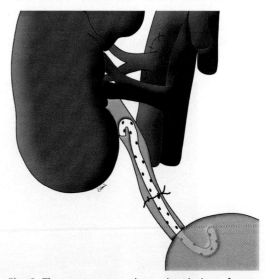

Fig. 9. The most commonly used technique for surgery in recipient: end to side anastomosis of vessels of donor kidney to the recipient's external iliac vessels. The cut end of donor's ureter is directly sutured to the bladder wall.

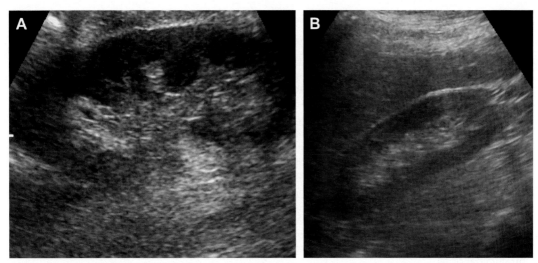

Fig. 10. (*A*) Transplanted right kidney showing a well-defined and hypoechoic peripheral parenchyma compared with the bright appearance of the echogenic renal sinus with easy differentiation of pyramids, as compared with the kidney appearance in a normal individual (*B*).

one in the native kidney or the recipient hepatic artery. Normally, it is a low-resistance waveform with the diastolic flow contributing up to nearly one half of the peak systolic value. Reduction in the diastolic flow is usually indicative of a pathologic process. In a case with adverse findings, it is usually advisable to perform Doppler studies every 24 to 48 hours in the early transplant period until the results are satisfactory.

The most frequently relied on Doppler indices are the pulsatility index (PI) and the resistive index (RI). With regard to the renal artery, peak systolic velocity up to 2.5m/s is considered normal [26–28]. The renal vein has no predefined value and it is simply assessed by the presence or absence of flow.

Complications and imaging considerations in recipients

Complications after renal transplant can be broadly classified into renal, urologic, vascular, and systemic. A list of preferred investigations is given in Table 4.

Early complications

Acute tubular necrosis versus acute rejection
Differentiating between acute tubular necrosis (ATN) and acute rejection is often difficult, considering the similarity of symptom presentation in the early posttransplant period. Ultrasound offers a limited role in diagnosis and usually, a histologic specimen of the transplanted kidney is required for diagnostic confirmation. Ultrasound is, however, the modality of choice for monitoring transplant dysfunction and assessing response to dialysis. Acute

rejection usually presents within 1 to 3 weeks and may be asymptomatic or associated with fever or upper respiratory symptoms (Fig. 11). The presence of acute rejection is, however, a poor prognostic indicator [29]. On the other hand, in ATN, the presence of other associated symptoms is usually rare.

B-mode ultrasound may reveal findings like reduction in corticomedullary differentiation and renal sinus echoes, increased cortical echogenicity, and initial increase in renal length and cross-sectional area. However, these findings are nonspecific and no longer relied on for prediction of acute rejection. Color Doppler, in combination with spectral Doppler, is more specific for assessment of the vessels and detection of RAS (Fig. 12). A PI greater than 1.8 and an RI greater than 0.7 are regarded as abnormal. However, Doppler has also failed to differentiate ATN from acute rejection; but the modality does provide a reasonable qualitative and quantitative evaluation of renal perfusion. Loss of diastolic flow with alteration in PI and RI can occur in ATN and acute rejection. Certain studies have revealed some encouraging results; for example, short acceleration time on day 1 was associated with longer duration of delayed function, whereas an acceleration time of less than 90 milliseconds at day 5 was associated with a high risk of rejection [30].

Ultrasound features, when correlated with clinical symptoms, are usually sufficient for a convincing diagnosis. Radionuclide study is the next in order; it may also be helpful in the diagnosis of acute rejection where an early normal postoperative phase study changes subsequently into an abnormal study. In cases of ATN, the renal excretion is

Table 4: **Common posttransplant complications and diagnostic investigations for recipient workup**

Complication	Ultrasonography/Doppler	Confirmatory investigation
	A. Early complications	
Acute tubular necrosis vs acute rejection	Nonconfirmatory: PI>1.8, RI>0.7, unable to differentiate	Radionuclide imaging/biopsy
	Vascular:	
Renal vein thrombosis (rare)	Confirmatory: dilatation of renal vein with thrombus with absent flow	—
Hemorrhage	Confirmatory: guided aspiration needed	(Re-exploration if significant)
	Perirenal collection:	
Hematoma, abscess	Confirmatory: guided aspiration needed	—
Ureteric obstruction (extrinsic compression by collection or intraluminal clots)	Detection of hydronephrosis by ultrasonography	Ultrasound-guided percutaneous nephrostomy if persistent
	B. Late complications	
Chronic rejection	Nonconfirmatory: decrease in kidney size and cortical echogenicity	Ultrasound-guided biopsy
RAS	Nonconfirmatory: PSV>2.5 m/s, RI>0.7 (confirmatory if RI>0.9)	Angiography (not needed if R.I >0.9), (MR angiography done in select places)
Arteriovenous fistula	Nonconfirmatory: arterial and venous flow on Doppler (small fistulae resolve on their own)	Angiography for confirmation if large and persistent

Abbreviation: PSV, peak systolic velocity.

abnormal but the perfusion phases are relatively well maintained (Fig. 13). MR imaging may show a diffuse increase in cortical intensity and loss of corticomedullary differentiation on T1-weighted scans, whereas an angiogram may show prolonged arterial phase, poor washout, and a patchy nephrogram.

Thrombosis   Renal vein thrombosis is rare, although more common than renal arterial thrombosis, and usually occurs between the third and eighth day of the posttransplant period. Characteristic features of renal vein thrombosis include a dilated transplanted renal vein containing a thrombus with absent venous flow, reversed diastolic flow, or a low-amplitude parvus tardus within the intrarenal arterial system and the transplant renal artery on Doppler imaging [31,32]. Arterial thrombosis, although rare, occurs in the early transplant period and shows complete absence of flow in the main transplant renal artery and intrarenal vasculature on color flow and spectral analyses [33].

Infections, obstruction, and perirenal collections   Indwelling urinary catheters are usually responsible

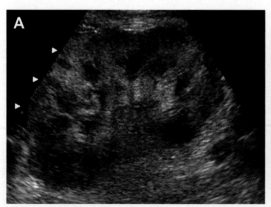
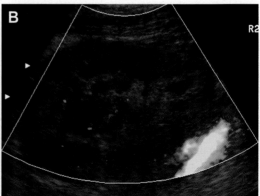

Fig. 11. (*A*) Acute rejection of transplanted right kidney showing increase in cortical echogenicity in a 46-year-old male recipient. (*B*) Marked reduction of renal perfusion is seen on power Doppler.

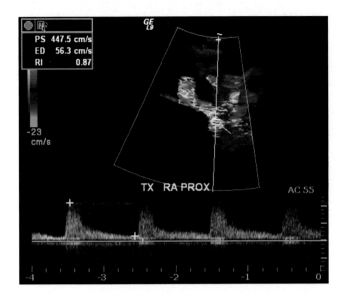

Fig. 12. Spectral Doppler analysis of a transplanted renal artery showing color aliasing, peak systolic (PS) velocity of 4.4m/s, and RI of 0.87, consistent with transplant artery stenosis.

for infections. The ultrasound picture may reveal echoes in the bladder and an associated thickening of the bladder wall but mostly the kidneys appear normal in early infection. Obstruction can be due to intraluminal blood clots secondary to surgery or extraluminal compression of the ureter by collections such as a lymphocele or hematoma. Hematoma mostly appears as a collection with septations and echoes, and is usually formed as

a result of bleeding from the skin excision of the vascular anastomosis itself (Fig. 14). The presence of a clearly anechoic collection or fluid with minimal echoes around the bladder, with reduction of urine output and increasing abdominal pain, is suggestive of an urinoma. In such cases, performing an isotope scan, cystogram, or an antegrade pyelography may prove useful for confirmation because communication between the extravesical and

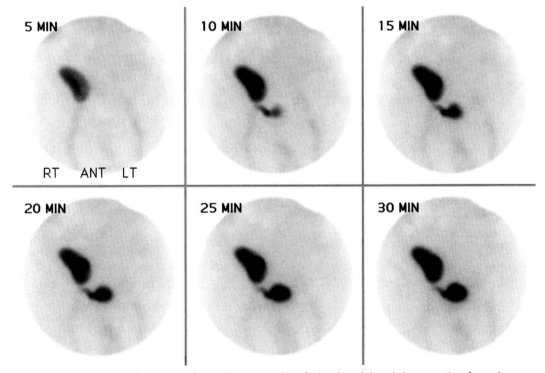

Fig. 13. Radionuclide scintigraphy study showing normal perfusion but delayed dye excretion from the transplanted right kidney, consistent with acute tubular necrosis.

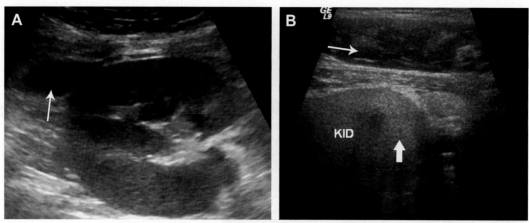

Fig. 14. (*A*) A small perinephric collection seen around the transplanted right kidney (*arrow*) in a 49-year-old female recipient. (*B*) A complex collection with echoes (*thin arrow*) seen in a 42-year-old male recipient above the transplanted right kidney (*thick arrow*), which shows an increase in cortical echogenicity consistent with acute rejection.

intravesical fluid can then be established. However, in such cases, ultrasound still remains the modality of choice for providing guidance to aspirate and drain these collections.

Early strictures are managed by balloon dilatation and stent placement for 1 to 12 weeks, which gives transient or permanent relief of obstruction in some patients.

However, in a case with presenting symptoms of urinary obstruction, ultrasound may fail to reveal the presence of a tiny calculus as its cause, in which case an unenhanced thin-section helical CT scan is the modality of choice. In a case with lymphoceles, scintigraphy demonstrates a photopenic area,

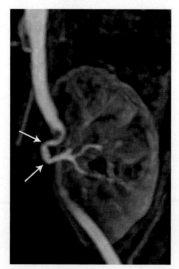

Fig. 15. MR angiogram showing kinking (*arrows*) of the renal artery of the transplanted left kidney in a 50-year-old male recipient.

which does not fill up with tracer on delayed images [34], whereas CT usually reveals a well-defined round or oval collection of 0 to 20 HU with no visible communication with the bladder lumen. Ultrasound usually serves as the initial modality of choice except in cases where visualization becomes difficult because of patient build or considerable postoperative skin edema, in which case CT or MR imaging is useful.

Late complications
Chronic rejection and drug toxicity Cyclosporine and tacrolimus have well-documented side effects on renal function and may lead to gradual failure of the transplanted kidney. At times it is difficult to distinguish gradual failure from chronic rejection. The strongest predisposing factor for chronic rejection is a history of repeated episodes of acute rejection. A generalized decrease in size of the transplanted kidney and increased echogenicity are some features of chronic rejection on ultrasound. However, the biopsy specimen provides the only means of confirmation, by revealing interstitial fibrosis and tubular atrophy.

Radionuclide studies show rapid uptake and washout. MR shows loss of corticomedullary differentiation, whereas MR spectroscopy shows altered levels of phosphate metabolites.

Vascular complications: renal artery stenosis and arteriovenous fistula The most common site of stenosis is at the site of anastomosis, followed by the postanastomotic transplant artery, mostly because of injury by the perfusion cannula. It is important to assess the recipient's iliac artery proximal to the anastomosis and ensure normal blood flow before the anastomotic region is assessed.

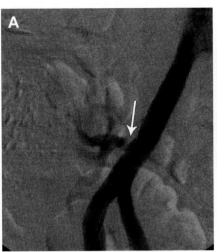 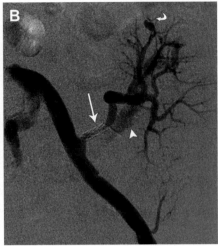

Fig. 16. (*A*) Angiogram showing RAS (*arrow*) in a 47-year-old female recipient. (*B*) RAS (*arrow*) in the region of the graft with immediate appearance of contrast in renal vein (*arrowhead*), consistent with arteriovenous fistula. An area of arteriovenous communication is also depicted (*curved arrow*).

Uncontrolled long-standing hypertension and deterioration of renal function following angiotensin converting enzyme inhibitor therapy are alarming signs and should raise suspicion for RAS. Early diagnosis before the setting of irreversible ischemia is crucial; angioplasty may salvage the transplant kidney and prevent host death. Stenosis can occur early, within a few months, most often caused by trauma to the donor's or recipient's vessel during clamping, or it may be delayed for few years, in which case atherosclerosis of the adjacent iliac artery is usually the cause. Kinking of the renal artery can occur when the transplant arterial length is longer than the vein, which usually occurs with the right-sided graft, raising clinical suspicion of RAS.

Doppler is preferred as the initial diagnostic modality. Most stenotic lesions, however, occur at, or close to, the anastomotic site and appear as focal aliasing on color flow imaging with peak systolic velocity greater than 2.5m/s on spectral flow [35]. Numerous twists and turns of the transplanted renal artery may contribute to defective Doppler angle correction on color flow imaging, in which case power Doppler may prove useful in providing a complete display of the renal vessel in question. The stenosis can be confirmed by angiography, which also provides a good estimate of the vessel extent and helps in the planning of percutaneous transluminal angioplasty.

Conventional angiography is invasive and poses an increased risk for thromboembolism leading to graft loss, groin hematoma pseudoaneurysms, and arteriovenous fistula. Contrast-induced nephropathy in the setting of a transplanted kidney and radiation dose issues are some important considerations that may make MR angiography preferable to CT and conventional angiography in the future. Nevertheless, conventional angiography has still retained its crucial role in diagnostic workup in most institutions. Doppler imaging can establish signs of RAS or venous thrombosis in the graft and is usually the first modality in the workup list because of its cost effectiveness, but MR imaging is usually done to confirm the findings of Doppler. MR imaging may be particularly helpful when a patient presents with signs of RAS despite normal Doppler findings; arterial kinks can be readily identified on MR imaging (Fig. 15). Surgical-clips, unless made of titanium, limit MR imaging because they may lead to artifacts, which can mimic RAS, in which case conventional angiography is done.

Formation of arteriovenous fistula is often a post-renal biopsy phenomenon and usually resolves on its own (Fig. 16) [36]. Spectral analysis reveals a focal pool of color flow containing arterial and venous components on spectral analysis; visualization of the pathologically increased flow of the fistula can be achieved by increasing the pulse repetition frequency.

Summary

MDCT provides greater accuracy and spatial resolution, a faster scan time, and better cost effectiveness when compared with MR imaging, which makes it, for most, the modality of choice for preoperative evaluation of renal donors. Although MR imaging shows accuracy similar to CT for evaluation of the renal vascular anatomy in renal donors, it has potential disadvantages, such as a longer scan time, higher cost, and inferior resolution, compared with MDCT. However, it is advisable to tailor the MDCT protocol for renal donors so that the protocol includes a precontrast phase, a late arterial phase of thin section acquisition, and thicker (8–10 mm) excretory phase acquisitions of the upper two thirds of the collecting system, which can reduce the overall radiation dose to these healthy patients compared with former protocols. Image postprocessing plays a vital role in CT and MR, where thick-volume MIPs and VR images can clearly demonstrate the renal vascular variants. Surgeons have welcomed these reconstructions because they help them choose the donor kidney and plan their laparoscopic versus open surgical approach.

Ultrasound and Doppler still remain the modalities of choice for assessment of posttransplant complications in recipients. They are useful as predictors of immediate complications like ATN and graft rejection and for diagnosing renal vascular pathologies. Ultrasound also facilitates the diagnosis of postoperative collections like hemorrhage, abscess, and urinoma. It is a preferred modality for guided diagnostic and therapeutic interventions pertaining to these complications. CT and MR imaging are preferred in patients where ultrasound imaging is difficult because of factors like increased skin thickness due to postoperative edema, and large patient size, but MR imaging is more accepted in a posttransplant setting because CT and conventional angiography pose risks of contrast-induced nephropathy. Radionuclide imaging plays an important role in demonstrating perfusion of the renal graft posttransplant and is usually preferred to confirm findings of ultrasound in the case of graft rejection and ATN. Angiography still retains its gold standard value in the diagnosis of vascular complications such as RAS and arteriovenous fistula but MR angiography has benefited from significant technologic advances.

References

[1] Rubin GD. MDCT imaging of the aorta and peripheral vessels [review]. Eur J Radiol 2003; 45(Suppl 1):S42–9.
[2] Flohr T, Stierstorfer K, Bruder H, et al. New technical developments in multislice CT–Part 1: approaching isotropic resolution with sub-millimeter 16-slice scanning. Rofo 2002;174(7): 839–45.
[3] Flowers JL, Jacobs S, Cho E, et al. Comparison of open and laparoscopic live donor nephrectomy. Ann Surg 1997;226(4):483–9 [discussion: 489–90].
[4] Urban BA, Ratner LE, Fishman EK. Three-dimensional volume-rendered CT angiography of the renal arteries and veins: normal anatomy, variants, and clinical applications. [review]. Radiographics 2001;21(2):373–86 [questionnaire: 549–55].
[5] Kawamoto S, Lawler LP, Fishman EK. Evaluation of the renal venous system on late arterial and venous phase images with MDCT angiography in potential living laparoscopic renal donors. AJR Am J Roentgenol 2005;184(2):539–45.
[6] Sahani DV, Rastogi N, Greenfield AC, et al. Multidetector row CT in evaluation of 94 living renal donors by readers with varied experience. Radiology 2005;235(3):905–10.
[7] Singh AK, Sahani DV, Kagay CR, et al. Semiautomated MIP images created directly on 16-section multidetector CT console for evaluation of living renal donors. Radiology 2007;244(2):583–90.
[8] Moritz M, Halpern E, Mitchell D, et al. Comparison of CT and MR angiography for evaluation of living renal donors. Transplant Proc 2001; 33(1–2):831–2 No abstract available.
[9] Toki K, Takahara S, Kokado Y, et al. Comparison of CT angiography with MR angiography in the living renal donor. Transplant Proc 1998;30(7): 2998–3000.
[10] Neimatallah MA, Dong Q, Schoenberg SO, et al. Magnetic resonance imaging in renal transplantation. J Magn Reson Imaging 1999;10(3):357–68.
[11] Israel GM, Lee VS, Edye M, et al. Comprehensive MR imaging in the preoperative evaluation of living donor candidates for laparoscopic nephrectomy: initial experience. Radiology 2002; 225(2):427–32.
[12] Kawamoto S, Montgomery RA, Lawler LP, et al. Multi-detector row CT evaluation of living renal donors prior to laparoscopic nephrectomy [review]. Radiographics 2004;24(2):453–66.
[13] Foley WD. Renal MDCT. Eur J Radiol 2003; 45(Suppl 1):S73–8.
[14] Hussain SM, Kock MC, IJzermans JN, et al. MR imaging: a "one-stop shop" modality for preoperative evaluation of potential living kidney donors. Radiographics 2003;23(2):505–20.
[15] Kim JK, Park SY, Kim HJ, et al. Living donor kidneys: usefulness of multi-detector row CT for comprehensive evaluation. Radiology 2003; 229(3):869–76.
[16] Singh AH, Sahani DV, Hahn PF, et al. Is a low dose (80 kVp) excretory phase scout image a viable alternative to thin section CT urography for accurate delineation of pyeloureteric anatomy of a kidney donor? [abstract 279]. In: Abstract book of American Roentgen Ray Society 106th annual meeting. Leesburg (VA): American Roentgen Ray Society; 2006. p. 73–4.
[17] Kalva SP, Sahani DV, Hahn PF, et al. Using the K-edge to improve contrast conspicuity and to lower radiation dose with a 16-MDCT: a phantom and human study. J Comput Assist Tomogr 2006;30(3):391–7.
[18] Rastogi N, Sahani DV, Blake MA, et al. Evaluation of living renal donors: accuracy of

three-dimensional 16-section CT. Radiology 2006;240(1):136–44 [Epub May 23, 2006].

[19] Rubin GD. 3-D imaging with MDCT [review]. Eur J Radiol 2003;45(Suppl 1):S37–41.

[20] Baxter GM. Ultrasound of renal transplantation [review]. Clin Radiol 2001;56(10):802–18.

[21] Pozniak MA, Dodd GD III, Kelcz F. Ultrasonographic evaluation of renal transplantation [review]. Radiol Clin North Am 1992;30(5): 1053–66.

[22] Brown ED, Chen MY, Wolfman NT, et al. Complications of renal transplantation: evaluation with US and radionuclide imaging [review]. Radiographics 2000;20(3):607–22.

[23] Hanto DW, Simmons RL. Renal transplantation: clinical considerations [review]. Radiol Clin North Am 1987;25(2):239–48.

[24] Shapiro R, Simmons RL. Renal transplantation. Atlas of organ transplantation. New York: Gower Medical; 1992.

[25] Oliver JH III. Clinical indications, recipient evaluation, surgical considerations and role of CT and MR in renal transplantation. Radiol Clin North Am 1995;33(3):435–46.

[26] Duda SH, Erley CM, Wakat J, et al. Posttransplant renal artery stenosis–outpatient intraarterial DSA versus color aided duplex Doppler sonography. Eur J Radiol 1993;16(2):95–101.

[27] Snider JF, Hunter DW, Moradian GP, et al. Transplant renal artery stenosis: evaluation with duplex sonography. Radiology 1989;172(3 Pt 2): 1027–30.

[28] Rigsby CM, Burns PN, Weltin GG, et al. Vascular complications in renal allografts: detection with duplex Doppler US. Radiology 1987;162(1 Pt 1): 31–8.

[29] Pirsch JD, Ploeg RJ, Gange S, et al. Determinants of graft survival after renal transplantation. Transplantation 1996;61(11):1581–6.

[30] Merkus JW, Hoitsma AJ, van Asten WN, et al. Doppler spectrum analysis to diagnose rejection during post transplant acute renal failure. Transplantation 1994;58(5):570–6.

[31] Baxter GM, Morley P, Dall B. Acute renal vein thrombosis in renal allografts: new Doppler ultrasonic findings. Clin Radiol 1991;43(2):125–7.

[32] Reuther G, Wanjura D, Bauer H. Acute renal vein thrombosis in renal allografts: detection with duplex Doppler US. Radiology 1989;170(2): 557–8.

[33] Sidhu PS, Baxter GM. Ultrasound of abdominal transplantation. Stuttgart (Germany): Thieme; 2002. p. 27–42.

[34] Kumar R, Bharathi Dasan J, Choudhury S, et al. Scintigraphic patterns of lymphocele in postrenal transplant. Nucl Med Commun 2003; 24(5):531–5.

[35] Baxter GM, Ireland H, Moss JG, et al. Colour Doppler ultrasound in renal artery stenosis: intrarenal waveform analysis. Br J Radiol 1996; 69(825):810–5.

[36] Merkus JW, Zeebregts CJ, Hoitsma AJ, et al. High incidence of arteriovenous fistula after biopsy of kidney allografts. Br J Surg 1993;80(3):310–2.

RADIOLOGIC
CLINICS
OF NORTH AMERICA

Radiol Clin N Am 46 (2008) 95–111

ELSEVIER
SAUNDERS

Cross-sectional Imaging Evaluation of Renal Masses

Srinivasa R. Prasad, MD*, Neal C. Dalrymple, MD,
Venkateswar R. Surabhi, MD

- ■ Cross-sectional imaging techniques
  Multidetector-row CT technique
  MR imaging technique
  MR imaging versus multidetector-row CT
- ■ Pattern-based approach to renal mass
  characterization: tumor morphology
  *Renal mass with predominant soft tissue
  component*
  *Renal mass with predominant macroscopic
  fat*
  *Renal mass with predominant (or
  exclusive) cystic component*
- ■ Pattern-based approach to renal mass
  characterization: tumor topography
- ■ Percutaneous biopsy of renal masses
- ■ Staging of renal cell carcinomas
- ■ Management of renal masses: knife,
  needle, or pills?
- ■ Follow-up imaging after surgery and
  ablative treatment
- ■ Summary
- ■ References

Most renal masses are neoplastic in nature. Infectious, inflammatory, and nonneoplastic masses constitute a small subset of renal masses. Many renal neoplasms demonstrate characteristic cell of origin, histology, and clinicobiologic behavior. Renal neoplasms may be primary or metastatic in origin. Primary renal tumors in adults are classified, based on histogenesis and histopathology, into renal cell, metanephric, mesenchymal, mixed epithelial and mesenchymal, and neuroendocrine neoplasms [1]. They are further categorized, based on tumor biology and histopathology, into benign and malignant neoplasms. The imaging characteristics of renal masses are protean; accurate distinction of benign and malignant neoplasms may not be possible because of overlap of imaging findings. A recent trend is toward percutaneous biopsy of renal masses in an attempt to characterize renal masses for the purpose of making treatment decisions.

The number of biopsies in patients who have advanced or multicentric renal neoplasms has increased, when a benign renal tumor is suspected, or in the presence of a known nonrenal primary or systemic malignancy [2].

Based on imaging findings, renal masses may be broadly classified into predominant soft tissue, adipose tissue, or cystic masses. Renal cell carcinoma (RCC) is by far the most common soft tissue mass in the kidney (Fig. 1). However, RCCs may demonstrate significant tumor heterogeneity and may appear entirely cystic or show a small proportion of macroscopic fat (Fig. 2) [3,4]. Other uncommon soft tissue renal masses in adults include oncocytomas, metanephric adenomas, benign and malignant mesenchymal neoplasms, and neuroendocrine neoplasms. Cystic renal lesions include kidney cysts (including hemorrhagic cysts), abscesses, and cystic neoplasms (multilocular cystic

Department of Radiology, University of Texas Health Science Center at San Antonio, 7703 Floyd Curl Drive, San Antonio, TX 78229, USA
* Corresponding author.
E-mail address: prasads@uthscsa.edu (S.R. Prasad).

doi:10.1016/j.rcl.2008.01.008

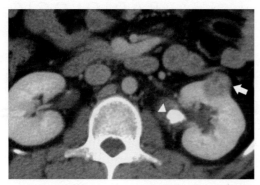

Fig. 1. RCC as soft tissue mass. A mildly enhancing soft tissue mass is partially exophytic from the anterior interpolar region of the left kidney (*arrow*). This finding was surgically proved to be RCC. Scan was performed to evaluate the renal pelvic stone (*arrowhead*).

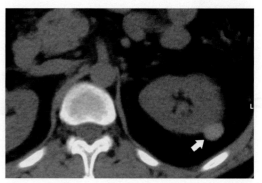

Fig. 3. Hemorrhagic renal cyst. Well-defined round lesion is predominantly exophytic from the lateral aspect of the left kidney (*arrow*). Uniform high attenuation and lack of enhancement on contrast-enhanced images (not shown) are consistent with a high-attenuation cyst, often called a hemorrhagic cyst.

RCC [MCRCC], cystic nephroma, and mixed epithelial and stromal tumor [MEST]) (Fig. 3). Most angiomyolipomas (AMLs) contain macroscopic fat and account for most renal masses with detectable adipose tissue (Fig. 4). However, up to 5% of AMLs may lack demonstrable fat on imaging techniques and are indistinguishable from other renal neoplasms (Fig. 5) [5]. In addition, a few RCCs may demonstrate macroscopic fat, either as a small intratumoral component or following engulfment of adjacent perinephric fat.

CT and MR imaging techniques constitute the mainstays of renal mass evaluation. They provide superior soft tissue discrimination and the spatial resolution necessary for detection, characterization, localization, and staging of renal masses. The imaging characteristics of some renal masses may be sufficient to suggest a pathologic diagnosis. However, the main roles of CT and MR are to define the location and extent of spread of the mass, and to monitor and assess response to treatment.

Cross-sectional imaging techniques

Multidetector-row CT technique

Recent advances in multidetector-row CT (MDCT) technology allow fast, multiphase, and high-resolution imaging of the abdominal viscera [6]. Subsecond gantry rotation and large detector size allow rapid volume coverage that not only facilitates multiphase scanning with short breath holds but also minimizes respiratory motion artifacts that can compromise lesion characterization. Retrospective thin-section data reconstruction permits routine acquisition of isotropic data that can be displayed in a multitude of multiplanar and three-dimensional formats, with minimal artifacts (Fig. 6) [6]. Scanning through the entire kidney is possible in less than 10 seconds, allowing for acquisition of thin-section images of the kidney during

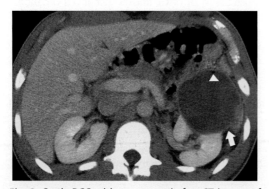

Fig. 2. Cystic RCC with macroscopic fat. CT image of this predominantly cystic mass shows mild irregular wall enhancement (*arrow*) and a trace amount of macroscopic fat (*arrowhead*). This finding was pathologically proved to be papillary RCC.

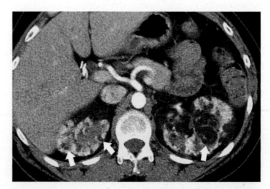

Fig. 4. Macroscopic fat within AMLs. Multiple fat attenuation lesions are present in both kidneys (*arrows*) in this patient who has tuberous sclerosis.

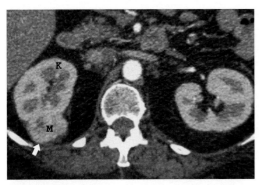

Fig. 5. AML with no detectable fat. A soft tissue mass (*arrow*) (M) is exophytic from the posterior aspect of the right kidney (K). Although this finding was pathologically proved to be an AML, no fat was detected at imaging, even on retrospective review.

the corticomedullary, nephrographic, and excretory phases, with little or no respiratory or patient-motion artifacts [7]. Multiphase imaging of the kidney thus permits not only high-resolution imaging of the renal parenchyma but also that of its vasculature and collecting systems [8].

Comprehensive evaluation of renal masses by CT requires a dedicated renal CT protocol. The various phases of CT imaging of the kidney include precontrast, arterial (15–25 second delay), corticomedullary (35–80 second delay), nephrographic (85–180 second delay) and excretory (3 minutes or more) phases [7]. Preliminary noncontrast scans are used to detect calcifications and allow quantification of enhancement on the postcontrast scans. However, unenhanced scans alone are inadequate for lesion characterization because no information exists regarding lesion vascularity/enhancement. In addition, the precontrast phase provides the lowest sensitivity for detecting renal masses.

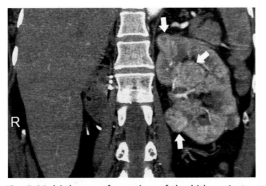

Fig. 6. Multiplanar reformation of the kidney. Isotropic scan acquisition and data reconstruction results in multiplanar image quality comparable to the source axial images. In this case of multicentric RCC, the distribution of three renal masses (*arrows*) can be seen on a single coronal image.

During the corticomedullary phase (CMP), contrast resides in the cortical capillaries, peritubular cells, proximal convoluted tubules, and columns of Bertin [9]. Optimal time delay for the CMP phase depends on the rate of injection, the amount of contrast material administered, and the patient's cardiac output. Advantages of the CMP include the differentiation of normal variants of renal parenchyma from renal masses and the better depiction of tumor hypervascularity [10–12]. Peak enhancement of renal vessels during early CMP also provides information on vascular anatomy and patency [7,9]. Two main disadvantages of the CMP are the difficulty in detecting small hypovascular lesions of the renal medulla (a low attenuation region during the CMP) (Fig. 7) and detecting small hypervascular tumors of the cortex (a high attenuation region during the CMP). Small hypervascular cortical RCCs may enhance to the same degree as the normal cortex, whereas hypovascular tumors of the medulla may not enhance during this phase [9–13].

The nephrographic phase is obtained during the passage of contrast material through the renal tubular system. During the nephrographic phase, which usually begins 80 to 120 seconds after contrast injection, the renal parenchyma enhances homogeneously. Although the duration of the nephrographic phase is not clearly defined, for practical reasons it may be divided into an early phase and a late phase, with the latter overlapping the excretory phase [7,9]. The nephrographic phase is considered the optimal phase for the detection and characterization of small renal masses [14]. The excretory phase begins when contrast material is excreted into the collecting system, 3 to 5 minutes after contrast administration. During this phase, the nephrogram remains homogeneous but its attenuation is diminished. A summary of the phases of renal enhancement for MDCT, including advantages and disadvantages, is shown in Table 1.

In many cases, the pattern of enhancement within a renal neoplasm is dense and irregular, and in such cases, subjective assessment for enhancement is sufficient. Even if enhancement is not particularly dense but is irregular or nodular within the mass, the mass is most likely neoplastic. However, in some cases of hypovascular masses, enhancement may be more subtle and uniform. In such cases, it is useful to compare attenuation measurements between the precontrast and each of the postcontrast phases. Because enhancement of the adjacent normal renal parenchyma results in some degree of beam hardening, attenuation measurements often drift upward slightly, even in proven simple cysts. This drift is more pronounced with smaller, predominantly intrarenal lesions,

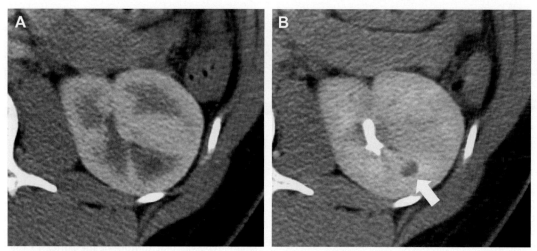

Fig. 7. Low attenuation medullary lesion in the CMP. (*A*) No renal abnormality is identified on the images acquired during the CMP. (*B*) A small simple cyst (*arrow*) is easily identified in the medullary region during the nephrographic phase.

because volume averaging and beam hardening have a higher statistical impact on the measurement within small lesions, particularly those less than 2 cm in diameter (a phenomenon known as "pseudoenhancement") [15,16]. As a rule, an increase in attenuation of 10 HU or more within a lesion between the pre- and postcontrast images, in a lesion measuring at least 2 cm in diameter, indicates enhancement. However, because pseudoenhancement may occur, only conclusive evidence of enhancement should be accepted as diagnostic. Although subtle areas of nodular enhancement can be convincing, lesions with no visual change that have an attenuation increase of 10 to 20 HU should be considered indeterminate, and further evaluation with ultrasound or MR imaging should

be considered [17]. It is often useful to use MR imaging to confirm the contrast enhancement, especially in small lesions.

Because the enhancement of renal masses is transient, washout of contrast can be as useful as the initial enhancement. Although it is usually not necessary to apply this principle with a multiphase protocol that includes precontrast images, it may be useful if only a single phase scan of the abdomen was performed and the abnormality is detected before the patient leaves the department. If this is the case, rescanning the kidneys permits assessment for "de-enhancement" [18,19]. If the area of enhancement decreases subjectively or quantitatively (with attenuation measurements of at least 10 HU), neoplasm is suspected (Fig. 8).

Table 1: **Phases of enhancement for multidetector-row CT of renal masses**

Phase	Delay	Advantages	Disadvantages
PCP	No injection	Detects calcifications; provides attenuation baseline for enhancement	Has low sensitivity and specificity
CMP	35–80 s	Provides good lesion enhancement;depicts vascular anatomy	May miss small hypervascular lesions in cortex
NP	85–180 s	Is optimal for detecting small lesions	May miss transient lesion enhancement
EP	3 min+	Defines relationship with collecting system (especially for planning nephron-sparing surgery)	Artifact from excreted contrast may obscure small medullary lesions May miss lesion enhancement

Abbreviations: EP, excretory phase; NP, nephrographic phase; PCP, precontrast phase.
Data from Yuh BI, Cohan RH. Different phases of renal enhancement: role in detecting and characterizing renal masses during helical CT. AJR Am J Roentgenol 1999;173:747–55.

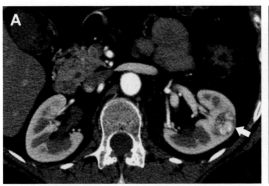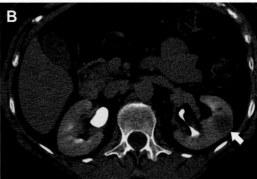

Fig. 8. De-enhancement of RCC. (*A*) Images acquired in the CMP demonstrate high attenuation within a centrally located lesion in the left kidney (*arrow*). Without precontrast images, the high attenuation could represent hypervascularity or calcification. (*B*) Repeat images in the excretory phase show loss of contrast enhancement, definitive for a hypervascular soft tissue mass.

MR imaging technique

Recent improvements in MR imaging hardware and software have enabled increased use of MR imaging for renal mass evaluation. Routine use of phased-array coils and parallel imaging allow fast– and high–spatial-resolution imaging of the kidneys [20,21]. Current MR scanners allow short breath hold, multiphase renal imaging without significant peristaltic, and respiratory motion artifacts. The physiologic principles behind the various dynamic postcontrast phases described in the MDCT section also hold true for dynamic MR imaging. A suggested MR imaging protocol for the evaluation of renal masses is summarized in Table 2.

Although patterns of renal mass enhancement (or nonenhancement) on MR imaging are similar to CT, the chemical-specific tissue characterization capabilities of MR imaging proves to be particularly valuable for several distinct types of renal lesion. Hemorrhagic cysts are an excellent example, because the lack of enhancement of a small, dense renal mass may be less than convincing on CT. On MR imaging, hemorrhagic cysts usually have high signal on T1-weighted images. Signal within

hemorrhagic or proteinaceous cysts on T2-weighted images is variable, ranging from low to mildly increased signal compared with renal parenchyma, but usually lower signal than seen in adjacent cerebrospinal fluid or other simple cysts. The combination of high signal on T1 and the lack of enhancement on MR imaging are diagnostic of a hemorrhagic renal cyst (Fig. 9).

MR imaging also has advantages over CT in the evaluation of complex renal cysts. Many of the septations within complex renal cysts that are vague or imperceptible on CT are readily apparent on MR imaging. Because fluid signal on T1-weighted MR images is usually darker than the low attenuation seen by CT, contrast enhancement within the septations is usually more apparent on MR than on CT (Fig. 10).

The macroscopic fat present in most AMLs allows accurate characterization by CT in most cases. However, in small lesions, volume averaging may hinder accurate attenuation measurements. MR imaging can help characterize small AMLs definitively in two ways: (1) frequency-selective chemical fat suppression will result in subjective signal loss

Table 2:	MR imaging protocol for evaluation of renal mass
Series	**Description**
1	Coronal T2-weighted single-shot turbo spin-echo sequence, serving as a localizer
2	Axial T2-weighted gradient and spin-echo sequence with fat suppression
3	Axial T1-weighted gradient-echo sequence, in phase and opposed phase (echo time 4.6 ms/ 2.3 ms), as a dual-echo sequence
4	Axial T1-weighted fat-suppressed gradient-echo sequence for dynamic imaging, using 20 mL intravenous gadolinium contrast; precontrast and postcontrast images in arterial, corticomedullary, and nephrographic phases are obtained
5	Coronal three-dimensional fast gradient-echo sequence with fat suppression, obtained immediately after the dynamic series for renal venous anatomy and for analysis of inferior vena cava for tumor thrombus

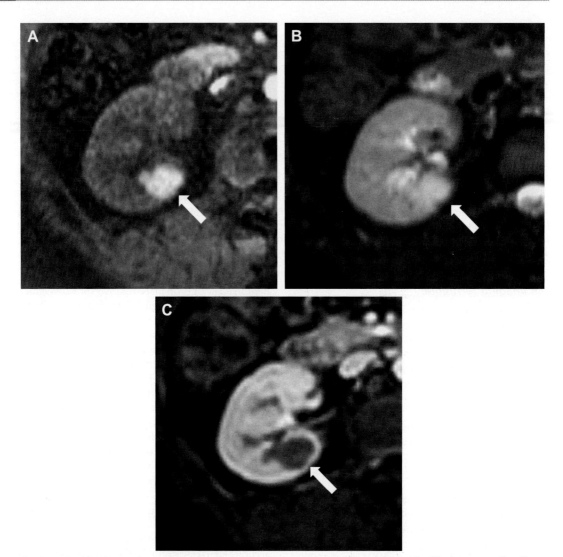

Fig. 9. Hemorrhagic renal cyst on MR imaging. (*A*) T1-weighted image performed with fat saturation shows a high signal intensity lesion in the posterior hilar lip of the right kidney (*arrow*). (*B*) T2-weighted image of the same lesion shows signal intensity nearly isointense to the adjacent renal parenchyma (*arrow*). (*C*) Postcontrast MR image demonstrates no enhancement within the lesion, consistent with a hemorrhagic cyst.

within fat-containing regions of the lesion, and (2) chemical shift artifact will result in India ink artifact at the interface between the lesion and the renal parenchyma (Fig. 11).

Contrast-enhanced CT is subject to the beam-hardening artifact and sometimes confounds the evaluation of small renal lesions. MR imaging is invaluable in this scenario, allowing confident assessment of enhancement. In such cases, subtraction techniques can help make enhancement (or the lack of it) more conspicuous, particularly if the signal is intermediate or high on precontrast T1-weighted images.

MR imaging versus multidetector-row CT

MR imaging is extremely versatile and, with appropriate pulse sequences, offers superior intrinsic soft tissue contrast and better demonstration of contrast enhancement. MR imaging requires no ionizing radiation or iodinated contrast material. CT is a less versatile, but often a more practical, modality in terms of accessibility and cost. CT provides excellent discrimination of fat from other tissues and is clearly superior to MR imaging for the evaluation of calcification. The CT examination requires less time, puts fewer demands on claustrophobic patients, is less prone to deleterious artifact from patient motion, and can be performed in patients who have implanted electric devices. Beer and colleagues [22] found no difference between MDCT and MR imaging in characterizing renal masses in 28 patients who had kidney lesions detected with sonography and requiring further evaluation. One

therapeutic decision making, ultrasound may be used reliably to direct biopsy.

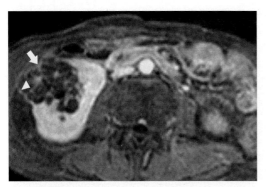

Fig. 10. Septal enhancement on MR imaging. Post-contrast T1-weighted images of the kidneys show irregular enhancement in the wall of the lesion (*arrow*) and enhancement of internal septations (*arrowhead*). This finding was proved to be cystic clear cell carcinoma.

reasonable approach for most cases is to use CT as the first imaging modality in a sequential diagnostic algorithm. If the mass is well demonstrated or is almost certain to be benign, no further imaging is necessary. If the mass is difficult to delineate from adjacent tissues, MR imaging can then be obtained. In many cases, information gleaned from the CT examination can help the radiologist determine an optimal protocol for the MR examination.

Although ultrasound is often useful to discriminate simple renal cysts from complex cystic or solid lesions, it has only a limited role in characterizing solid renal masses. When a solid renal neoplasm is identified by ultrasound, CT or MR imaging must be performed because ultrasound lacks the soft tissue discrimination and specificity needed for tumor staging. In cases where percutaneous tissue biopsy of a renal mass is desired to facilitate

Pattern-based approach to renal mass characterization: tumor morphology

Renal mass with predominant soft tissue component

RCC is by far the most common solid renal mass. RCC is the most lethal urologic cancer, responsible for approximately 12,890 deaths in the United States in 2007. RCC is composed of different histologic subtypes with variable histology, tumor biology, and prognosis (Box 1). Clear cell RCC is the most common histologic subtype of RCC. Combined, clear cell, papillary, and chromophobe RCC subtypes constitute approximately 90% to 95% of all RCCs in adults.

Clear cell RCC (also referred to as conventional RCC) is the most common histologic subtype of RCC, accounting for up to 75% of RCCs [23]. Multicentric and bilateral clear cell RCCs are found in patients who have von Hippel-Lindau (VHL) syndrome, an autosomal dominant, multisystem hereditary tumor syndrome characterized by the inactivation of the tumor-suppressor (VHL) gene. Inactivating mutations of the VHL gene are seen in approximately 60% to 75% of sporadic clear cell RCCs [1]. Clear cell RCCs typically appear as variegated, expansile, cortical masses with areas of necrosis, hemorrhage, and cystic changes [1,24]. The characteristic presence of intratumoral, microscopic fat may be established by chemical shift T1-weighted MR imaging. Calcification is seen in up to 15% of tumors [1].

Clear cell RCCs typically show hypervascularity on contrast-enhanced CT and MR imaging, presumably because of up-regulation of the vascular and

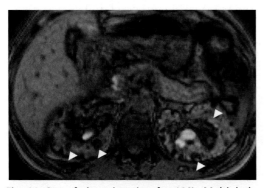

Fig. 11. Out-of-phase imaging for AML. Multiple lesions with high signal on in-phase images (not shown) are outlined with dark India ink artifact on out-of-phase T1-weighted image (*arrowheads*). With small lesions, the artifact makes the entire lesion low signal.

> **Box 1:** **Histologic subtypes of renal cell carcinoma**
>
> Clear cell RCC
> Multilocular clear cell RCC
> Papillary RCC
> Chromophobe RCC
> Collecting duct carcinoma
> Renal medullary carcinoma
> Translocation carcinomas
> RCC associated with neuroblastoma
> Mucinous tubular and spindle cell carcinoma
> RCC unclassified
>
> *Data from* Eble JN, Sauter G, Epstein JI, et al, editors. World Health Organization classification of tumors. Pathology and genetics of tumors of the urinary system and male genital organs. Lyon (France): IARC Press; 2004.

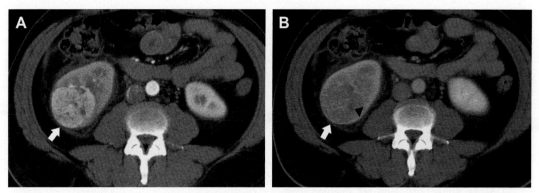

Fig. 12. Clear cell RCC. (*A*) Axial CT images during the CMP of enhancement shows dense enhancement of a right renal mass (*arrow*), typical of clear cell RCC. (*B*) Enhancement decreased significantly during the nephrographic phase (*arrow*). A small central area of low attenuation (*black arrowhead*) likely represents early necrosis.

somatic growth factors associated with the loss of VHL gene function (Fig. 12) [24,25]. Clear cell RCCs commonly show hematogenous metastatic dissemination to the lungs, liver, and bones. The propensity of clear cell RCC for lymphatic, and late and unusual sites of, metastasis is also well known [1].

Papillary RCC, characterized by papillary or tubulopapillary histologic architecture, accounts for 10% to 15% of sporadic RCCs [23]. Papillary RCC is more often multicentric than other RCC subtypes, especially in the setting of acquired renal cystic disease and hereditary papillary carcinoma syndrome [24,26].

Papillary RCCs commonly appear as homogeneous, soft tissue cortical masses with foci of calcification [24,26]. Papillary RCCs are often hypovascular and typically show a lesser degree of contrast enhancement than clear cell RCCs on contrast-enhanced CT and MR imaging (Fig. 13) [24,26]. Papillary RCCs frequently show areas of hemorrhage and necrosis. The low signal intensity

of papillary RCCs on T2-weighted MR images has been ascribed to the presence of hemosiderin [27]. A small subset of papillary RCCs may show a small focus of macroscopic fat that corresponds to cholesterol-laden macrophages on histology [1,4].

Chromophobe RCCs represent 5% of renal cell cancers and are histologically characterized by large, pale ("chromophobe") cells with prominent cell membranes [1]. Most chromophobe RCCs occur as solitary renal cortical masses. Bilateral, multicentric chromophobe RCCs are found in association with oncocytomas and "hybrid" tumors in patients who have Birt-Hogg-Dubé syndrome, an autosomal dominant genodermatosis syndrome [28].

Chromophobe RCCs typically appear as well circumscribed, homogenous renal masses with a cortical epicenter. In contradistinction to clear cell RCCs, but akin to papillary RCCs, chromophobe RCCs demonstrate a uniform and lesser degree of contrast enhancement, even in large tumors (Fig. 14) [24,29]. Chromophobe RCCs are commonly hypovascular at catheter angiography, possibly related to

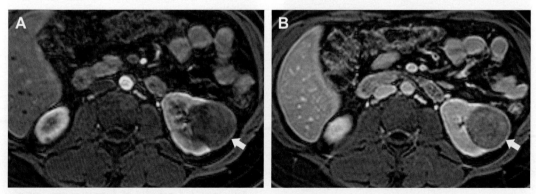

Fig. 13. Papillary RCC. Post–gadolinium-injection T1-weighted MR images of the kidneys. Mild internal enhancement of the lesion is seen during the CMP (*arrow*) (*A*), becoming slightly more conspicuous during the nephrographic phase (*arrow*) (*B*).

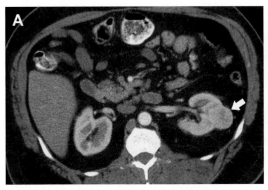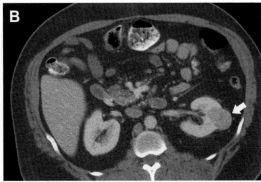

Fig. 14. Chromophobe RCC. Axial postcontrast CT images of the kidneys. (*A*) Image acquired during the CMP shows lesion enhancement (*arrow*) similar to that of the adjacent renal cortex. (*B*) During the nephrographic phase, contrast washout results in a lesion (*arrow*) that is slightly lower in attenuation than the renal cortex.

the presence of thick-walled, hyalinized blood vessels; however, a spoke-wheel pattern of vascularity has recently been described in the urology literature [1,30]. The other histologic subtypes of RCCs and renal tumors in familial or hereditary RCC syndromes shown in Table 3 are rare; a detailed discussion is beyond the scope of this article.

Renal oncocytoma is a benign renal epithelial neoplasm comprising 3% to 5% of all primary epithelial neoplasms that occur in the adult kidney [31]. Oncocytomas are histologically composed of large cells (oncocytes) with mitochondria-rich cytoplasm [1].

Most oncocytomas occur as well circumscribed, unencapsulated, solitary, solid renal cortical tumors. The characteristic central scar is seen in up

to one third of large oncocytomas (Fig. 15) [1]. Bilateral and multifocal oncocytomas are seen in patients who have renal oncocytosis and Birt-Hogg-Dubé syndrome [32]. Oncocytomas are typically hypervascular at catheter angiography, with a characteristic spoke-wheel pattern of feeding arteries [33]. However, oncocytomas are indistinguishable from RCCs by imaging studies alone.

Metanephric adenoma (MA) is a rare benign renal neoplasm that is histologically characterized by a monotonous population of small, embryonal (metanephric) cells. MA most commonly occurs as an incidental finding in patients during their fifth or sixth decades [34].

MAs commonly manifest as well circumscribed, homogenous, solid tumors of the kidney (Fig. 16). Large MAs show heterogeneity due to hemorrhage, necrosis, and calcification. MAs demonstrate hypovascularity and delayed, minimal enhancement following contrast administration [35,36].

Table 3: **Select hereditary renal tumor syndromes**

Syndrome	Gene	Tumor
von Hippel-Lindau	VHL (3p25)	Clear cell RCC
Tuberous sclerosis	TSC1, TSC2	Angiomyolipoma Clear cell RCC
Hereditary papillary RCC	c-MET	Papillary type 1 RCC
Hereditary leiomyoma RCC	FH	Papillary type 2 RCC
Birt-Hogg-Dubé	BHD	Chromophobe RCC Oncocytoma, hybrid tumors, other RCC types
Constitutional chromosome 3 translocation	Responsible gene not found	Clear cell RCC
Familial renal carcinoma	Gene not identified	Clear cell RCC

Data from Refs. [24,26,28,47,58].

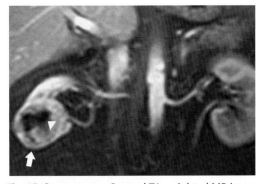

Fig. 15. Oncocytoma. Coronal T1-weighted MR image acquired following the injection of intravenous contrast media shows an enhancing mass in the inferior pole of the right kidney (*arrow*). The low-signal central scar (*arrowhead*) is typical of oncocytoma but in most cases cannot be differentiated from the central necrosis often seen with RCC.

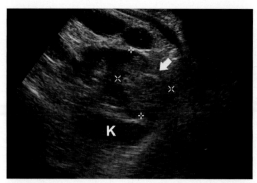

Fig. 16. Metanephric adenoma. Ultrasound image of the left kidney (K) shows a heterogeneous, solid left renal mass (*arrow, cursors*). Surgical specimen was shown to be metanephric adenoma.

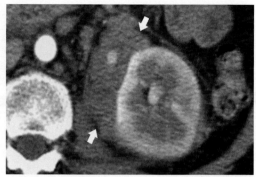

Fig. 17. Perirenal lymphoma. Axial CT image shows abnormal soft tissue surrounding the left kidney, most pronounced medial to the kidney (*arrows*).

Renal leiomyomas are rare, benign mesenchymal neoplasms that commonly arise from the capsule of the kidney [1,37]. Leiomyomas typically appear as expansile, well-defined, solid, peripheral renal tumors that show an exophytic growth pattern [37]. However, renal leiomyomas, particularly larger tumors, may show variegated morphology [38]. Leiomyomas commonly derive their blood supply from the capsular vessels [37].

Renal lymphoma usually describes renal involvement in the presence of systemic disease, although in some cases, the kidneys may be the only documented site of involvement. Renal involvement is more common with non–Hodgkin's disease than Hodgkin's disease and is more often bilateral. Renal involvement by lymphoma is often asymptomatic and routinely discovered at staging CT.

Although autopsy series show renal involvement in approximately 38% of patients who have lymphoma [39], only 3% to 8% of lymphoma patients have renal abnormalities detectable by imaging [40]. The most common pattern of renal lymphoma detected at imaging is that of multiple bilateral renal masses [41]. Other less common forms of involvement include solitary mass, direct invasion of renal parenchymal involvement from retroperitoneal and renal hilar lymphadenopathy, and a perirenal rind of soft tissue (Fig. 17). Although the presence of multiple homogeneous, hypovascular solid renal masses in a patient who has a known diagnosis of lymphoma is not a diagnostic dilemma, solitary renal mass in a lymphoma patient can be more problematic. A percutaneous biopsy may be necessary to differentiate between an RCC (more common renal tumor in the general population) and lymphomatous involvement in the kidney [2,42].

Renal metastases are rare and can occur from either hematogenous or lymphangitic dissemination. Renal metastases are frequently asymptomatic at presentation. Although hematogenous spread usually presents with bilateral, multiple renal masses, lymphangitic spread presents with perirenal and renal masses. Hematogenous renal metastases may occur with various primary neoplasms, including the lung, breast, malignant melanoma, malignancies of the gastrointestinal tract, and hematologic malignancies [43]. Lymphangitic spread is common with melanoma and lung cancer. In most cases, metastatic lesions show only mild enhancement and are multifocal, although solitary metastases may occur (Fig. 18). Metastases from lung, breast and colon carcinomas are the most likely to result in large solitary metastases that are difficult to distinguish from RCC [43]. As with suspected cases of renal lymphoma, image-guided percutaneous biopsy may be necessary to discriminate between primary renal malignancy and lesions metastatic to the kidney, because the primary renal malignancies usually require surgical intervention or ablation, whereas the metastases are treated with systemic therapy.

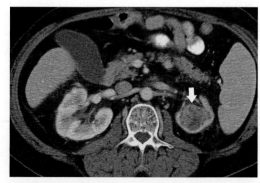

Fig. 18. Renal metastasis. Axial CT image shows a solitary mass within an atrophic left kidney (*arrow*). Biopsy confirmed a solitary metastasis in this patient who has known colon carcinoma.

Renal mass with predominant macroscopic fat

AML is a benign, triphasic mesenchymal neoplasm consisting of adipose tissue, smooth muscle cells, and thick-walled blood vessels, in varying proportions [1,44]. Based on a putative common cell of origin, AMLs are now grouped under a family of tumors characterized by the proliferation of perivascular epithelioid cells (PEComas) [44,45]. Bilateral, multiple renal AMLs are seen in patients who have tuberous sclerosis, an autosomal dominant phakomatoses syndrome [1].

Tuberous sclerosis–associated AMLs are mostly asymptomatic and occur in young patients aged between 25 and 35 years. They do not have a specific sex predilection. On the other hand, non-TS AMLs are frequently symptomatic and are more common in women in the fourth and the fifth decades [1,46].

Classic AML, the most common mesenchymal renal neoplasm, may originate from the cortex or the medulla. Renal AML commonly appears as a large, heterogeneous renal mass with varying proportions of macroscopic fat, intralesional aneurysms, and hypervascular soft tissue (see Fig. 4) [47]. Macroscopic fat is readily identified by noncontrast CT and frequency-selective, fat-suppressed MR imaging [45]. However, the intratumoral fat content may be variable and AMLs with minimal fat cannot be distinguished from other renal tumors by imaging criteria (see Fig. 5) [48]. Hemorrhage and renal failure are notable complications of renal AMLs, particularly in patients who have tuberous sclerosis [47].

Renal mass with predominant (or exclusive) cystic component

Bosniak [49,50] introduced a radiologic taxonomic system (first proposed in 1986, revised in 1993) to facilitate surveillance and management of patients who have renal cysts and cystic masses. The current

Bosniak renal cyst classification is based on CT findings and enables a cystic lesion to be categorized into one of five groups (categories I, II, IIF, III, and IV) (Table 4). Although the Bosniak renal cyst classification was developed and based on CT findings, it is commonly applied to other imaging modalities, including ultrasound and MR imaging [51]. The internal characteristics of renal cystic lesions, such as septations, solid or mural components, intralesional hemorrhage, and degree of contrast enhancement are better evaluated by dedicated renal CT and MR imaging. Image subtraction CT with MR imaging is a useful technique to assess the degree of contrast enhancement. Pseudoenhancement of renal cystic lesions may result from beam hardening and partial volume effects on CT. However, current MDCT scanners, by permitting thin-section acquisition, allow more accurate Hounsfield measurements. A lesion that exhibits 10 to 20 HU enhancement following contrast administration is assumed to be a neoplasm.

Most renal cystic lesions are benign and may be either diagnosed with certainty or monitored by serial imaging studies. Renal cystic lesions that warrant either conservative (including interventional radiology techniques) or surgical management include abscess, and cystic neoplasms such as cystic nephroma, MCRCC, and mixed epithelial and stromal tumor.

Renal abscess usually occurs as a complication of acute pyelonephritis. Predisposing factors for the development of abscess include repeated urinary tract infections, vesicoureteral reflux and diabetes mellitus. In other cases, hematogenous seeding of the kidney occurs as a result of bacterial endocarditis or other pyogenic infections such as diverticulitis. Renal abscess may appear as a homogeneous low attenuation region of the kidney or as a complex cystic lesion. Abscesses are often multiple and are associated with pyelonephritis and

---

Table 4: **Summary of the Bosniak classification of renal cysts**

Category	Features
I	A simple water-attenuation cyst with a hairline-thin wall, without septa, calcification, or solid components; no contrast enhancement
II	Bosniak type I with a few thin septa or fine calcification in the wall or septa Sharply marginated, nonenhancing, uniformly high-attenuation lesions of <3 cm
IIF	Bosniak type II cystic lesion with minimal enhancement of a hairline-thin septum or wall or minimal thickening of the septum or wall; the cyst might contain calcification that might be nodular and thick but there is no contrast enhancement Uniformly high-attenuation lesions of >3 cm
III	Bosniak type IIF cystic lesion with thickened irregular walls or septa, and contrast enhancement
IV	Enhancing soft tissue components or mural nodules

Data from Bosniak MA. The current radiological approach to renal cycts. Radiology 1986;158:1–10; and Israel GM, Bosniak MA. An update of the Bosniak renal cyst classification system. Urology 2005;66:484–8.

inflammatory stranding (Fig. 19). Temporal changes in morphology and size of the renal abscess within a short interval of time are also characteristic and these characteristics are sometimes helpful for distinguishing renal abscess from an atypical renal tumor. A confident diagnosis can usually be made based on imaging features in conjunction with clinical and laboratory findings. If necessary, percutaneous aspiration can be diagnostic and therapeutic.

MESTs of the kidney are uncommon benign renal tumors that are seen almost exclusively in perimenopausal women [52,53]. Previously referred to by several names, including hamartoma and adult mesoblastic nephroma, the nomenclature of MEST was introduced by Michal and Syrucek [54] in 1998. MEST is believed to be a hormonally dependent neoplasm.

MESTs are characterized by variegated imaging patterns including complex cysts, and mixed solid-cystic masses that show delayed and heterogeneous contrast enhancement (Fig. 20) [55]. The degree of delayed enhancement and hypointense signal on T2-weighted MR imaging depend on the proportion and cellularity of the stromal component [55].

Cystic nephromas are rare, benign renal neoplasms that show a marked female preponderance (the female/male ratio is 8:1) [56]. Most patients are asymptomatic and tumors are usually discovered incidentally. Cystic nephromas are predominantly unilateral, well-circumscribed cystic lesions with thin septations (Fig. 21). Hemorrhage or urinary obstruction may be caused by the "prolapse" of the cystic mass into the renal pelvis [57].

MCRCC is a recently described, rare subtype of RCC [3]. The term "MCRCC" is used exclusively to identify a cystic RCC with a small volume (25%

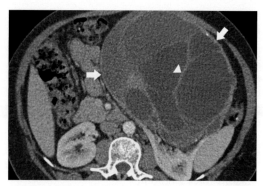

Fig. 20. MEST. CT image acquired during the CMP of enhancement shows low-level enhancement of the wall (*arrows*) and septations (*arrowhead*) of this complex cystic mass.

or less) of neoplastic clear cells in the cyst walls [3]. MCRCCs typically manifest as multiseptated cystic masses with thin septations on imaging (see Fig. 10). Distinction from other cystic masses on imaging studies is difficult [3].

Pattern-based approach to renal mass characterization: tumor topography

Recent advances in pathology have shed fresh light on the nosology of many renal neoplasms. It is believed that certain renal tumors arise from, or show differentiation toward, specific epithelium of different segments of the nephrons [29]. Most neoplasms of the kidney, including most RCCs and oncocytomas, arise from the renal cortex; however, the renal medulla may be the site of origin of a multitude of renal neoplasms such as transitional carcinoma, collecting duct carcinoma, medullary carcinoma, and hemangioma. Although the clear cell RCC and papillary RCC differentiate toward the

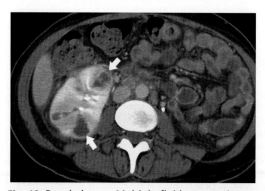

Fig. 19. Renal abscess. Multiple fluid-attenuation regions within the right kidney (*arrows*) are associated with an abnormal nephrogram and inflammatory changes in the fat surrounding the kidney. The clinical findings of fever, pyuria, and bacteremia confirm the diagnosis of renal abscesses, which resolved following treatment with antibiotics.

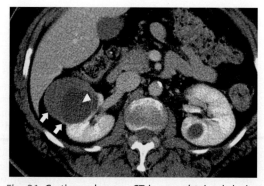

Fig. 21. Cystic nephroma. CT image obtained during the nephrographic phase of enhancement shows subtle irregular enhancement of the lateral wall (*arrows*). Mild enhancement is also seen within a septation (*arrowhead*).

epithelium of proximal convoluted tubule, the chromophobe RCC and oncocytoma recapitulate the epithelium of the cortical collecting ducts [58]. Thus, most RCC subtypes (clear cell, papillary, and chromophobe variants) arise from the cortex, and rare RCC subtypes such as collecting duct and medullary carcinomas have a medullary origin [59] (Fig. 22). Cystic nephroma and MESTs are cystic renal masses that may herniate into the renal pelvis. Most renal leiomyomas typically arise from the capsule of the kidney and most kidney hemangiomas arise from the renal sinus region. However, the medullary origin of neoplasms may be difficult to ascertain in large renal masses. Nonetheless, the epicenter of the mass, tumor composition, and patient demographics may provide additional clues to accurate characterization of renal masses.

Percutaneous biopsy of renal masses

A significant proportion of benign renal masses are either incidentally discovered in asymptomatic patients at imaging or diagnosed at pathology following surgery for presumed RCC. Kutikov and colleagues [60] found that approximately one sixth of benign masses were diagnosed among 143 patients who underwent partial nephrectomy for presumed solitary RCCs. Other studies have also found that a significant proportion of solid renal masses are histologically benign [61–63]. Accurate differentiation of RCC from benign renal lesions may not be feasible on imaging studies [64]. In an effort to characterize indeterminate renal masses definitively, percutaneous renal mass biopsy is being increasingly performed [2,61,62]. A recent study by Beland and colleagues [61] showed that imaging-guided biopsy of a solid enhancing renal mass was diagnostic in 90% of biopsies and the diagnosis

of a benign lesion was made in 27% of diagnostic biopsies. In select cases, ultrasound or CT-guided renal mass biopsy is a useful technique that can be performed with minimal morbidity and complications (Fig. 23). Recent advances in histopathology, immunocytochemistry, and cytogenetics permit accurate characterization of most renal masses and help guide optimal patient management.

Staging of renal cell carcinomas

MDCT and MR imaging are commonly used for staging of the RCC. Studies have shown that CT has a staging accuracy of up to 91% [65], making it the imaging method of choice for most patients. Two main limitations of MDCT are in distinguishing T2 and T3a lesions (presence of perirenal stranding does not always indicate perirenal fat invasion, because it can be seen secondary to inflammation, edema, and vascular engorgement) and in imaging the superior extent of tumor thrombus [66].

MR imaging has a similar accuracy to CT for staging RCC [66]; as with CT, the correct identification of tumoral spread into perinephric tissues remains problematic. MR imaging remains the method of choice for determining caval extension of tumor thrombus, because it can accurately obtain optimal venous opacification and differentiate bland from tumor thrombus better than CT. Therefore, MR imaging remains the imaging test of choice for delineating tumor thrombus (Fig. 24) [67].

Management of renal masses: knife, needle, or pills?

Radical nephrectomy has long been considered the standard of care for the treatment of RCC. The

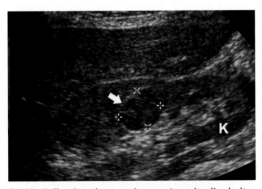

Fig. 22. Collecting duct carcinoma. Longitudinal ultrasound image of the right kidney (K) demonstrates a solid, hypoechoic mass located deep within the parenchyma of the kidney (*arrow, cursors*). This location is typical for collecting duct carcinoma and medullary renal carcinoma.

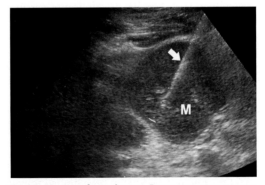

Fig. 23. Biopsy of renal mass. Percutaneous core-needle biopsy (*arrow*) of a mass (M) in the inferior pole of the left kidney was performed in a patient presenting with lesions in the lung, adrenal glands, bones, and kidney. The large infiltrating renal mass was shown to be urothelial carcinoma.

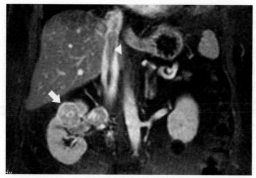

Fig. 24. MR imaging for staging RCC. Coronal post-contrast MR image of the kidneys demonstrates an enhancing renal mass in the superior pole of the right kidney (*arrow*). An apparent lobulation of the mass medially is actually tumor thrombus within the right renal vein. The tumor thrombus is seen to extend into the intrahepatic inferior vena cava (*arrowhead*).

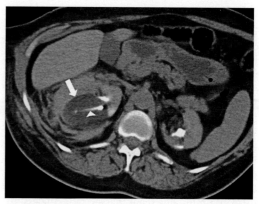

Fig. 25. Cryoablation of RCC. Noncontrast CT image acquired during performance of cryoablation of a right renal mass. Low attenuation (*arrow*) defines the "ice ball" created by cryoablation of a RCC. The probe is still seen within the ablation site (*arrowhead*). (*Courtesy of* Ronald J. Zagoria, MD, Winston-Salem, NC.)

diagnosis of RCC as small asymptomatic tumors has created a management dilemma. Small (less than 4 cm) renal tumors have a slow growth rate (0.2–1.2 cm/year) [68]. This relatively indolent early course, combined with the frequent diagnoses in elderly patients, has prompted the exploration of less invasive treatments. Renal-sparing surgery (partial nephrectomy) has now become a widely accepted method for removing small renal cancers. The introduction of laparoscopic radical and partial nephrectomy has decreased the recovery time but remains technically difficult.

Recently, interest has increased in percutaneous ablation of RCC as an even less invasive alternative to conventional or laparoscopic surgery or ablation. Image-guided ablative therapies are being used increasingly to treat renal cancers (Fig. 25). In 1997, the first use of the radio frequency modality for renal tumor ablation as an intraoperative technique was reported [69]. The first description of percutaneous radio frequency ablation of a renal tumor was reported the following year [70]. Recently, several clinical series have become available demonstrating the safety and short-term efficacy of radio frequency ablation for routine clinical use [71–73]. Patients who do not have comorbid conditions and have life expectancies of longer than 10 years, and patients who have metastatic disease, are generally excluded. The goals for radio frequency ablation are twofold: to treat patients who are otherwise at high risk for surgery and to preserve renal function in patients who have limited reserve or multifocal RCC [74]. The early clinical results with ablation of RCC are promising. In general, central tumors near the renal hilum are more difficult to ablate completely, compared with peripheral exophytic tumors. Because of the proximity of

central renal tumors to the renal pelvis (blood flow in the large hilar blood vessels causes a cooling "heat-sink" effect), these must be approached with more care to avoid damage to the pelvis and ureter [68]. As expected, the local recurrence rate, or incomplete treatment rate, is higher for central than for peripheral RCC [68]. As strategies to help protect the renal pelvis continue to evolve and as more powerful RF devices become available, this number is expected to decrease.

Until recently, the only effective treatment for metastatic RCC was cytokine therapy with interferon-alpha or interleukin-2 (IL-2). However, the characterization of the von Hippel-Lindau (*VHL*) tumor suppressor gene and of its role in up-regulating growth factors in RCCs (particularly hereditary and sporadic clear cell RCCs) helped define a series of potential targets for novel therapeutic approaches. Several agents now show promising activity in this disease and are changing patient management.

Follow-up imaging after surgery and ablative treatment

MDCT or MR imaging may be performed for surveillance following surgery or ablation treatment. The frequency and type of imaging modality used are institution specific. On follow-up imaging after the ablation procedure, the tumor should not show enhancement or interval increase in size. However, periablational enhancement (thin, symmetric, concentric enhancement) can last up to 6 months secondary to inflammation associated with the thermal injury. Irregular peripheral

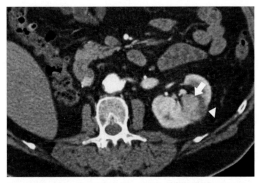

Fig. 26. Recurrent RCC following cryoablation. CT image of the kidney performed in follow-up following cryoablation of papillary RCC of the left kidney. Although peripheral portions of the tumor show low attenuation (*arrowhead*), the central region enhances (*arrow*), consistent with local tumor recurrence.

nodular enhancement or residual enhancement within the tumor itself is concerning for residual or recurrent tumor (Fig. 26). Most cases of incomplete treatment become manifest during the first year after therapy.

In addition, complications related to surgery or ablative therapies, such as hematoma, urinomas, and abscess formation can also be detected on follow-up imaging (Fig. 27).

Summary

Current imaging techniques (particularly MDCT and MR imaging) challenge the radiologist to participate in an increasingly sophisticated process of characterizing and managing renal masses. Once

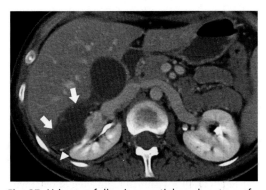

Fig. 27. Urinoma following partial nephrectomy for RCC. CT image of the kidneys acquired in the excretory phase shows a fluid collection (*arrow*) extending from the site of partial nephrectomy. A thin line of high attenuation seen posteriorly within the collection (*arrow*) was not present on precontrast images and indicates leak of contrast-opacified urine (*arrowhead*) into the urinoma.

considered a relatively simple, although usually devastating, entity of "hypernephroma," current understanding of RCC reveals a complex and diverse group of renal tumors. The broad category of hereditary and sporadic forms of renal tumors includes indolent, benign lesions, slow-growing neoplasms, and aggressive malignancies. The combination of early diagnosis (due, in part, to increased availability of imaging and the common incidental discovery of a renal mass) and innovative surgical and ablative techniques has resulted in a range of therapeutic options to match the spectrum of disease. CT and MR imaging remain the cornerstones of diagnosis, characterization, and staging of RCCs at present. We are only beginning to stratify the imaging characteristics of renal masses in a manner to predict tumor activity accurately, and further refinement and innovation are necessary to facilitate the tailored therapeutic approaches available today and the more targeted therapies on the horizon.

References

[1] Eble JN, Sauter G, Epstein JI, et al, editors. World Health Organization classification of tumors. Pathology and genetics of tumors of the urinary system and male genital organs. Lyon (France): IARC press; 2004.

[2] Silverman SG, Gan YU, Mortele KJ, et al. Renal masses in the adult patient: the role of percutaneous biopsy. Radiology 2006;240:6–22.

[3] Nassir A, Jollimore J, Gupta R, et al. Multilocular cystic renal cell carcinoma: a series of 12 cases and review of the literature. Urology 2002;60: 421–7.

[4] Lesavre A, Correas JM, Merran S, et al. CT of papillary renal cell carcinomas with cholesterol necrosis mimicking angiomyolipomas. AJR Am J Roentgenol 2003;181:143–5.

[5] Kim JK, Park SY, Shon JH, et al. Angiomyolipoma with minimal fat: differentiation from renal cell carcinoma at biphasic helical CT. Radiology 2004;230:677–84.

[6] Coppenrath EM, Mueller-Lisse UG. Multidetector CT of the kidney. Eur Radiol 2006;16: 2603–11.

[7] Yuh BI, Cohan RH. Different phases of renal enhancement: role in detecting and characterizing renal masses during helical CT. AJR Am J Roentgenol 1999;173:747–55.

[8] Smith PA, Ratner LE, Lynch FC, et al. Role of CT angiography in the preoperative evaluation for laparoscopic nephrectomy. Radiographics 1998; 18:589–601.

[9] Schreyer HH, Uggowitzer MM, Ruppert-Kohlmayr A. Helical CT of the urinary organs. Eur Radiol 2002;12:575–91.

[10] Birnbaum BA, Jacobs JE, Ramchandani P. Multiphasic renal CT: comparison of renal mass enhancement during the corticomedullary

and nephrographic phases. Radiology 1996;200: 753–8.

[11] Cohan RH, Sherman LS, Korobkin M, et al. Renal masses: assessment of corticomedullary-phase and nephrographic-phase CT scans. Radiology 1995;196:445–51.

[12] Kopka L, Fischer U, Zoeller G, et al. Dual-phase helical CT of the kidney: value of the corticomedullary and nephrographic phase for evaluation of renal lesions and preoperative staging of renal cell carcinoma. AJR Am J Roentgenol 1997;169: 1573–8.

[13] Zhang J, Lefkowitz RA, Bach A. Imaging of kidney cancer. Radiol Clin North Am 2007;45: 119–47.

[14] Szolar DH, Kammerhuber F, Altziebler S, et al. Multiphasic helical CT of the kidney: increased conspicuity for detection and characterization of small (<3-cm) renal masses. Radiology 1997; 202:211–7.

[15] Abdulla C, Kalra MK, Saini S, et al. Pseudoenhancement of simulated renal cysts in a phantom using different multidetector CT scanners. AJR Am J Roentgenol 2002;179:1473–6.

[16] Birnbaum BA, Maki DD, Chakraborty DP, et al. Renal cyst pseudoenhancement: evaluation with an anthropomorphic body CT phantom. Radiology 2002;225:83–90.

[17] Israel GM, Bosniak MA. How I do it: evaluating renal masses. Radiology 2005;236:441–50.

[18] Macari M, Bosniak MA. Delayed CT to evaluate renal masses incidentally discovered at contrast-enhanced CT: demonstration of vascularity with deenhancement. Radiology 1999;213: 674–80.

[19] Zagoria RJ, Gasser T, Leyendecker JR, et al. Differentiation of renal neoplasms from high-density cysts: use of attenuation changes between the corticomedullary and nephrographic phases of computed tomography. J Comput Assist Tomogr 2007;31:37–41.

[20] Koyama T, Tamai K, Togashi K. Current status of body MR imaging: fast MR imaging and diffusion-weighted imaging. Int J Clin Oncol 2006; 11:278–85.

[21] Rofsky NM, Lee VS, Laub G, et al. Abdominal MR imaging with a volumetric interpolated breath-hold examination. Radiology 1999;212:876–84.

[22] Beer AJ, Dobritz M, Zantl N, et al. Comparison of 16-MDCT and MR imaging for characterization of kidney lesions. AJR Am J Roentgenol 2006;186:1639–44.

[23] Renshaw AA. Subclassification of renal cell neoplasms: an update for the practising pathologist. Histopathology 2002;41:283–300.

[24] Prasad SR, Humphrey PA, Catena JR, et al. Common and uncommon histologic subtypes of renal cell carcinoma: imaging spectrum with pathologic correlation. Radiographics 2006;26: 1795–806 [discussion: 1806–10].

[25] Soyer P, Dufresne A, Klein I, et al. Renal cell carcinoma of clear type: correlation of CT features with tumor size, architectural patterns, and pathologic staging. Eur Radiol 1997;7:224–9.

[26] Choyke PL. Imaging of hereditary renal cancer. Radiol Clin North Am 2003;41:1037–51.

[27] Roy C, Sauer B, Lindner V, et al. MR imaging of papillary renal neoplasms: potential application for characterization of small renal masses. Eur Radiol 2007;17:193–200.

[28] Schmidt LS. Birt-Hogg-Dubé syndrome, a genodermatosis that increases risk for renal carcinoma. Curr Mol Med 2004;4:877–85.

[29] Prasad SR, Narra VR, Shah R, et al. Segmental disorders of the nephron: histopathological and imaging perspective. Br J Radiol 2007;80(956): 593–602.

[30] Kondo T, Nakazawa H, Sakai F, et al. Spoke-wheel-like enhancement as an important imaging finding of chromophobe cell renal carcinoma: a retrospective analysis on computed tomography and magnetic resonance imaging studies. Int J Urol 2004;11:817–24.

[31] Amin MB, Crotty TB, Tickoo SK, et al. Renal oncocytoma: a reappraisal of morphologic features with clinicopathologic findings in 80 cases. Am J Surg Pathol 1997;21:1–12.

[32] Perez-Ordonez B, Hamed G, Campbell S, et al. Renal oncocytoma: a clinicopathologic study of 70 cases. Am J Surg Pathol 1997;21:871–83.

[33] Quinn MJ, Hartman DS, Friedman AC, et al. Renal oncocytoma: new observations. Radiology 1984;153:49–53.

[34] Davis CJ Jr, Barton JH, Sesterhenn IA, et al. Metanephric adenoma. Clinicopathological study of fifty patients. Am J Surg Pathol 1995;19: 1101–14.

[35] Imamoto T, Furuya Y, Ueda T, et al. Metanephric adenoma of the kidney. Int J Urol 1999;6:200–2.

[36] Fielding JR, Visweswaran A, Silverman SG, et al. CT and ultrasound features of metanephric adenoma in adults with pathologic correlation. J Comput Assist Tomogr 1999;23:441–4.

[37] Lee SY, Hsu HH, Chang CT, et al. Renal capsular leiomyoma–imaging features on computed tomography and angiography. Nephrol Dial Transplant 2006;21:228–9.

[38] Nagar AM, Raut AA, Narlawar RS, et al. Giant renal capsular leiomyoma: study of two cases. Br J Radiol 2004;77:957–8.

[39] Miyake O, Namiki M, Sonoda T, et al. Secondary involvement of genitourinary organs in malignant lymphoma. Urol Int 1987;42:360–2.

[40] Reznek RH, Mootoosamy I, Webb JA, et al. CT in renal and perirenal lymphoma: a further look. Clin Radiol 1990;42:233–8.

[41] Sheth S, Ali S, Fishman E. Imaging of renal lymphoma: patterns of disease with pathologic correlation. Radiographics 2006;26:1151–68.

[42] Rybicki FJ, Shu KM, Cibas ES, et al. Percutaneous biopsy of renal masses: sensitivity and negative predictive value stratified by clinical setting and size of masses. AJR Am J Roentgenol 2003;180: 1281–7.

[43] Choyke PL, White EM, Zeman RK, et al. Renal metastases: clinicopathologic and radiologic correlation. Radiology 1987;162:359–63.

[44] Hornick JL, Fletcher CD. PEComa: what do we know so far? Histopathology 2006;48:75–82.

[45] Prasad SR, Mino-Kenudson M, Narra VR, et al. Neoplasms of the perivascular epithelioid cell involving the abdomen and the pelvis: cross-sectional imaging findings. J Comput Assist Tomogr 2007;31(5):688–96.

[46] Eble JN. Angiomyolipoma of kidney. Semin Diagn Pathol 1998;15:21–40.

[47] Casper KA, Donnelly LF, Chen B, et al. Tuberous sclerosis complex: renal imaging findings. Radiology 2002;225:451–6.

[48] Jinzaki M, Tanimoto A, Narimatsu Y, et al. Angiomyolipoma: imaging findings in lesions with minimal fat. Radiology 1997;205:497–502.

[49] Bosniak MA. Problems in the radiologic diagnosis of renal parenchymal tumors. Urol Clin North Am 1993;20:217–30.

[50] Bosniak MA. The current radiological approach to renal cysts. Radiology 1986;158:1–10.

[51] Israel GM, Bosniak MA. An update of the Bosniak renal cyst classification system. Urology 2005;66:484–8.

[52] Adsay NV, Eble JN, Srigley JR, et al. Mixed epithelial and stromal tumor of the kidney. Am J Surg Pathol 2000;24:958–70.

[53] Michal M. Benign mixed epithelial and stromal tumor of the kidney. Pathol Res Pract 2000;196:275–6.

[54] Michal M, Syrucek M. Benign mixed epithelial and stromal tumor of the kidney. Pathol Res Pract 1998;194:445–8.

[55] Park HS, Kim SH, Kim SH, et al. Benign mixed epithelial and stromal tumor of the kidney: imaging findings. J Comput Assist Tomogr 2005;29:786–9.

[56] Jevremovic D, Lager DJ, Lewin M. Cystic nephroma (multilocular cyst) and mixed epithelial and stromal tumor of the kidney: a spectrum of the same entity? Ann Diagn Pathol 2006;10:77–82.

[57] Kural AR, Obek C, Ozbay G, et al. Multilocular cystic nephroma: an unusual localization. Urology 1998;52:897–9.

[58] Polascik TJ, Bostwick DG, Cairns P. Molecular genetics and histopathologic features of adult distal nephron tumors. Urology 2002;60:941–6.

[59] Prasad SR, Humphrey PA, Menias CO, et al. Neoplasms of the renal medulla: radiologic-pathologic correlation. Radiographics 2005;25:369–80.

[60] Kutikov A, Fossett LK, Ramchandani P, et al. Incidence of benign pathologic findings at partial nephrectomy for solitary renal mass presumed to be renal cell carcinoma on preoperative imaging. Urology 2006;68:737–40.

[61] Beland MD, Mayo-Smith WW, Dupuy DE, et al. Diagnostic yield of 58 consecutive imaging-guided biopsies of solid renal masses: should we biopsy all that are indeterminate? AJR Am J Roentgenol 2007;188:792–7.

[62] Maturen KE, Nghiem HV, Caoili EM, et al. Renal mass core biopsy: accuracy and impact on clinical management. AJR Am J Roentgenol 2007; 188:563–70.

[63] Vasudevan A, Davies RJ, Shannon BA, et al. Incidental renal tumours: the frequency of benign lesions and the role of preoperative core biopsy. BJU Int 2006;97:946–9.

[64] Jinzaki M, Tanimoto A, Mukai M, et al. Double-phase helical CT of small renal parenchymal neoplasms: correlation with pathologic findings and tumor angiogenesis. J Comput Assist Tomogr 2000;24:835–42.

[65] Catalano C, Fraioli F, Laghi A, et al. High-resolution multidetector CT in the preoperative evaluation of patients with renal cell carcinoma. AJR Am J Roentgenol 2003;180:1271–7.

[66] Hallscheidt PJ, Bock M, Riedasch G, et al. Diagnostic accuracy of staging renal cell carcinomas using multidetector-row computed tomography and magnetic resonance imaging: a prospective study with histopathologic correlation. J Comput Assist Tomogr 2004;28:333–9.

[67] Hallscheidt P, Pomer S, Roeren T, et al. [Preoperative staging of renal cell carcinoma with caval thrombus: is staging in MR imaging justified? Prospective histopathological correlated study]. Urologe A 2000;39:36–40 [in German].

[68] Boss A, Clasen S, Kuczyk M, et al. Image-guided radiofrequency ablation of renal cell carcinoma. Eur Radiol 2007;17:725–33.

[69] Zlotta AR, Wildschutz T, Raviv G, et al. Radiofrequency interstitial tumor ablation (RITA) is a possible new modality for treatment of renal cancer: ex vivo and in vivo experience. J Endourol 1997; 11:251–8.

[70] McGovern FJ, Wood BJ, Goldberg SN, et al. Radio frequency ablation of renal cell carcinoma via image guided needle electrodes. J Urol 1999; 161:599–600.

[71] Farrell MA, Charboneau WJ, DiMarco DS, et al. Imaging-guided radiofrequency ablation of solid renal tumors. AJR Am J Roentgenol 2003;180: 1509–13.

[72] Roy-Choudhury SH, Cast JE, Cooksey G, et al. Early experience with percutaneous radiofrequency ablation of small solid renal masses. AJR Am J Roentgenol 2003;180:1055–61.

[73] Zagoria RJ, Traver MA, Werle DM, et al. Oncologic efficacy of CT-guided percutaneous radiofrequency ablation of renal cell carcinomas. AJR Am J Roentgenol 2007;189:429–36.

[74] Schiller JD, Gervais DA, Mueller PR. Radiofrequency ablation of renal cell carcinoma. Abdom Imaging 2005;30(4):442–50.

R A D I O L O G I C
C L I N I C S
O F N O R T H A M E R I C A

Radiol Clin N Am 46 (2008) 113–132

ELSEVIER
SAUNDERS

Imaging of Hematuria

Owen J. O'Connor, MD, MRCSI[a,b],
Sean E. McSweeney, MB, MRCSI, FFR(RCSI)[a,b],
Michael M. Maher, MD, FRCSI, FFR(RCSI), FRCR[a,b],*

Hematuria may have a number of causes, the more common being urinary tract calculi, urinary tract infection (UTI), urinary tract neoplasms (including renal cell carcinoma and urothelial tumors), trauma to the urinary tract, and renal parenchymal disease [1–5]. Hematuria is broadly divided into macroscopic and microscopic varieties [6]. Hematuria is described as macroscopic or frank when blood is visible within the urine [7,8]. A diagnosis of microscopic (occult) hematuria requires the detection of three to five red cells per high powered view, or greater than five red blood cells per 0.9 mm^3 of urine [5,9]. The prevalence of microscopic hematuria in asymptomatic individuals is approximately 2.5% [10].

Investigation of hematuria

The investigation of hematuria should begin with a search for bacteriuria or pyuria. If either is present,

a urine culture should be ordered to confirm UTI. In the absence of infection, the next step is to distinguish glomerular and nonglomerular sources of hematuria. If the findings suggest a glomerular source of bleeding, no urologic evaluation is necessary, at least initially, and referral to a nephrologist is indicated [11]. Indeed, there is a body of opinion that suggests that patients aged less than 40 years and presenting with hematuria can be investigated initially by a nephrologist, as the risk of urologic malignancy is low [6]. The results of a recent study by Edwards and colleagues [6] support this policy.

If a glomerular source is excluded in those with risk factors for urologic disease, urologic referral is advised [12]. Risk factors include smoking history, occupational exposure to chemicals or dyes, history of macroscopic hematuria, age greater than 40 years, previous urologic history, symptoms of irritative voiding, UTIs, analgesic abuse, cyclophosphamide intake, and history of pelvic irradiation.

[a] Department of Radiology, Cork University Hospital, Wilton, Cork, Ireland
[b] Mercy University Hospital and University College Cork, Cork, Ireland
* Corresponding author. Department of Radiology, Cork University Hospital, Wilton, Cork, Ireland.
E-mail address: m.maher@ucc.ie (M.M. Maher).

doi:10.1016/j.rcl.2008.01.007

Most experts agree that a complete urologic evaluation should include imaging of the upper urinary tract and cytoscopic examination of the urinary bladder. The role of urine cytology is controversial, as a negative cytology can never completely exclude the presence of a bladder tumor [12]. The goal of imaging is to detect neoplasms, including renal cell carcinoma (RCC), and the less prevalent transitional cell carcinoma (TCC), of the renal pelvis and ureters, urinary tract calculi, renal cystic disease, and obstructive lesions [11].

This article discusses the current status of imaging of patients suspected of having urologic causes of hematuria. The imaging of posttraumatic hematuria, of patients with UTI, and patients with glomerular causes of hematuria is beyond the scope of this review. The role of all modalities, including plain radiography, intravenous urography or excretory urography, retrograde pyelography, ultrasonography, multidetector computed tomography (MDCT), including MDCT urography (MDCTU) and magnetic resonance (MR) urography, is discussed. In recent years, MDCTU has undergone significant development and has been the subject of research and investigation as a new technique for evaluation of patients with urinary tract pathology [13,14]. Evidence is accumulating, which suggests that this technique is now ready to play a pivotal role in imaging of patients presenting with hematuria. This article highlights the current status of MDCTU in imaging of patients with hematuria, and discusses various—often controversial—issues, such as optimal protocol design, accuracy of the technique in imaging of the urothelium, and the significant issue of radiation dose associated with MDCTU.

Common urologic causes of hematuria

Urinary tract calculi

Urolithiasis is associated with idiopathic hypercalciuria, secondary hypercalciuria, and hyperuricosuria [15]. Stones are most commonly composed of calcium oxalate and phosphate (34%), calcium oxalate (33%), calcium phosphate (6%), mixed struvite and apatite (15%), uric acid (8%), and cystine (3%) [3]. Nephrocalcinosis is characterized by the formation of calculi within renal tubules and interstitium, leading to impaired renal function [16]. Nephrocalcinosis is associated with medullary sponge kidney, renal tubular acidosis, and hyperparathyroidism, and may present with hematuria [16,17]. Urinary tract calculi frequently present with ureteric colic caused by obstruction of the urinary collecting system. With regard to the association of urinary tract calculi with development of microscopic hematuria, a recent study by Edwards and colleagues [6] showed a prevalence of urinary

tract calculi of 7.8% in adult patients with microscopic hematuria and 8.8% in patients with macroscopic hematuria.

Malignancy

The most common malignant conditions associated with hematuria in adults are renal cell carcinoma, transitional cell carcinoma, prostate carcinoma, and less commonly, squamous cell carcinoma, which can result from chronic inflammatory conditions [18–20].

RCC is the most common malignant neoplasm of the kidney, representing up to 90% of renal neoplasms and up to 3% of all neoplasms [18,21]. RCC is more common in men than women, has a peak incidence at 60 to 70 years of age, and is associated with smoking, obesity, and antihypertensive therapy [22]. In recent years, the triad of flank pain, hematuria, and a palpable mass is less frequently the mode of presentation for RCC, because over 50% of lesions are identified by cross-sectional imaging, either incidentally or when performed for vague and apparently unrelated symptoms. This is not surprising, as systemic symptoms, such as anorexia and weight loss, are commonly associated with RCC [23].

Urothelial tumors account for 10% of upper urinary tract neoplasms [24]. Although urothelial malignancies are most likely to occur in the bladder, the ureters have been reported to be involved in 2%, and the renal pelvis (extrarenal pelvis in preference to infundibulocalyceal regions) in 5% of cases [19,25]. The multifocal and bilateral nature of TCC makes this a challenging condition for the radiologist [23]. Synchronous tumors occur in up to 2% of renal and 9% of ureteric lesions, with metachronous lesions typically occurring within the bladder in up to 50% of cases with upper ureteric tumors on presentation [26,27]. Therefore, imaging is required for primary diagnosis of TCC but is also very commonly used for detection of synchronous and metachronous lesions [23].

Bladder neoplasia is the fifth most common malignancy in Europe and the fourth most common cancer in the United States [28]. TCC of the bladder occurs more commonly in men than women, is associated with smoking (fourfold greater than in nonsmokers), exposure to chemicals such as benzene and 2-naphtylamine, and structural abnormalities (horseshoe kidney) [29,30]. Squamous cell carcinoma and adenocarcinoma are significantly less common in the bladder than TCC [31]. Greater than 70% of bladder cancers are superficial and 25% invade muscle at the time of diagnosis [32]. Bladder cancer most frequently presents with hematuria but can be associated with more nonspecific signs, such as urinary frequency and urgency, dysuria, and suprapubic pain [23].

Macroscopic and microscopic hematuria and prevalence of urologic disease

Both macroscopic and microscopic hematuria are associated with an increased likelihood of carcinoma. A recent study by Edwards and colleagues [6] reported the results of a prospective analysis of the diagnostic yield from the attendance of over 4,000 patients presenting at a protocol-driven hematuria clinic. This study was unique in its detailed dissection of the largest volume of prospectively recorded, consecutive, contemporary data derived in a diagnostic protocol in the setting of hematuria. Of the patients presenting, 1,950 had microscopic hematuria (48.5%) and 2,073 had macroscopic hematuria (51.5%). Of the 1,950 patients with microcopic hematuria, 153 had urinary tract calculi (7.8%), 19 had RCC (1.0%), 3 had upper tract TCC (0.2%), 73 (3.7%) had bladder TCC, while 87.3% had no cause for hematuria detected. The overall prevalence of malignancy in patients with microscopic hematuria was 4.8%. For the 2,073 patients presenting with macrocopic hematuria, 183 (8.8%) had urinary tract calculi, 41 (2.0%) had RCC, 10 (0.5%) had upper tract TCC, 342 (16.5%) had bladder TCC, while 1,497 (72.2%) had no cause identified for their hematuria. The overall prevalence of malignancy in patients with macroscopic hematuria was 18.9%. There was a higher prevalence of malignant disease detected in males compared with females (14% versus 9%). Of note, no upper tract malignancies were detected in patients less than 30 years, with no upper tract TCC detected in those patients less than 50 years. Most upper tract TCC presented with microscopic hematuria, whereas for those with RCC, the mode of presentation was equivalent between microscopic and macroscopic hematuria [6]. One of the most interesting findings of this study was that the prevalence of urinary tract tumors in this study was four times greater than that of the largest previous series [6,33]. Two possible explanations that were proposed included occult variations in patient population or the increasing usage of CT, where ultrasound (US) and intravenous urography (IVU) findings were equivocal. If the increased prevalence of urinary tract tumors reported in this study is a result of increased use of CT, this finding highlights the importance of the appropriate choice of imaging modality in patients presenting with microscopic hematuria.

Imaging of hematuria

The issue of how best to image patients with clinical history of hematuria has always been controversial and remains controversial, particularly in recent years with the development and continued refinement of MDCTU [13,14].

Conventional radiography

Plain radiography, being a widely available, inexpensive, reproducible examination, familiar both to urologists and nephrologists, has long been the mainstay of screening and quantifying the burden of urolithiasis [34]. However, conventional radiography has only 60% sensitivity for the detection of renal and ureteric calculi [35]. Since Smith's initial report of 97% sensitivity and 96% specificity for detection of urinary tract calculi with nonspiral CT, several reports have confirmed these findings, with sensitivities ranging from 98% to 100% and specificities of 92 to 100% [36–39]. Therefore, for the definitive detection of urinary tract calculi and for the characterization of calcifications in the anatomic distribution of the urinary tract as calculi, plain film radiography does not compare favorably with MDCT. The major factors that prevent the abandonment of plain radiography and its replacement with MDCT are the expense, limited availability of CT in comparison with plain radiography at most centers, and most importantly the significantly increased radiation dose associated with MDCT [40–45]. Protocol development focused on optimizing radiation dose in an era of rapidly improving MDCT technology may result in diagnostic quality "stone protocol" MDCT at substantially lower radiation doses, thus removing one of the most compelling current arguments for continued use of plain radiography.

Plain radiography typically has little value in the detection of TCC; calcifications occur in approximately 7% of TCC lesions [26]. These tumors may obstruct the collecting system and can mimic urinary calculi [46]. Renal cell carcinoma is only rarely detectable on plain radiography when calcified (8%–18%) [23], or when the tumor has reached sufficient size to cause displacement of bowel loops or normal soft tissue structures or fat stripes. Therefore, when tumors of the kidney or urothelium are suspected, plain radiography is of little value, and in patients characterized as "high risk" by the American Urological Association Best Practice criteria, plain radiography should be avoided when further upper urinary tract imaging is required [12,26].

Intravenous urography and excretion urography

The urinary tract was first imaged in 1923 when it was noticed by Osborne and colleagues [47] that 10% sodium iodide injected intravenously, as part of the treatment of syphilis, was excreted in urine. This discovery precipitated efforts to minimize iodine toxicity and led to the first IVU in 1929, using uroselectan, a mono-iodinated compound [48]. Since then, IVU or excretory urography has undergone many changes and refinements in protocol, and the switch from ionic monomers to non-ionic monomers reduced the risk of contrast reactions and also resulted in less osmotic diuresis and higher urinary tract opacification [49]. With the development of ultrasound and MDCT, and more recently MDCTU, there has been a significant reduction in use of IVU. In 1975, an estimated 10,000,000 urograms were performed annually in the United States. By 1995, the number of IVUs had dropped to approximately 600,000 per year [50]. Accompanying this reduced use, there is undoubtedly cause for concern at many centers regarding reduced quality of IVU studies being performed because of decreasing skills of radiographers and technologists in the performance of IVU, quality of equipment in IVU suites, and skills of radiologists in the interpretation of IVU [34].

A full IVU, including nephrotomograms and totaling an average of 11.6 films, has been calculated to yield an effective dose between 5 mSv and 15 mSv [51]. Reducing the number of films acquired directly affects the dose imparted [51,52]. A mean effective dose of 3 mSv has been reported when an average of 9.3 films are acquired [52]. Three-phase MDCTU examinations yield a mean effective dose of 15 mSv plus or minus 9 mSv (155 mAs–200 mAs at 120 kV, 1 mm–2.5 mm collimation), corresponding to a radiation dose 1.5 times higher than conventional urography [51]. Interestingly, the mean skin dose of conventional urography has been reported to be 2.7 times that of MDCTU. This is because of an exponential decrease in radiation dose between entrance and exit sites, unlike MDCTU, which administers a more uniform exposure. Caoili and colleagues [35] found doses to range from 25 mSv to 35 mSv for four phase examinations. Therefore, in many studies MDCTU has been reported to be associated with much higher radiation dose than IVU, and careful assessment of pretest probability of risk of significant pathology should be calculated before MDCTU is performed [53].

In the investigation of suspected urolithiasis, IVU is gradually being replaced by CT. The rationale for this change in practice is CT's unsurpassed diagnostic accuracy for detection of urinary tract calculi [54]. Many reports have suggested that IVU fails to detect urinary tract calculi in 31% to 48% of cases, compared with reported sensitivities of 100% for unenhanced MDCT [50]. IVU requires the use of intravenous contrast, is time consuming (requiring at least 30 minutes to perform), and occasionally requires delayed radiographs taken up to 24 hours after intravenous contrast administration to define the level of obstruction [13,34].

One of the factors that contributed to the continued referral of patients to radiology for IVU was the perception that pelvicaliceal morphology could be better evaluated with IVU than with ultrasound or MDCT. Experience with IVU had defined characteristic imaging features in conditions, such as medullary sponge kidney and papillary necrosis [55]. However, increasing experience with MDCTU and improving capability for three-dimensional reconstruction should allow these characteristic findings to be appreciated at MDCTU [13].

When performed alone, IVU has limited sensitivity in detecting renal masses, when compared with US and MDCT [12]. For masses confirmed and characterized by CT, the sensitivity of IVU is only 21%, 52%, and 85% for masses less than 2 cm, 2 cm to 3 cm, and greater than 3 cm, respectively [56]. In addition, masses detected by IVU inevitably require further imaging for lesion confirmation and characterization by either US, MDCT, or more recently by MR imaging.

Many urologists and some radiologists believe that IVU is still the "gold-standard" examination for evaluating the urothelium [57]. This belief is maintained, in spite of reports in the literature of detection rates for urothelial neoplasms with IVU of only 43% to 64% [35]. In the early stages, these neoplasms are seen on IVU as subtle filling defects or focal mural thickening. TCC tends to appear as fixed, smooth, or irregular, single, or multiple filling defects within the renal collecting systems. On IVU, a papillary lesion may absorb contrast into its interstitium, resulting in a stipple sign [26]. However, although frequently associated with TCC, this radiologic sign is not specific for TCC and can be produced by other pathologic processes, such as fungal lesions and blood clots [58]. An obstructed infundibulum occurs in 26% of cases [26]. This can produce a phantom calyx that may fill either early, late, or not at all because of the presence of a TCC [59].

Traditionally, retrograde pyelogram has been utilized to demonstrate an amputated calyx, which might not be demonstrated by IVU [26]. Sometimes subtle in appearance, a delayed nephrogram because of longstanding pelviureteric junction obstruction and atrophy occurs in 13% of cases [26,55]. Acute hydronephrosis with renal enlargement may also occur. Signs of ureteric TCC include the presence of a nonfunctioning kidney (46%), fixed wall thickening that can be either eccentric or circumferential, filling defects, hydronephrosis (36%) with or without hydroureter, and irregular ureteric narrowing with proximal shouldering (goblet sign) [26,60]. One of the difficulties in the interpretation of IVU or MDCTU is that a filling defect in the renal pelvis or ureter can be caused by a primary neoplasm, metastases (Fig. 1), calculus, blood clot, mycetoma, or vascular impression. Unlike MDCTU, IVU or retrograde ureterography only demonstrate the lumen of the ureter and do not allow direct visualization of extrinsic abnormalities that involve the ureter. The ability to evaluate renal parenchyma in the vicinity of a pelvicaliceal abnormality or the wall or tissues surrounding the ureter can yield important diagnostic information, which can aid in characterization of imaging appearances suspicious for TCC. MDCTU has shown increased sensitivity and specificity for detecting urothelial tumors, compared with retrograde ureterography, an imaging test assumed to be superior to intravenous pyelogram (IVP) in evaluating the collecting system and ureters [53].

Caoili and colleagues [61] reported 89% sensitivity with MDCTU in detection of malignant upper tract urothelial lesions (confirmed by surgery or endoscopic biopsy) in a study population of 18 subjects, and Tsili and colleagues [62] detected seven of seven foci of upper tract malignancy and nine of ten urinary bladder malignancy with MDCTU. Therefore, early evidence in small case series suggests that MDCTU is a promising technique in imaging the urothelium, and further studies in larger groups of subjects are awaited to definitively answer whether MDCTU can replace the role of IVU

in imaging the urothelium. The attractiveness of MDCTU over IVU is its potential to act as a "one-stop" imaging study assessing renal parenchyma and urothelium, whereas IVU will always need to be supplemented with US or CT for evaluation of the renal parenchyma [12].

Retrograde pyelography

Retrograde pyelography is indicated to further characterize filling defects or lesions in the renal pelvis or ureters identified at IVU or MDCTU. In the era before MDCTU was developed, opacification of the urinary tract was frequently very poor with IVU in patients with diminished renal function (even with double dose of iodinated contrast), and retrograde pyelography was then the only available method of visualizing the pelvicaliceal system and ureters. The development of MDCTU has facilitated excellent pelvicaliceal and ureteric visualization because of the modality's ability to easily trace the anatomic course of the ureter. Furthermore, the excellent contrast resolution of MDCT facilitates evaluation of an opacified ureter, even with diminished renal function or in obese patients. MR urography is another option in these patients, and this has the advantage of not requiring the use of iodinated contrast administration [63]. The improved ability to visualize the ureters in

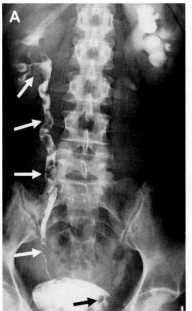

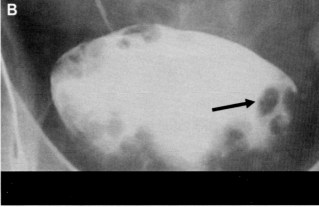

Fig. 1. A 32-year-old female with metastatic melanoma presenting with hematuria. (*A*) Intravenous urogram showing multiple filling defects within the right collecting system, ureter (*white arrows*) and bladder. On the left side, there is a delayed nephrogram with hydronepnosis and hydroureter to the level of the ureterovesical junction. (*B*) The left ureteric obstruction, at this level, was caused by a metastatic deposit in the bladder at the ureterovesical junction (*black arrow*).

obese patients, compared with IVU, is therefore no longer a major indication for retrograde pyelography. Retrograde pyelography is still used to further evaluate filling defects detected on other modalities, such as US, MDCT, IVU, and MR urography (Fig. 2). However, a recent study by Cowan and colleagues [53] was performed to validate quantitatively the use of MDCTU for diagnosing upper urinary tract urothelial tumor. This study compared retrograde ureteropyelography (RUP) and MDCTU in subjects with suspected urothelial tumors [53]. The results of the study showed that RUP shared similar diagnostic sensitivities and specificities for diagnosis of upper urinary tract urothelial tumors, leading to the recommendation that MDCTU should replace US, IVU, and RUP for investigating patients with hematuria, and RUP should be reserved for patients in which findings on MDCTU are equivocal and in whom the increased radiation is not justifiable [53]. Further studies with larger patient numbers are required to determine the remaining role of retrograde pyelography in the era of MDCTU.

Ultrasound

In patients with hematuria, US is a safe method of examining for urolithiasis, particularly in pediatric patients, thus avoiding the use of radiation [64,65]. Ultrasound is inferior to plain radiography and MDCT for the quantification of stone burden [66]. In comparison with MDCT, US has reported sensitivities as low as 24% for the detection of calculi [67]. Conventional radiography in combination with US increases sensitivity for stone detection to 70%, but this level of sensitivity does not approach MDCT for detection of urinary tract calculi [68].

Before the development of CT, renal tumors less than 3 cm represented 5% of renal lesions [69]. With increasing usage of CT, the number of detected renal lesions less than 3 cm has increased to between 9% and 38% of lesions detected [69]. In 1988, a study by Warshauer and colleagues [56] documented the relative insensitivity of intravenous urography and ultrasound for renal masses detected by CT. For lesions less than 3 cm, IVU was much less sensitive than US (50% versus 82%). For lesions less than 2 cm, IVU was also less sensitive than US (13% versus 60%) and these differences in sensitivity were also present for lesions less than 1 cm (13% versus 26%). One of the most worrisome findings in this study was the poor sensitivity of ultrasound in detecting renal masses less than 2 cm [56]. Additional studies have reported data that suggest that CT is more sensitive than US for detection of small renal masses (less than 1.5 cm) [70].

Ultrasound is very useful in determining internal architecture of renal lesions detected on other modalities, such as CT. The findings on US in this setting can be useful in determining the Bosniak grade of cystic lesions, which is vital to guiding future management. Cystic lesions may be effectively examined using US for the presence of wall thickening and internal septations, and so assist in classification [26,56]. Category 1 and 2 lesions are considered benign; lesions with wall and septal thickening or solid areas are categorized as 3 or 4. Ultrasound is very useful in the evaluation of

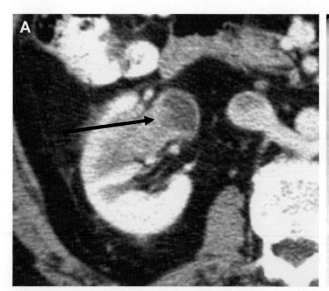
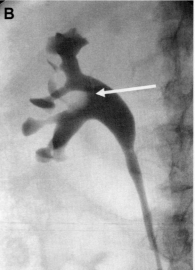

Fig. 2. A 65-year-old male with painless hematuria. (*A*) MDCT performed in nephrographic phase shows filling defect within the right collecting system (*black arrow*). (*B*) Retrograde pyelogram shows corresponding filling defect in right collecting system (*white arrow*) suspicious for TCC. This was confirmed at surgery to be TCC of the collecting system.

hyperattenuating renal lesions detected on MDCT, to determine whether they represent hyperdense cysts (Bosniak 2) or solid lesions.

The combination of US and CT findings has been shown to improve characterization of renal masses, particularly in the case of renal lesions greater than 1 cm, when compared with interpretation based on each modality alone [70]. One potential pitfall when characterizing renal lesions with US is that internal echoes or artifacts can sometimes give such lesions a solid appearance at US. In this scenario, further evaluation by renal mass protocol CT or MR imaging can be helpful and is usually indicated. Renal mass protocol CT comprises two or three-phase CT scans to assess for definitive enhancement or de-enhancement when nephrographic phase images are compared with unenhanced and delayed phase images (5 minutes) [13,71]. Density measurements in Hounsfield units, can be made before and after contrast, and an assessment can be made for unequivocal enhancement, which is indicative of solid mass and neoplasm [71]. The issue of definitive or unequivocal contrast enhancement at MDCT is defined later in this article and is indicative of solid lesion [13,71]. Overall, however, US is not as sensitive as MDCT in identifying or characterizing renal masses when performed using optimized protocol [55].

On sonography, most RCCs are solid but can be appreciated at sonography as hypoechoic, isoechoic, or hyperechoic lesions. The majority of RCCs are isoechoic and smaller numbers of lesions are hypoechoic or echogenic. Two recent articles have suggested that smaller lesions are more likely to be echogenic, with between 61% and 77% of lesions less than 3 cm being found to be echogenic relative to normal kidney [23]. This poses a challenge to the radiologist, as the distinction between small RCC and angiomyolipoma can be difficult.

The main disadvantage in using ultrasound as a screening test in patients with hematuria is its inability to thoroughly evaluate the urothelium for TCC [55]. The use of US alone, therefore, is not considered appropriate for the evaluation of microscopic hematuria in high-risk patients, although the development of endoluminal US may change this [72]. Ultrasound has poor sensitivity in detecting urothelial lesions in the pelvicaliceal system and also in the ureters [55]. One possible solution, suggested by many investigators, is that US should be performed in combination with IVU for patients believed to be at high risk for upper urinary tract neoplasm, as the combination of these two modalities ensures a more comprehensive evaluation of the renal parenchyma and the urothelium for malignant causes of hematuria than is possible with the use of US or IVU alone [6,11].

When TCC of the renal pelvis is detected during US examination, it typically appears as a central soft tissue mass in the echogenic renal sinus, with or without hydronephrosis [23,55]. The presence of fat within the renal sinus frequently makes detection and exclusion of TCC in this region very difficult [55]. The appearance of TCC on sonography can be variable, depending on tumor morphology, location, and size, and small nonobstructing TCCs may be impossible to visualize [23]. Frequently, TCC is slightly hyperechoic relative to surrounding renal parenchyma and may cast a subtle posterior acoustic shadow, though not as impressive as that cast by calculi [55]. When central, these lesions can be impossible to differentiate from blood clots, sloughed papilla, or fungus ball [23]. The use of MDCTU can be helpful in making this distinction and the interpretation of both studies together can be very helpful. Occasionally, high-grade TCC may show areas of mixed echogenicity. Infundibular tumors may cause focal hydonephrosis. Although lesions may extend into the renal cortex and cause focal contour distortion, typically TCC is infiltrative and does not cause renal contour distortion [55].

Ultrasound has a very limited role in the evaluation of ureteric TCC, as the ureters are rarely visualized in their entirety, even if dilated [55]. Most TCCs of the ureter are found in the lower third [23]. On sonography, the most common positive finding is hydronephrosis and hydroureter, and if ureteric TCCs are directly visualized, these tumors are seen as intraluminal soft tissue masses with proximal ureteric distension [55].

Bladder TCCs occur most frequently at the trigone and along the lateral and posterior walls of the bladder. Sonographic detection of bladder TCC is excellent, with sensitivities of greater than or equal to 95% being reported. The typical appearance of bladder TCC is of a focal nonmobile mass or area of urothelial thickening. These findings, however, are not specific to TCC of the bladder and must be confirmed by cystoscopy and biopsy to exclude conditions that can mimic TCC, including cystitis, wall thickening secondary to bladder outlet obstruction, blood clot, postoperative change, prostate carcinoma, lymphoma, neurofibromatosis, and endometriosis [23].

Multidetector CT urography

The advent of multidetector computed tomography has made evaluation of the entire urinary tract possible during a single breath-hold, with reduction in respiratory mis-registration and partial-volume effect [13,71]. In addition, the acquisition of multiple thin overlapping slices of optimally distended and opacified urinary tract potentially provides excellent two-dimensional (2D) and three-dimensional (3D) reformations of the urinary tract [73]. The concept of multidetector CT urography has emerged from the combination of these technical improvements [13,71].

Multidetector CT urography may be defined as the examination of the urinary tract by MDCT in the excretory phase, following intravenous contrast administration. The range of indications for MDCTU has rapidly expanded and MDCTU has replaced intravenous urography at many institutions for almost all indications. There is a large volume of research currently focused on the refinement of MDCTU protocols, and this subject remains controversial and is still a work-in-progress, with a variety of protocols being used at different centers [14]. Protocol design has required input from experts in MDCT technology but has also relied heavily on "old tricks" learned initially by uroradiologists while optimizing IVU for general usage and also for specific indications. Most CT urography protocols performed for the evaluation of hematuria resemble IVU, providing unenhanced images of the urinary tract for detection of calcifications and for subsequent quantification of lesion enhancement following intravenous contrast administration, a nephrographic phase for renal parenchymal evaluation, and delayed imaging in the pyelographic phase for evaluation of the urothelium [14].

Indications for multidetector CT urography

Proponents of MDCTU describe it as a comprehensive test, which can be performed as a substitute "one-stop" imaging test for a number of imaging studies, thereby saving time, hospital visits, and cost, and potentially shortening the duration of diagnostic evaluation for urinary tract pathology [8,14]. It has been established unequivocally that currently, MDCT is the most sensitive and specific test for the diagnosis of urinary tract calculi and also for the detection and characterization of renal masses [14]. The major controversy surrounding MDCTU is the question of whether this modality is as accurate as IVU for the evaluation of the urothelium in patients presenting with hematuria, and this still represents the "final major hurdle" facing MDCTU before it will be universally accepted by radiologists and urologists as a replacement for IVU [9,13,14].

Many studies published in the early years of this decade are showing very encouraging sensitivities for MDCTU in detection of upper tract TCC, with MDCTU outperforming IVU and even retrograde pyelography in many of these studies [53]. Once the use of MDCTU for evaluation of the urothelium in patients with hematuria is validated unequivocally, its potential as a "one-stop" imaging study

will be realized. MDCTU will then simultaneously confirm or exclude urinary tract calculi and also evaluate the renal parenchyma, ureters, and bladder for neoplasms, thus eliminating the need for a combination of imaging tests as occurs currently with ultrasound and IVU [13,36,74]. The second major concern, which may limit universal acceptance of MDCTU, is the radiation dose associated with the procedure [14]. Radiation dose with MDCTU clearly significantly exceeds IVU [14,35]. However, radiation dose can be reduced by adapting scanning parameters for each phase of MDCTU and by reduction of number of phases [51,71].

Imaging protocol

Noncontrast CT

Noncontrast CT scans are obtained initially to locate the kidneys, visualize anomalies, evaluate for urinary tract calcifications including calculi, detect hematoma, and obtain baseline attenuation of renal masses [71]. Unenhanced CT is accepted as the primary imaging investigation to detect urinary tract calculi. The rationale for the use of unenhanced CT scanning for this indication is its unsurpassed accuracy for detection of urinary tract calculi [54]. Since Smith's initial report of 97% sensitivity and 96% specificity for detection of urinary tract calculi with nonspiral CT, several reports have confirmed these findings with sensitivities ranging from 98% to 100% and specificities of 92% to 100% [36–39]. This compares with much poorer sensitivities of 60% reported for plain radiography and other studies reporting that up to 48% of urinary calculi can be missed on IVU [71]. Other advantages of MDCT, when compared with IVU, are the speed at which MDCTU can detect calculi and accurately determine the level of obstruction [54]. In addition, MDCTU enjoys another advantage over IVU, namely the ability to exclude extraurinary pathologies that may mimic calculi in clinical presentation (Fig. 3) [75]. With IVU, determining the level of obstruction can depend on delayed imaging at up to 24 hours following contrast administration. MDCT eliminates the need for the administration of iodinated contrast material (required for IVU) in almost all cases, and thus eliminates associated risks of nephrotoxicity [13].

Unenhanced helical CT reliably detects urinary tract calculi, including those containing uric acid, in the collecting system by direct visualization, because calculi are of sufficient density to be visualized by CT [13]. At most institutions, the "stone protocol" component of MDCTU comprises 3-mm to 5-mm thick images from the upper poles of the kidneys to the symphysis pubis. In general, high attenuation oral contrast should be avoided

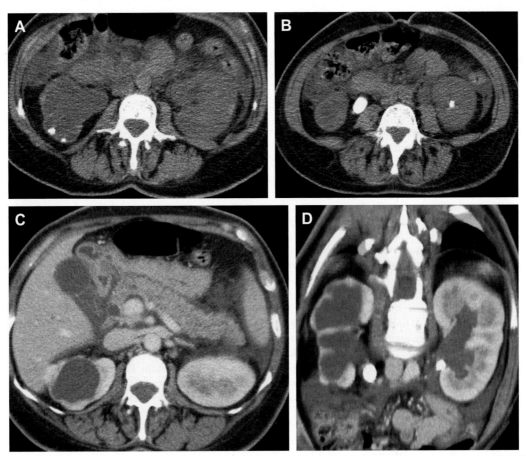

Fig. 3. A 50-year-old female presenting with abdominal pain and hematuria presumed to represent ureteric colic with background primary hyperparathyroidism. (*A, B*) "Stone protocol" CT demonstrates bilateral renal and ureteric calculi with bilateral hydronephrosis. There is severe global cortical loss in the right kidney, suggesting long-standing obstruction. Incidental note was made of fluid in the both anterior pararenal spaces and significant pancreatic swelling and peripancreatic fat "stranding." (*C*) Contrast enhanced MDCT was performed and confirmed acute pancreatitis without acute pancreatic necrosis. Surgical referral was advised and acute pancreatitis was confirmed. (*D*) Coronal oblique multiplanar reformation (MPR) confirms bilateral hydronephrosis with bilateral ureteropelvic stones. The MPR shows preservation of cortex on the left. There is marked cortical loss on the right suggesting long-standing obstruction.

in evaluation of urolithiasis, as dense oral contrast can be problematic and can make detection of ureteral stones more difficult [13,71].

MDCT can detect calculi in unusual positions, such as in calyceal diverticulae, and is more accurate than IVU for detecting presence, size, and location of urinary tract calculi [13]. The two known exceptions are stones of protease inhibitors, such as indinavir sulfate, or mucoid matrix stones, which are of low attenuation similar to soft tissue and frequently, therefore, are not visible directly by CT [76,77].

Following the initial introduction of MDCT for investigation of patients with urinary tract calculi, skeptics argued against MDCT because it lacked IVU's advantage of demonstrating physiologic information, gained from the degree of delayed excretion, which was considered an index of severity of obstruction [14]. However, study of MDCT findings in cases of obstructing urinary tract calculi has demonstrated reliable secondary signs of obstructing calculi [13]. These include hyronephrosis, hydroureter, ipsilateral renal enlargement, perinephric and periureteral fat stranding, perinephric fluid, "ureter rim sign," and ureterovesical edema [13,36]. The combination of hydronephrosis, hydroureter, and perinephric stranding has a positive predictive value of 90% for obstructing urinary tract calculi [13]. Recent studies have proposed that the extent of perinephric edema on unenhanced CT images can be used to accurately predict the degree of acute ureteral obstruction in ureterolithiasis [71,78]. However, at times, nonobstructing ureteral calculi may be indistinguishable from phleboliths on unenhanced MDCT [13,71]. The presence of the "soft-tissue rim sign," namely a circumferential rim of soft tissue attenuation surrounding an abdominal or pelvic calcification, is a reliable indicator that the calcification in question represents a calculus within the ureter [79]. Calculi associated with the "soft-tissue rim sign" have a mean size of 4 mm [80,81]. Conversely, a "comet-tail sign," namely a linear or curvilinear soft-tissue structure extending from an abdominal or pelvic calcification, has been reported as an important indicator that a suspicious calcification represents a phlebolith, whereas its absence suggests indeterminate calcification [71,80–82]. Coll and colleagues [83] have documented the relationship of spontaneous passage of ureteral calculi to stone size and location as revealed by unenhanced helical CT. Spontaneous passage rate for ureteric calculi was 76% for 2-mm to 4-mm calculi, 60% for 5-mm to 7-mm calculi, 48% for 7-mm to 9-mm stones, and less than 25% for stones greater than 9 mm [83].

The administration of iodinated contrast is rarely necessary for investigation of patients with suspected urinary tract calculi. Rarely, intravenous contrast administration followed by imaging in the pyelographic phase may be helpful when uncertainty exists as to whether a calcification is within or external to the urinary tract. Contrast can also be helpful in attempting to distinguish parapelvic cysts from hydronephrosis, a distinction that may also be difficult on ultrasound examination [13].

Contrast-enhanced CT
In the 10-year period since the initial description of CT urography, many innovative modifications have been employed to optimize protocols; currently there is no consensus as to which is the most appropriate protocol [13,14]. Differences exist at every stage of performance of MDCTU including:

Techniques of intravenous contrast injection (ie, a single or "split-bolus" of intravenous contrast),
Number of phases of CT scanning (ie, single, two-phase, three-phase, or four-phase),
The use of imaging with MDCT alone versus hybrid techniques (ie, CT combined with conventional intravenous urography or MDCTU supplemented with CT digital radiography images during the excretory phase),
Patient positioning during MDCTU (ie, prone versus supine versus combination of prone and supine for different imaging phases),
The use of compression techniques,
The additional administration of saline or low-dose diuretics during the procedure, and
The timing of CT scanning for pyelographic phase imaging [13,14,84].

Common protocol variations
The most commonly used MDCTU protocol comprises a three-phase protocol, which typically consists of an initial, unenhanced phase, as described above, a second phase acquired following the administration of nonionic contrast material (100 mL–150 mL of 300 mg/mL iodine concentration at a rate of 2 mL–4 mL per second); this is also known as the nephrographic phase, which is acquired following a delay of 90 to 100 seconds [13,71]. Typically, during this phase, CT scanning (2.5-mm to 5-mm slice thickness) is confined to the kidneys [13,71]. This phase is employed to evaluate the renal parenchyma for masses; the nephrographic phase has been shown to have the highest sensitivity for the detection of renal masses and comparison of nephrographic phase with unenhanced-phase images is required for assessment of unequivocal enhancement within detected renal lesions [13]. This phase is then followed by the pyelographic phase, typically taken 5 to 15 minutes following contrast administration, to evaluate the urothelium from the pelvicaliceal system to the bladder [14]. One of the disadvantages of MDCTU when compared with IVU is encountered in patients with asymmetric excretion. This is most commonly seen in patients with unilateral obstruction, and the lack of sequential imaging with MDCTU can result in suboptimal opacification in the pyelographic phase on the obstructed side [14].

A three-phase protocol is used at most institutions, as it allows a thorough evaluation of the urinary tract for the most common urologic causes of hematuria: that is, urinary tract calculi, renal neoplasms, and urothelial tumors. Caoili and colleagues [85] described a four-phase protocol (two excretory phases at 5 minutes and 7.5 minutes) in an effort to optimize ureteric distension and opacification. Subsequently, Caoli's group has reverted to a three-phase protocol, with the excretory phase being acquired at 12 minutes [84].

The major disadvantages of three and four-phase techniques are high radiation dose, time-consuming technique, and increased number of images for review by the radiologist. In an effort to tackle these important issues, which impact patient safety, Chai and colleagues [86] proposed the use of a split-bolus technique in place of a single intravenous injection to facilitate a two-phase protocol, namely an unenhanced series of images, and a second phase in which nephrographic and pyelographic phases are simultaneously acquired: the "nephropyelographic phase". With this protocol, after the initial noncontrast examination, 30-ccs of nonionic contrast material are infused intravenously and the patient is removed from the CT table. If feasible, the patient is encouraged to walk about for 10 minutes. At 10 to 15 minutes postintravenous contrast administration, the patient is again placed on the CT table in the prone position. A dynamic contrast-enhanced study is then performed following the administration of an additional 100 cc of nonionic contrast material (300 mg/mL, injected at 2 cc per second), following a delay of 100 seconds [13]. Thus, in a single "nephropyelographic phase" acquisition, the renal parenchyma (nephrographic phase) and the collecting system, ureters, and bladder (pyelographic phase) are assessed (Fig. 4) [13].

A variation of this technique, again using a split bolus technique to achieve a two-phase technique, was described by Chow and colleagues [87] in 2007. Potential disadvantages of the "split bolus" approach have been suggested, including a small volume of contrast distending and opacifying the collecting systems and ureters, and the potential for streak artifacts from opacified collecting systems during the nephropyelographic phase, which could impact assessment of renal parenchyma [13,86,88]. The authors have used Chai's technique extensively and have investigated means of optimizing opacification and distension of the ureters and collecting system with various maneuvers, including supine and prone imaging and additional intravenous administration of saline. Subjective and objective evaluations of images acquired with these protocols during these trials suggested satisfactory technique, and the potential

disadvantages suggested above did not significantly impact study quality [89].

Most experts in the field agree, however, that regardless of the protocol being used, there will always be segments of the ureters that are suboptimally opacified and distended [13,71,86]. Concerns exist that suboptimal opacification and distension may lead to failure to detect urothelial lesions within unopacified segments [14]. This is not a universally held view, however, as some investigators believe that urothelial neoplasms in the ureters almost always manifest as filling defects or obstruction [62]. Tsili's study [62] showed a negative predictive value of 100% of the nonopacified ureter for the presence of urothelial lesions, supporting the latter belief.

Techniques to improve urinary tract distension and opacification

Comprehensive evaluation of the urothelium is widely believed to be dependent on adequate opacification and distension of the pelvicaliceal system and ureters [13]. Over the past few years, protocol design and modifications have focused on these factors [14,85]. Many of the techniques developed for IVU have been employed as part of these efforts.

Compression Lower abdominal compression is a well-established technique in intravenous urography for improving distension of the upper urinary tract [90]. Various investigators have shown that it is possible to successfully use compression

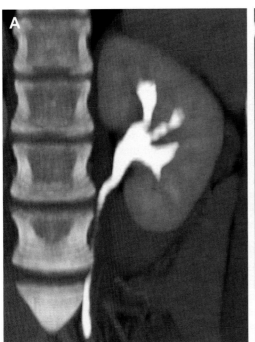
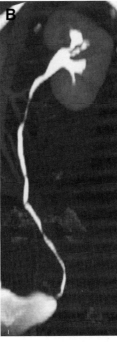

Fig. 4. A 53-year-old patient with microscopic hematuria. Nephropyelographic phase image showing excellent anatomic detail of the left kidney, pelvicaliceal system, and ureter. (*A*) Coronal MPR image showing normal left renal parenchyma, collecting system, and proximal ureter. (*B*) Coronal oblique 3D maximum intensity projection (MIP) image showing entire left urinary tract in a single image.

techniques in CT urography [85,91,92]; however, there is variation in the ways in which compression is incorporated into MDCTU protocols. One method results in excretory phase-CT scanning being split into two ranges, one scan from the diaphragm to the iliac crests with compression, and the second range (postrelease of compression) from the iliac crests to the symphysis [14,73]. Another protocol has been described which acquires two excretory-phase scans, each including the whole urinary tract—one scan with compression and one after release of compression [85]—but this obviously adds an extra phase with an associated increase in radiation dose, examination time, and number of images for review.

External compression is not recommended in patients with abdominal pain or in patients with history of urinary tract obstruction, radical cystectomy, recent surgery, and aortic aneurysm [14]. As to the effectiveness of abdominal compression in improving ureteric distension and opacification, two separate reports by McNicholas and colleagues [91] and Heneghan and colleagues [92] suggested a positive impact on ureteric distension as a result of abdominal compression. In a subsequent study, Caoili and colleagues [85] showed improved opacification scores with compression, compared with controls, for all segments of the urinary tract. However, analysis of the data suggested that the percentage of nonvisualized segments reached up to 25% with compression, which was not significantly different from CT urography without compression. In the authors' practice, we remain unconvinced of the benefits of compression, and feel that the benefits are outweighed by added inconvenience and discomfort for the patient. The authors have not incorporated compression into their MDCTU protocol.

Saline infusion   Another method used to optimize ureteric distension at MDCTU is the addition of intravenous saline infusion to MDCTU protocols. However, theoretically at least, additional intravenous saline administration can result in reduced opacification of the urinary tract because of the dilutional effect of saline on endoluminal iodinated contrast. This would almost certainly be a major disadvantage for IVU [14]. However, with MDCT, because of the technique's superior contrast resolution in comparison with IVU, overzealous opacification of the collecting system can result in streak and beam-hardening artifact, and thus the dilutional effect can counter these effects and potentially, may even be advantageous. Numerous reports have investigated the value of infusion of 100 cc to 250 cc of saline infused either before or immediately after the administration of nonionic contrast [85,93]. The data from these studies show some conflicting findings, with Caoili and colleagues [85] and McTavish and colleagues [93] showing improved opacification following saline infusion; however, the segments in which improved opacification was observed were significantly different in the two studies. However, Sudakoff and colleagues [94] found that saline infusion did not significantly improve ureteric distension or opacification, and suggested that saline infusion may stimulate ureteric peristalsis in certain cases, potentially having a deleterious effect [42,94]. The authors' group also evaluated the impact of the addition of 100 cc of intravenous saline administration on ureteric distension and opacification in the split-bolus two-phase technique, described above, and found no significant effect [89]. The ineffectiveness of saline infusion in this study was attributed by some commentators to the fact that 100 cc was an insufficient volume to positively impact ureteric distension and opacification at MDCTU [14].

Diuretic administration   There are only very few reports of the use of intravenous low-dose diuretic to optimize MDCTU. Proponents of low-dose diuretic administration have recommended that the diuretic be administered 1 minute before contrast administration. The administration of intravenous diuretic has been reported to increase ureteric distension and also to dilute contrast [14]. However, as discussed above, because of MDCT's excellent inherent contrast resolution in comparison to IVU, this is not a particular disadvantage and may be actually be advantageous.

Patient positioning   As previously described, distension and opacification of the mid- and especially the distal ureters is frequently suboptimal with MDCTU. McNicholas and colleagues [91] reported that MDCTU performed with the patient in the prone position achieved higher opacification of the mid- and distal ureters than supine scanning, reaching statistical significance only for the mid ureters. The study reported by McTavish and colleagues [93] suggested that prone positioning did not significantly impact opacification of the distal ureters. In spite of conflicting and equivocal supporting evidence, we routinely employ prone positioning for the nephropyelographic phase of the "split-bolus" two-phase technique.

Image interpretation

As previously discussed, interpretation of MDCTU involves review of a large number of images, which includes thorough comparison of unenhanced and enhanced images for presence of calculi and for assessment of degree of contrast enhancement, which is particularly important for characterization of renal masses. The importance of state-of-the-art, user-friendly workstations cannot be over emphasized. When MDCTU was initially introduced, the importance of 3D reformation was stressed [13,71]. There is no doubt that 3D reconstruction was hugely important in convincing urologists initially of the acceptability of this technique, as 3D images most closely resembled conventional IVU [13,71]. MPR and MIP images are most commonly used and are still very useful in the evaluation of the ureter and in localizing the exact level of the abnormality [13,71]. These reformats are also useful in the characterization of some urinary tract anomalies [13]. One other very important point worth emphasizing is that the liberal usage of wide window settings in the evaluation of delayed pyelographic phase images is very useful to reduce potential for obscuration of intraluminal filling defects by artifacts from excessively dense endoluminal contrast material within the ureters [13,71].

Current status of multidetector CT urography in the evaluation of the patient with hematuria

There is little doubt that MDCTU is an appropriate imaging test for detection and characterization of renal masses. The initial unenhanced CT is obtained to serve as the baseline for measurements of enhancement on nephrographic-phase images [13]. Most renal cell cancers are solid, with attenuation values greater than 20 Hounsfield units (HU) on unenhanced CT [95]. Lesion enhancement greater than 10 HU following intravenous contrast also suggests a solid lesion, and enhancement greater than 20 HU is considered highly suspicious of malignant lesion. Small lesions (less than 3 cm) are usually homogenous in appearance, but large lesions are more likely to be heterogenous secondary to hemorrhage or necrosis (Fig. 5). Confirmation of unequivocal enhancement within a small lesion can be impacted by volume averaging, and can also be difficult in larger lesions that have necrotic components [96].

The location of the tumor may be helpful in the diagnosis and characterization of solid renal masses. Renal cell carcinoma is frequently located at the periphery or near the corticomedullary junction of the kidney, as it originates in the renal cortex, whereas transitional cell carcinoma and other tumors arise from the urothelium, and thus extend into the kidney from the renal pelvicaliceal system and occur more centrally in the kidney, usually displacing surrounding renal sinus fat [97,98].

Transitional cell carcinoma is the most common malignant neoplasm of the urothelium. TCC is 30 to 50 times more common in the bladder than in the ureters and renal pelvis, and is often multifocal

[99]. Many urologists believe that intravenous urography is still the "gold-standard" for evaluating the urothelium [57]; however, as previously described, intravenous urography has been reported in the literature to have detection rates for urothelial neoplasms of only 43% to 64% [35]. In the early stages, these neoplasms are seen as subtle filling defects or focal mural thickening. A filling defect in the renal pelvis or ureter can be caused by a neoplasm, calculus, blood clot, mycetoma, or vascular impression. MDCTU has shown increased sensitivity and specificity for detecting urothelial tumor compared with retrograde ureterography, an imaging test assumed to be superior to IVP in evaluating the collecting system and ureters [53]. One of the main advantages of MDCTU over intravenous urography includes identification and characterization of intrinsic and extrinsic causes of ureteric obstruction, including mural thickening with short segment malignant strictures, retroperitoneal masses or lymphadenopathy, retroperitoneal fibrosis, benign ureteric strictures, and iatrogenic causes [13,71].

Results of recent studies evaluating the ability of MDCTU to detect urothelial tumors in the renal collecting system or in the ureter have reported very promising data [13]. One recent study suggests that MDCTU can detect urothelial tumors in up to 89% of cases [61]. Another recent study suggests that MDCTU is an accurate means for detection and staging of upper urinary tract TCC, with accuracy for prediction of peritumoral invasion with positive and negative predictive values of 88.8% and 87.5%, respectively [100].

Cowan and colleagues [53] validated quantitatively the use of MDCTU for diagnosing upper urinary tract urothelial tumor with sensitivity of 0.97, a specificity of 0.93, and a positive predictive value (PPV) of 0.79 and negative predictive value (NPV) of 0.99. In the same study, retrograde ureteropyelography (RUP) had a sensitivity of 0.97, specificity of 0.93, and PPV and NPV of 0.79 and 0.99 [53]. Therefore, MDCTU and RUP shared similar diagnostic sensitivities and specificities for diagnosis of upper urinary tract urothelial tumors, leading to the recommendation that MDCTU should replace ultrasound, IVU, and RUP for investigating patients with hematuria, and RUP should be reserved for patients in which MDCTU is equivocal and in whom the increased radiation is justifiable [53].

Cystoscopy remains the "gold-standard" for evaluation of the urinary bladder, but MDCTU is playing an increasing role in the detection of bladder urothelial neoplasms [101]. As with other urinary tract tumors, assessment for bladder tumor requires contrast-enhanced examination with optimum distention and opacification of the urinary bladder for detection of abnormalities. In cases where

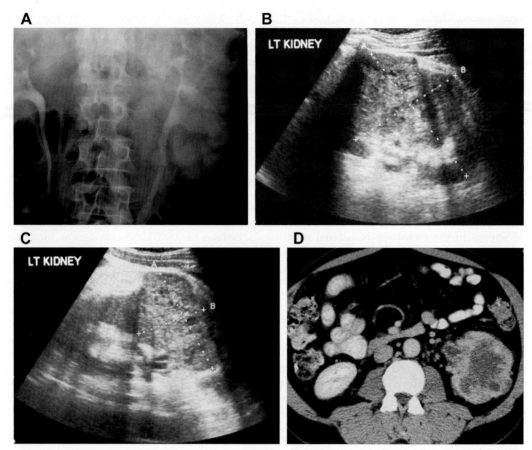

Fig. 5. A 70-year-old male with frank hematuria. (*A*) Image from IVU showing distorted and extrinsically compressed pelvicaliceal and collecting system at mid- and lower pole of left kidney. (*B, C*) Two images from subsequent renal ultrasound confirm large mass in left kidney at mid- and lower pole. (*D*) MDCT performed in nephrographic phase shows large enhancing mass with low attenuation centrally, suggesting necrosis. Imaging features suggested RCC, and this was confirmed at surgery.

bladder neoplasm is suspected, the two-phase MDCTU technique can be modified with additional further delayed images (5–10 minutes after the nephropyelographic phase) to obtain a more densely opacified and more distended bladder [13]. As with urothelial tumors of the upper urinary tract, bladder neoplasms present as a filling defect, a focal mass, or an area of focal bladder wall thickening (Fig. 6) [101]. Turney and colleagues [102] reported a sensitivity of 93% and a specificity of 99% for MDCTU in detecting bladder neoplasms, when compared with cystoscopy. Dillman and colleagues [101] alluded to data from an unpublished study, which found a sensitivity for MDCTU for diagnosis of bladder tumors of 89% when compared with cystoscopy. A very interesting finding of this study was that four lesions located in the bladder base and dome were detected at MDCTU but were not seen at cystoscopy [101]. Overall the sensitivity of MDCTU for detecting bladder TCC is comparable

or very slightly inferior than published sensitivities for ultrasound [23].

With regard to protocol design, noncontrast images of the bladder are again important to detect focal areas of mural calcification that can be associated with transitional cell or squamous cell carcinoma of the bladder [13,35]. Other causes of bladder wall calcification include cyclophosphamide-induced cystitis, prior radiation treatment, schistosomiasis, or tuberculosis [71]. Mural filling defects or focal bladder wall thickening, when associated with increased bladder wall enhancement, also suggests carcinoma, whereas diffuse or uniform bladder wall thickening is usually secondary to cystitis or changes related to obstructive uropathy [35].

MR urography

One of the main advantages of MDCTU in the evaluation of patients with hematuria, is its ability to

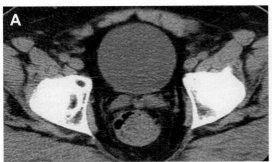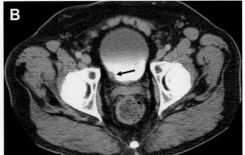

Fig. 6. A 75-year-old man with frank hematuria. (*A*) Noncontrast MDCT of pelvis shows normal bladder, seminal vesicles and rectum. (*B*) Further MDCT of bladder was performed 5 to 10 minutes after contrast administration, showing a partially contrast-filled bladder with filling defect on right posterolateral wall of bladder (*black arrow*) and subtle contiguous thickening of the posterior bladder wall suspicious for TCC. This was confirmed at cystoscopy with biopsy.

display and thoroughly evaluate the entire urinary tract, including renal parenchyma, pelvicaliceal systems, ureters, and the bladder using a single imaging study [13,71]. The alternative imaging studies, including ultrasonography and IVU, alone, do not offer equivalent coverage [13]. Magnetic resonance urography (MRU) is the only alternative study that can thoroughly image all the anatomic components of the urinary tract in a single test [103]. MRU, using either heavily T2-weighted pulse sequences or gadolinium-enhanced T1-weighted sequences, has shown potential to detect, localize, and characterize collecting system abnormalities [104]. Because neither iodinated intravenous contrast nor ionizing radiation is used, it is safe in patients with contraindication to iodinated contrast media, in young patients, and without contrast in the pregnant patient [57]. However, with MRU, contrast is usually required to evaluate the renal parenchyma, especially for renal masses [105].

The main disadvantages of MR urography, which have hindered its widespread usage in the evaluation of the urinary tract, is its limited ability to reliably detect urinary tract calcifications and air, limited availability in comparison to MDCTU, and limited experience in interpretation of images [103]. With regard to detection of calcifications and urinary calculi, these appear as filling defects or signal voids on both heavily T2-weighted and gadolinium enhanced T1-weighted MR urograms (Fig. 7). Recent analysis have reported sensitivities of 94% to 100% in diagnosing ureteral stones in the setting of obstruction [57]. However, the visualisation of nonobstructing stones is much more difficult. Another disadvantage of MRU is that spatial resolution of MRU does not approach MDCTU or IVU, and therefore, subtle ureteric or collecting system abnormalities could potentially be missed [57].

How should we image the patient with hematuria in 2008?

In 2001, the American Urological Association published the Best Practice Policy on evaluation of adults with microscopic hematuria [12]. It would appear that there was no representation from the subspeciality of uroradiology among the coauthors of this report. With regard to imaging, this report concluded that no data was available at that time, which demonstrated the impact of IVU, US, CT or MR imaging on the treatment of patients with asymptomatic microscopic hematuria, and that evidence based guidelines could not be formulated. The potential role of CT was considered, without discussion of specific protocols such as MDCTU, although the use of imaging with MDCT and hybrid techniques—that is, additional scout or kidneys-ureter-bladder (KUB) following contrast enhanced MDCT—was suggested. However, this report suggested that IVU or CT should be considered the methods of choice and that CT protocols should be modified to diagnostic goals [12]. These guidelines did suggest that for low-risk patients, KUB and US could replace IVU and CT. It is interesting that radiation dose was not a major consideration in the choice of imaging modality at the time.

Since then, MDCTU has undergone major refinement in an attempt to optimize ureteric distension and opacification to guarantee optimal evaluation of the urothelium [13,14,71]. A systematic review in Health Technology Assessment, published in 2006, evaluated diagnostic tests and algorithms used for the investigation of hematuria [5]. In spite of a growing literature supporting the use of MDCTU for evaluation of the urothelium, this systematic review concluded that the evidence from studies included in the review was insufficient to draw any firm conclusions regarding the

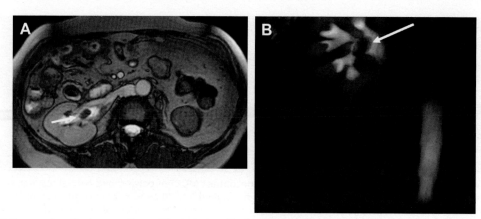

Fig. 7. Pregnant patient presenting with ureteric colic. (*A, B*) MR image with MR urogram shows presence of large signal void, suggesting filling defect (*white arrow*) in right renal pelvis consistent with a large stone.

diagnostic accuracy of imaging studies in determining the cause of hematuria. This conclusion reflects the low level of current evidence, mostly derived from case-series, and the lack of randomized controlled studies or meta-analyses. The lack of studies with higher levels of evidence is a common problem in the radiology literature. Economic analyses suggested that US followed by CT in the case of a negative result with persisting hematuria may be cost-effective [5]. Once again, CT was considered without discussion of specific protocols such as MDCTU or "stone protocol CT."

The low-level evidence currently available suggests that MDCTU offers excellent sensitivity (89%–100%) and specificity for detection of both pelvicaliceal and ureteric TCC [62]. In addition, it is already widely accepted that MDCTU outperforms all other modalities, including US, IVU, and plain radiography in the evaluation of the renal parenchyma for masses and the urinary tract for calculi [13,56,71]. These data have prompted leading investigators in the field to conclude that MDCTU is more sensitive and specific than IVU and retrograde pyelography for detection of urothelial tumors, and that MDCTU should be considered as a first-line investigation in patients with hematuria when risk of disease outweighs risk of radiation exposure (ie, patients at high-risk of urologic cancer) [53]. Clearly therefore, in the opinion of many radiologists, additional radiation exposure with MDCTU in selected patients has replaced concern regarding sensitivity in detecting urothelial tumors, as the major obstacle to replacing IVU with MDCTU in the investigation of patients with hematuria.

The identification of patients in which risk of disease outweighs risk of radiation exposure associated with MDCTU will require further study. The study of over 4,000 patients with hematuria, reported by Edwards and colleagues [6],

highlighted a few important findings which may aid in answering this question. No upper tract neoplasms were detected in patients less than 30 years. RCCs but no upper tract TCCs were diagnosed in patients less than 50 years. Upper tract TCC was twice as common in men as women. Most upper tract TCCs presented with macroscopic hematuria, whereas with RCC the mode of presentation was equivalent. The investigators reported a prevalence of upper tract neoplasms, four times that of previous series, and suggested that the increased prevalence could be the result of increased usage of CT when US and IVU findings were equivocal [6]. The investigators concluded that US should be used in most patients presenting with hematuria, and that IVU should be confined to those patients with macroscopic hematuria or in men aged greater than 50 years. With the currently available evidence, in patients less than 50 years upper tract imaging could be performed by US to detect RCC and could be supplemented by ultralow-dose CT, as described by Kluner and colleagues [43], to detect urinary tract calculi. An advantage of US in this setting is that the bladder could be evaluated for TCC but could be supplemented by cystoscopy when deemed necessary. In patients, greater than 50 years-old, especially if male, MDCTU should be considered because of its potential as a "one-stop" imaging test, simultaneously evaluating the urinary tract for calculi, the renal parenchyma and urothelium for neoplasms, and could be supplemented by cystocopy. Efforts at optimising MDCTU protocols need to be focused on radiation-dose optimization. These questions currently are controversial and require careful discussion by a multdisciplinary group from the fields of urology, uroradiology, nephrology, family practice, pathology/cytology public health, and health technology assessment.

Summary

MDCTU protocols have undergone refinement in an effort to optimize contrast opacification and distension to allow thorough evaluation of the urothelium in patients with hematuria. Recent studies have shown encouraging data validating MDCTU usage in the evaluation of the urothelium for neoplasms, including transitional cell carcinoma. Future efforts in continued refinement of these protocols must focus on radiation dose optimization and radiation dose reduction, which will likely be achieved by reducing the number of imaging phases and by using emerging technologies for radiation dose reduction at MDCT. If efforts to optimize radiation dose results in acceptable radiation dosages comparable with IVU, MDCTU would appear to be the most likely imaging study to offer comprehensive "one-stop" imaging of the urinary tract.

References

[1] Bjerklund Johansen TE. Diagnosis and imaging in urinary tract infections. Curr Opin Urol 2002;12(1):39–43.

[2] Belldegrun A, Dekernion JB. Renal tumours. In: Walsh PC, Retik AB, Vaughan DE, et al, editors. Campbell's urology. Philadelphia: WB Saunders Co; 1998. p. 2283–326.

[3] Dunnick RN, Sandler CM, Newhouse JH, et al, editors. Nephrocalcinosis and nephrolithiasis. In: Textbook of uroradiology 3rd edition. Philadelphia: Lippincott Williams & Wilkins; 2001. p. 178–194.

[4] McInnis MD, Newhouse IJ, von Duvillard SP, et al. The effect of exercise intensity on hematuria in healthy male runners. Eur J Appl Physiol Occup Physiol 1998;79(1):99–105.

[5] Rodgers M, Nixon J, Hempel S, et al. Diagnostic tests and algorithms used in the investigation of haematuria: systematic reviews and economic evaluation. Health Technol Assess 2006;10(18):1–276.

[6] Edwards TJ, Dickinson AJ, Natale S, et al. A prospective analysis of the diagnostic yield resulting from the attendance of 4020 patients at a protocol-driven haematuria clinic. BJU Int 2006;97(2):301–5 [discussion: 305].

[7] Malmstrom PU. Time to abandon testing for microscopic haematuria in adults? BMJ 2003; 326(7393):813–5.

[8] Kawashima A, Vrtiska TJ, LeRoy AJ, et al. CT urography. Radiographics 2004;24:S35–54.

[9] Feldstein MS, Hentz JG, Gillett MD, et al. Should the upper tracts be imaged for microscopic hematuria? BJU Int 2005;96:612–7.

[10] Ritchie CD, Bevan EA, Collier SJ. Importance of occult hematuria found at screening. Br Med J (Clin Res Ed) 1986;292:681–3.

[11] Cohen RA, Brown RS. Clinical practice. Microscopic hematuria. N Engl J Med 2003;348(23): 2330–8.

[12] Grossfeld GD, Litwin MS, Wolf JS, et al. Evaluation of asymptomatic microscopic hematuria in adults: the American Urological Association best practice policy—part I: definition, detection, prevalence, and etiology. Urology 2001; 57(4):599–603.

[13] Maher MM, Kalra MK, Rizzo S, et al. Multidetector CT urography in imaging of the urinary tract in patients with hematuria. Korean J Radiol 2004;5:1–10.

[14] Nolte-Ernsting C, Cowan N. Understanding multislice CT urography techniques: many roads lead to Rome. Eur Radiol 2006;16:2670–86.

[15] Dyer RB, Chen MY, Zagoria RJ. Abnormal calcifications in the urinary tract. Radiographics 1998;18:1405–24.

[16] Pressler CA, Heinzinger J, Jeck N, et al. Late-onset manifestation of antenatal Bartter syndrome as a result of residual function of the mutated renal Na+-K+-2Cl- co-transporter. J Am Soc Nephrol 2006;17(8):2136–42.

[17] Joffe SA, Servaes S, Okon S, et al. Multi-detector row CT urography in the evaluation of hematuria. Radiographics 2003;23(6):1441–55.

[18] Pantuck AJ, Zisman A, Belldegrun AS. The changing natural history of renal cell carcinoma. J Urol 2001;166:1611–23.

[19] Hardeman SW, Perry A, Soloway MS. Transitional cell carcinoma of the prostate following intravesical therapy for transitional cell carcinoma of the bladder. J Urol 1988;140(2): 289–92.

[20] Winalski CS, Lipman JC, Tumeh SS. Ureteral neoplasms. Radiographics 1990;10(2):271–83.

[21] European network of cancer registries. Eurocim version 4.0. European incidence database V2.3, 730, ICD Dictionary. Lyon (France): IARC; 2001.

[22] Bergstrom A, Hsieh CC, Lindblad P, et al. Obesity and renal cell cancer—a quantitative review. Br J Cancer 2001;85(7):984–90.

[23] Thurston W, Wilson SR. The urinary tract. In: Rumack CM, Wilson SR, Charbonneau JW, editors. Diagnostic ultrasound. 3rd edition. St. Louis (MI): Elsevier Mosby; 2005. p. 321–93.

[24] Kirkali Z, Tuzel E. Transitional cell carcinoma of the ureter and renal pelvis. Crit Rev Oncol Hematol 2003;47(2):155–69.

[25] American Cancer Society. Cancer facts and figures. Atlanta (GA): American Cancer Society; 2004. p. 3329–4251.

[26] Wong-You-Cheong JJ, Wagner BJ, Davis CJ Jr. Transitional cell carcinoma of the urinary tract: radiologic-pathologic correlation. Radiographics 1998;18(1):123–42.

[27] Keeley FX, Kulp DA, Bibbo M, et al. Diagnostic accuracy of ureteroscopic biopsy in upper tract transitional cell carcinoma. J Urol 1997; 157(1):33–7.

[28] Jensen OM, Esteve J, Moller J, et al. Cancer in the European community and its member states. Eur J Cancer 1990;26:1167–77.

[29] Clavel J, Cordier S, Boccon-Gibod L, et al. Tobacco and bladder cancer in males. Increased risk for inhalers and smokers of black tobacco. Int J Cancer 1984;44:605–10.

[30] Lee TY, Ko SF, Wan YL, et al. Unusual imaging presentations in renal transitional cell carcinoma. Acta Radiol 1997;38(6):1015–9.

[31] Dawson C, Whitfield H. ABC of urology. Urological malignancy–II: urothelial tumours. BMJ 1996;312(7038):1090–4.

[32] Stein JP. Choosing earlier therapy for muscle-invasive bladder cancer. Rev Urol 2005;7(3):190–2.

[33] Khadra MH, Pickard RS, Charlton M, et al. A prospective analysis of 1,930 patients with hematuria to evaluate current diagnostic practice. J Urol 2000;163:524–7.

[34] Vrtiska TJ. Quantitation of stone burden: imaging advances. Urol Res 2005;33:398–402.

[35] Caoili EM, Cohan RH, Korbkin M, et al. Urinary tract abnormalities: initial experience with multi-detector row CT urography. Radiology 2002;222:353–60.

[36] Fielding JR, Silverman SG, Rubin GD. Helical CT of the urinary tract. AJR Am J Roentgenol 1999;172:1199–206.

[37] Smith RC, Verga M, McCarthy S, et al. Diagnosis of acute flank pain: value of unenhanced helical CT. AJR Am J Roentgenol 1996;166:97–101.

[38] Chen MY, Zagoria RJ. Can noncontrast helical computed tomography replace intravenous urography for evaluation of patients with acute urinary tract colic? J Emerg Med 1999;17: 299–303.

[39] Niall O, Russell J, MacGregor R, et al. A comparison of noncontrast computerized tomography with excretory urography in the assessment of acute flank pain. J Urol 1999;161:534–7.

[40] Eikefjord EN, Thorsen F, Rorvik J. Comparison of effective radiation doses in patients undergoing unenhanced MDCT and excretory urography for acute flank pain. AJR Am J Roentgenol 2007;188(4):934–9.

[41] Wall BF, Hart D. Revised radiation doses for typical X-ray examinations. Report on a recent review of doses to patients from medical X-ray examinations in the UK by NRPB. Br J Radiol 1997;70:437–9.

[42] Kalra MK, Maher MM, D'Souza RV, et al. Detection of urinary tract stones at low-radiation-dose CT with z-axis automatic tube current modulation: phantom and clinical studies. Radiology 2005;235(2):523–9.

[43] Kluner C, Hein PA, Gralla O, et al. Does ultra-low-dose CT with a radiation dose equivalent to that of KUB suffice to detect renal and ureteral calculi? J Comput Assist Tomogr 2006;30(1):44–50.

[44] Katz SI, Saluja S, Brink JA, et al. Radiation dose associated with unenhanced CT for suspected renal colic: impact of repetitive studies. AJR Am J Roentgenol 2006;186(4):1120–4.

[45] Jackman SV, Potter SR, Regan F, et al. Plain abdominal x-ray versus computerized tomography screening: sensitivity for stone localization after nonenhanced spiral computerized tomography. J Urol 2000;164(2):308–10.

[46] Daniel WW Jr, Hartman GW, Witten DM, et al. Calcified renal masses. A review of ten years experience at the Mayo Clinic. Radiology 1972;103(3):503–8.

[47] Osborne ED, Sutherland CG, Scholl AJ. Roentgenography of the urinary tract during excretion of sodium iodide. JAMA 1923;80: 368–73.

[48] Swick M. Darstellung der niere und harnwege in roentgenbild durch intravenose einbringung neuen kontraststoffes: des uroselectans. Klin Wochenschr 1929;8:2087–9.

[49] Stacul F. Reducing the risks for contrast-induced nephropathy. Cardiovasc Intervent Radiol 2005;28(Suppl 2):S12–8.

[50] Dalla Palma L. What is left of IV urography? Eur Radiol 2001;11(6):931–9.

[51] Nawfel RD, Judy PF, Schleipman AR, et al. Patient radiation dose at CT urography and conventional urography. Radiology 2004;232: 126–32.

[52] Yakoumakis E, Tsalafoutas IA, Nikolaou D, et al. Differences in effective dose estimation from dose are product and entrance surface dose measurements in intravenous urography. Br J Radiol 2001;74:727–34.

[53] Cowan NC, Turney BW, Taylor NJ, et al. Multi-detector computed tomography urography for diagnosing upper urinary tract urothelial tumour. BJU Int 2007;99:1363–70.

[54] Kenney PJ. CT evaluation of urinary lithiasis. Radiol Clin North Am 2003;41(5):979–99.

[55] Browne RF, Meehan CP, Colville J, et al. Transitional cell carcinoma of the upper urinary tract: spectrum of imaging findings. Radiographics 2005;25(6):1609–27.

[56] Warshauer DM, McCarthy SM, Street L, et al. Detection of renal masses: sensitivities and specificities of excretory urography/linear tomography, US, and CT. Radiology 1988; 169(2):363–5.

[57] Kawashima A, Glockner JF, King BF Jr. CT urography and MR urography. Radiol Clin North Am 2003;41:945–61.

[58] McLean GK, Pollack HM, Banner MP. The "stipple sign"—urographic harbinger of transitional cell neoplasms. Urol Radiol 1979;1(2): 77–9.

[59] Brennan RE, Pollack HM. Nonvisualized ("phantom") renal calyx: causes and radiological approach to diagnosis. Urol Radiol 1979; 1(1):17–23.

[60] Batata MA, Whitmore WF, Hilaris BS, et al. Primary carcinoma of the ureter: a prognostic study. Cancer 1975;35(6):1626–32.

[61] Caoili EM, Cohan RH, Inampudi P, et al. MDCT urography of upper tract urothelial neoplasms. AJR Am J Roentgenol 2005;184(6):1873–81.

[62] Tsili AC, Efremidis SC, Kalef-Ezra J, et al. Multi-detector row CT urography on a 16-row CT scanner in the evaluation of urothelial tumors. Eur Radiol 2007;17(4):1046–54.

[63] Nolte-Ernsting C, Adam GB, Gunther RW. MR urography: examination techniques and clinical applications. Eur Radiol 2001;11:355–72.

[64] Greenfield SP, Williot P, Kaplan D. Gross hematuria in children: a ten-year review. Urology 2007;69(1):166–9.

[65] Hulton SA. Evaluation of urinary tract calculi in children. Arch Dis Child 2001;84(4):320–3.

[66] Vrtiska TJ, Hattery RR, King BF, et al. Role of ultrasound in medical management of patients with renal stone disease. Urol Radiol 1992;14:131–8.

[67] Fowler KA, Lochen JA, Duchesne JH, et al. US for detecting renal calculi with nonenhanced CT as a reference standard. Radiology 2002;222:109–14.

[68] Levine JA, Neitlich J, Verga M, et al. Ureteral calculi in patients with flank pain: correlation of plain film radiography with unenhanced helical CT. Radiology 1997;204:27–31.

[69] Curry NS. Small renal masses (lesions smaller than 3 cm): imaging evaluation and management. AJR Am J Roentgenol 1995;164(2):355–62.

[70] Jamis-Dow CA, Choyke PL, Jennings SB, et al. Small (< or = 3-cm) renal masses: detection with CT versus US and pathologic correlation. Radiology 1996;198(3):785–8.

[71] Kalra MK, Maher MM, Sahani DV, et al. Current status of multidetector computed tomography urography in imaging of the urinary tract. Curr Probl Diagn Radiol 2002;31:210–21.

[72] Hadas-Halpern I, Farkas A, Patlas M, et al. Sonographic diagnosis of ureteral tumors. J Ultrasound Med 1999;18(9):639–45.

[73] Chow LC, Sommer FG. Multidetector CT urography with abdominal compression and three-dimensional reconstruction. AJR Am J Roentgenol 2001;177:849–55.

[74] Urban BA. The small renal mass: what is the role of multiphasic helical scanning? Radiology 1997;202:22–3.

[75] Sourtzis S, Thibeau JF, Damry N, et al. Radiologic investigation of renal colic: unenhanced helical CT compared with excretory urography. Am J Roentgenol 1999;172:1491–4.

[76] Blake SP, McNicholas MM, Raptopoulos V. Nonopaque crystal deposition causing ureteric obstruction in patients with HIV undergoing indinavir therapy. AJR Am J Roentgenol 1998;171:717–20.

[77] Pfister SA, Deckart A, Laschke S, et al. Unenhanced helical computed tomography vs intravenous urography in patients with acute flank pain: accuracy and economic impact in a randomized prospective trial. Eur Radiol 2003;13:2513–20.

[78] Boridy IC, Kawashima A, Goldman SM, et al. Acute ureterolithiasis: nonenhanced helical CT findings of perinephric edema for prediction of degree of ureteral obstruction. Radiology 1999;213:663–7.

[79] Kawashima A, Sandler CM, Boridy IC, et al. Unenhanced helical CT of ureterolithiasis: value of the tissue rim sign. AJR Am J Roentgenol 1997;168:997–1000.

[80] Bell TV, Fenlon HM, Davison BD, et al. Unenhanced helical CT criteria to differentiate distal ureteral calculi from pelvic phleboliths. Radiology 1998;207:363–7.

[81] Guest AR, Cohan RH, Korobkin M, et al. Assessment of the clinical utility of the rim and comet-tail signs in differentiating ureteral stones from phleboliths. AJR Am J Roentgenol 2001;177:1285–91.

[82] Boridy IC, Nikolaidis P, Kawashima A, et al. Ureterolithiasis: value of the tail sign in differentiating phleboliths from ureteral calculi at nonenhanced helical CT. Radiology 1999;211:619–21.

[83] Coll DM, Varanelli MJ, Smith RC. Relationship of spontaneous passage of ureteral calculi to stone size and location as revealed by unenhanced helical CT. AJR Am J Roentgenol 2002;178:101–3.

[84] Noroozian M, Cohan RH, Caoili EM, et al. Multislice CT urography: state of the art. Br J Radiol 2004;77:S74–86.

[85] Caoili EM, Inampudi P, Cohan RH, et al. Optimization of multi-detector row CT urography: effect of compression, saline administration, and prolongation of acquisition delay. Radiology 2005;235:116–23.

[86] Chai RY, Jhaveri K, Saini S, et al. Comprehensive evaluation of patients with haematuria on multi-slice computed tomography scanner: protocol design and preliminary observations. Australas Radiol 2001;45:536–8.

[87] Chow LC, Kwan SW, Olcott EW, et al. Split-bolus MDCT urography with synchronous nephrographic and excretory phase enhancement. AJR Am J Roentgenol 2007;189:314–22.

[88] Sussman SK, Illescas FF, Opalacz JP, et al. Renal streak artifact during contrast enhanced CT comparison of high versus low osmolality contrast media. Abdom Imaging 1993;18:180–5.

[89] Maher MM, Jhaveri K, Lucey J, et al. Does the administration of saline flush during CT urography (CTU) improve ureteric distension and opacification? Radiology 2001;221:500.

[90] Hattery RR, Williamson B Jr, Hartman GW, et al. Intravenous urographic technique. Radiology 1988;167:593–9.

[91] McNicholas MMJ, Raptopoulos VD, Schwartz RK, et al. Excretory phase CT urography for opacification of the urinary collecting system. AJR Am J Roentgenol 1998;170:1261–7.

[92] Heneghan JP, Kim DH, Leder RA, et al. Compression CT urography: a comparison with IVU in the opacification of the collecting system and ureters. J Comput Assist Tomogr 2001;25:343–7.

[93] McTavish JD, Jinaki M, Zou KH, et al. Multidetector CT urography: analysis of techniques and comparison with IVU. Radiology 2000;225:783–90.

[94] Sudakoff GS, Dunn DP, Hellman RS, et al. Opacification of the genitourinary collecting system during MDCT urography with enhanced CT digital radiography: nonsaline versus saline bolus. AJR Am J Roentgenol 2006;186:122–9.

[95] Sheth S, Scatarige JC, Horton KM, et al. Current concepts in the diagnosis and management of renal cell carcinoma: role of multidetector CT and three-dimensional CT. Radiographics 2001;21:S237–54.

[96] Silverman SG, Lee BY, Seltzer SE, et al. Small (< or = 3 cm) renal masses: correlation of spiral CT features and pathologic findings. AJR Am J Roentgenol 1994;163:597–605.

[97] Kocakoc E, Bhatt S, Dogra VS. Renal multidector row CT. Radiol Clin North Am 2005;43:1021–47.

[98] Zagoria RJ. Imaging of small renal masses: a medical success story. AJR Am J Roentgenol 2000;175:945–55.

[99] Anderson EM, Murphy R, Rennie AT, et al. Multidetector computed tomography urography (MDCTU) for diagnosing urothelial malignancy. Clin Radiol 2007;62:324–32.

[100] Fritz GA, Schoellnast H, Deutschmann HA, et al. Multiphasic multidetector-row CT (MDCT) in detection and staging of transitional cell carcinomas of the upper urinary tract. Eur Radiol 2006;16:1244–52.

[101] Dillman JR, Caoili EM, Cohan RH. Multidetector CT urography: a one-stop renal and urinary tract imaging modality. Abdom Imaging 2007;32:519–29.

[102] Turney BW, Willatt JM, Nixon D, et al. Computed tomography urography for diagnosing bladder cancer. BJU Int 2006;98(2):345–8.

[103] Maher MM, Prassad TA, Fitzpatrick JM, et al. Spinal dysraphism at MR Urography: Initial experience. Radiology 2000;216:237–41.

[104] Nolte-Ernsting C, Staatz G, Wildberger J, et al. MR urography and CT urography: principles, examination techniques, applications. Rofo 2003;175:211–22.

[105] Silverman SG, Mortele KJ, Tuncali K, et al. Hyperattenuating renal masses: etiologies, pathogenesis, and imaging evaluation. Radiographics 2007;27(4):1131–43.

ELSEVIER
SAUNDERS

RADIOLOGIC
CLINICS
OF NORTH AMERICA

Radiol Clin N Am 46 (2008) 133–147

Imaging the Male Reproductive Tract: Current Trends and Future Directions

Jurgen J. Fütterer, MD, PhD[a],*, Stijn W.T.P.J. Heijmink, MD[a],
J. Roan Spermon, MD, PhD[b]

The male reproductive system encompasses several organs: the testes, ejaculatory ducts, seminal vesicles, prostate, and penis. The function of this system is to accomplish reproduction. The testes are outside the abdominal cavity within the scrotal sac. This keeps the testes from the regular body temperature and at an optimal temperature for sperm. The main role of the prostate gland is to produce and secrete an alkaline fluid. This helps to energize and protect the sperm during intercourse in the vaginal canal.

The male reproductive tract is a common site for diseases. Diagnostic imaging modalities, such as ultrasound (US), CT, MR imaging, and positron emission tomography (PET), increasingly are used to evaluate these diseases. The purpose of this review is to provide an overview of the use of imaging techniques in the male reproductive tract and to discuss current trends and future directions in prostate and testicular imaging. This review focuses on the prostate and scrotum.

Prostate

The prostate changes and commonly enlarges with age. The most frequent types of prostate disease are prostatitis, benign prostatic hyperplasia (BPH), and prostate cancer. Prostate cancer is the most common malignancy in men [1]. Imaging of the prostate remains a challenging endeavor.

Anatomy of the prostate

The prostate is a small gland and situated directly caudal to the bladder. The prostate gland envelops the prostatic urethra and the ejaculatory ducts. The seminal vesicles are paired grapelike pouches filled with fluid that are located caudolateral to the corresponding deferent duct, between the bladder and rectum. The prostate is divided into apex and base (directed upward to the inferior border of the bladder). On the basis of its embryologic origins, the prostate is divided anatomically into

[a] Department of Radiology (667), University Medical Centre Nijmegen, Geert Grooteplein 10, 6500 HB Nijmegen, The Netherlands
[b] Department of Urology, University Medical Centre Nijmegen, Geert Grooteplein 10, 6500 HB Nijmegen, The Netherlands
* Corresponding author.
E-mail address: j.futterer@rad.umcn.nl (J.J. Fütterer).

0033-8389/08/$ – see front matter © 2008 Elsevier Inc. All rights reserved.   doi:10.1016/j.rcl.2008.01.005
radiologic.theclinics.com

three zones that are located eccentrically around the urethra (the transition zone is the innermost zone, the central zone, and the outermost peripheral zone). In elderly patients, the transition and central zones cannot be distinguished radiologically because of compression of the central zone by BPH in the transition zone and, therefore, is called the central gland. Seventy percent of all prostate cancers are located in the peripheral zone, whereas 20% emerge from the transition zone, and 10% in the central zone. The neurovascular bundle courses bilaterally along the posterolateral aspect of the prostate and is a preferential pathway of tumor spread.

Acute and chronic prostatitis

The prevalence of prostatitis (ie, chronic pelvic pain syndrome) ranges between 2% and 16% [2]. Prostatitis may occur in any age and in any race; however, its incidence increases with age. Perineal pain and increased frequency of (painful) voiding are the most common symptoms in chronic prostatitis, whereas in acute prostatitis, symptoms of acute onset of fever and severely tender prostate are in the foreground. Prostatitis detection on imaging remains a challenge.

Transrectal US (TRUS) is the imaging modality used most widely for the prostate. Advantages of TRUS over other modalities, such as MR imaging, are wider availability, lower costs, potential use by urologists and radiologists, and ability to visualize the prostate in real time.

In acute bacterial prostatitis, an area of hypoechogenicity can be found with high Doppler signal within and around the lesion [3]. TRUS can be used for treatment follow-up by determining whether or not the prostate volume decreases [4,5]. In some institutions, however, TRUS is used only to exclude prostate abscesses. Increased enhancement of contrast agent can be found in patients who have chronic prostatitis.

With MR imaging, it is difficult to differentiate chronic prostatitis from prostate cancer, because both diseases demonstrate low signal intensity areas on T2-weighted imaging [6]. In a study by Shukla-Dave and colleagues [6], MR imaging demonstrated indeterminate focal low signal intensity that was not nodular (ie, contour deforming) in 58% of chronic prostatitis lesions (greater than 6 mm in largest diameter). Spectroscopic MR imaging demonstrated metabolic abnormalities from the regions of chronic prostatitis, which appeared similar to those for cancer [6].

Benign prostate hyperplasia

Worldwide, 30 million men have symptoms related to BPH. According to the National Institutes of Health, BPH affects more than 50% of men over age 60 and as many as 90% of men over age 70.

BPH is a benign disease of the prostate gland and consists of nodular hypertrophy of the fibrous, muscular, and glandular tissue within the periurethral and transition zones. The exact pathophysiology of BPH in the prostate is unknown. It probably is associated with hormonal changes that occur as men age.

Many symptoms caused by BPH are related to mechanical obstruction or compression of the urethra and altered bladder function. Obstructive symptoms of BPH include incomplete bladder emptying, dribbling after voiding, difficulty initiating, and stopping urination and a weak urinary stream.

Generally, TRUS of the prostate is performed to assess prostate volume and to rule out prostate cancer. TRUS is not indicated, however, for the evaluation of BPH. CT and MR imaging have no specific place in the evaluation of BPH. Nevertheless, MR imaging has high tissue contrast, which can be used to determine the histologic type (glandular and fibromuscular BPH) [7].

Prostate cancer

Despite a slight decrease in incidence in 2007, prostate cancer is is the most common malignancy among Western men. In 2007, an estimated 218,890 new cases of prostate cancer will have been diagnosed in the United States, and an estimated 27,050 men will have died of the disease [1]. In an early stage, prostate cancer commonly is asymptomatic because most cancers are located in the peripheral zone (70%). Few patients have symptoms of the lower urinary tract resulting from obstruction. Prostate cancer patients rarely present with symptoms of hematuria or hematospermia. Prostate cancer is suspected in patients who have elevated prostate-specific antigen (PSA) values. The urologic work-up in patients who have elevated PSA consists of a digital rectal examination, TRUS, and TRUS-guided biopsies. Imaging plays a central role in the detection, localization, staging, and local recurrence detection in patients who have prostate cancer.

Gray-scale imaging

Gray-scale imaging has improved by application of higher frequency probes (up to 10 MHz) and new signal reception techniques, such as tissue harmonic imaging. Currently, the main use of gray-scale TRUS is the guidance of prostate biopsies. Before the advent of PSA as a biomarker for prostate cancer, the pathognomonic feature of prostate cancer on TRUS was the hypoechoic nodule (Fig. 1) [8]. Currently, because of PSA screening, prostate cancer is detected at an earlier stage, and many cancer foci are isoechoic compared with healthy prostate tissue [9].

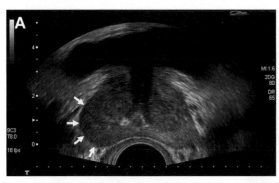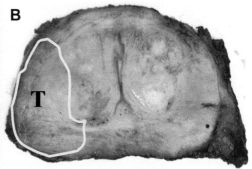

Fig. 1. (*A*) Gray-scale US imaging (Aplio, Toshiba Medical Systems, Tokyo, Japan) of the prostate in a 65-year-old man who had a PSA level of 19.02 ng/mL revealed a marked hypoechoic area in the right peripheral zone (*arrows*). (*B*) Step-section histopathology after radical prostatectomy confirmed the presence of a large Gleason score 3 + 4 cancer focus (yellow outline, T).

Therefore, a systematic biopsy strategy of all six sextants of the prostate (apex, midgland, and base on both sides) was adopted and has been the standard of reference in prostate cancer detection for nearly 2 decades [10]. Many institutions have performed variants of this systematic sextant biopsy protocol. These variants included extension of the number of randomly taken biopsies in general or, based on prostate volume, addition of more laterally directed biopsies and augmentation with bilateral central gland biopsies [11–14].

Because of the use of PSA in screening, a stage migration has occurred toward less aggressive, organ-confined cancer [15]. Staging sensitivities in two more recent studies using gray-scale TRUS varied between 30% and 50% with specificities between 77% and 96% [16,17]. In particular, use of 3-D TRUS aided in the assessment of extracapsular extension and seminal vesicle invasion [18–20].

Urologists and radiation oncologists most often use a combination of the PSA level and digital rectal examination to detect local disease recurrence [21,22]. Consensus exists that biopsy proof of recurrence is necessary only in case local salvage therapeutic treatment is planned. Thus, the application of TRUS in local recurrence detection is limited. Most local recurrences appear hypoechoic compared with healthy tissue near the anastomosis and isoechoic compared with the vesicourethral anastomosis and bladder neck [23–26]. It is difficult to distinguish fibrotic tissue from recurrent cancer on gray-scale TRUS, leading to a high number of false-positive findings [27]. In the large studies encompassing at least 100 patients, sensitivities ranged from 66% to 92% with relatively low specificities (29%–66%) [28–31].

Doppler transrectal ultrasound

Prostate cancer has an increased microvessel density compared with healthy prostatic tissue. Thereby,

Doppler visualization of streaming blood within the vasculature may aid in detecting and localizing prostate cancer (Fig. 2). Cancer grade correlates positively with the degree of Doppler signal [32]. Few studies have compared Doppler-guided and systematic biopsies directly [33], with one study achieving a detection rate of 40% [34].

Increased capsular flow on color Doppler imaging has been applied as a criterion for capsular penetration [35]. The only study that performed Doppler TRUS staging revealed a sensitivity of 59% for detecting locally advanced disease [36].

In detecting local recurrence, addition of Doppler imaging to gray-scale TRUS in two studies with small patient populations was deemed to aid in differentiating fibrotic tissue from recurrence [37,38].

Contrast-enhanced transrectal ultrasound

Visualization of the cancer microvasculature can be improved by means of contrast-enhanced TRUS. New contrast agents constantly are being developed; however, not all are approved by the Food and Drug Administration or European Medicines Agency and few have been applied in prostate research. The contrast agents used most widely in prostate cancer are Levovist (Schering, Berlin, Germany) and SonoVue (Bracco, Milan, Italy). Contrary to MR imaging contrast agents, these 2- to 8-μm molecules remain within the vasculature, thus acting as blood pool agents.

Several signal reception techniques may be applied to contrast agents. First, conventional Doppler imaging may be enhanced by the microbubbles. This increases the signal received from the vasculature. The main disadvantage, however, is the high-energy output by the US probe (ie, the high mechanical index [MI]). Although microbubbles remain intact at low MIs, at higher MIs, the bubbles expand beyond their limits and are destroyed. Therefore, scanning with high MIs decreases the half-life of the contrast agent considerably.

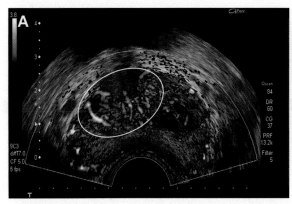 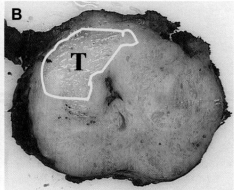

Fig. 2. (*A*) Power Doppler US imaging (Aplio, Toshiba Medical Systems, Tokyo, Japan) of the prostate in a 56-year-old man who had a PSA level of 4.8 ng/mL. In the ventral part of the right central gland a large area with substantial Doppler signal compared with the rest of the prostate was observed. (*B*) Step-section histopathology after radical prostatectomy revealed a large ventral cancer focus (yellow outline, T) with Gleason score 3 + 4.

Second, new low-MI signal reception techniques can be applied that use the nonlinear resonance properties of microbubbles. Microbubbles that are within the plane of the US probe do not have an equal rate of expansion and contraction and send back various frequencies to the probe, among which frequencies that are multiples (ie, harmonics) of the frequency transmitted by the probe. Because prostatic tissue transmits these frequencies to a much lesser extent, the contrast-to-noise ratio for visualization of the vasculature using contrast-harmonic imaging is high (Fig. 3).

Third, the MI can be changed intermittently. By briefly applying a high MI, the microbubbles within the plane of the probe are destroyed. Switching back to low MI, the first pass inflow of microbubbles can be mimicked, allowing repeated analysis of contrast agent inflow at different levels of the prostate. This technique is referred to as intermittent scanning [39].

A recent systematic review compared systematic biopsy and contrast-enhanced targeted biopsy of patients at risk for prostate cancer [33]. Contrast-enhanced targeted biopsy consistently detected an equal number of patients with half the number of biopsies necessary, thereby significantly improving the positive per core percentage (10.4%–32.6%) compared with systematic biopsy (5.7%–17.9%). Thus, a biopsy core taken with contrast-enhanced targeted biopsy was 2.6 times more likely to detect cancer than a systematic biopsy core [35]. Furthermore, the cancer foci detected by contrast-enhanced targeted biopsies had significantly higher mean Gleason scores [34]. A biopsy core taken with contrast-enhanced targeted biopsy was 2.6 times more likely to detect cancer than a systematic biopsy core [35]. Sensitivities of contrast-enhanced targeted biopsy varied widely between 40% and 94% with specificities between 40% and 88%

[36]. Disadvantages of applying US contrast agents are the longer duration and higher degree of invasiveness of the examination. Adverse events, however, usually are minor [39].

Sonoelastography
US signal transmission and backscattering also can be used to analyze small displacements of tissue during application of compression [40]. From these data, the compression characteristics of the prostatic tissue can be determined. Malignant tissue was deemed to have lower compression ability [41] and cancer foci would be more solid. Few studies of prostate sonoelastography are published.

In a population of 404 men at risk for prostate cancer, the detection rate by means of real-time sonoelastography targeted biopsies was 37.4% [42]. If the patients detected solely by means of systematic biopsy were included in the analysis, sonoelastography detected 84.1% of all positive cases. A preliminary study comparing sonoelastography imaging with systematic biopsy revealed a sensitivity and specificity of localizing prostate cancer of 86% and 72%, respectively [43]. In a study by Pallwein and colleagues [44–50], direct comparison of systematic biopsy with sonoelastography targeted biopsy revealed similar results as contrast-enhanced targeted biopsy: a similar per-patient detection rate (25%–30%), with a significantly higher per core detection rate (12.7%) compared with systematic biopsy (5.6%). A current difficulty of prostate sonoelastography is standardization of the applied pressure to provide optimal and reproducible compression.

MR imaging
MR imaging is a powerful method to image the prostate with high spatial resolution, which provides excellent soft tissue contrast. MR imaging is

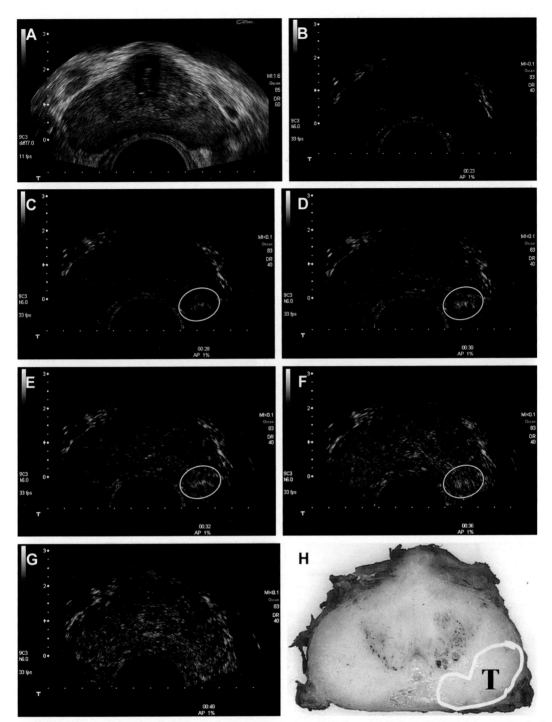

Fig. 3. US imaging (Aplio, Toshiba Medical Systems, Tokyo, Japan) of the prostate in a 55-year-old man who had a PSA level of 6.89 ng/mL. (*A*) No abnormality was observed on gray-scale imaging. (*B–H*) Contrast harmonic imaging was performed. (*B*) Until 28 seconds after bolus injection of 2.4 mLSonoVue (Bracco, Milan, Italy), no enhancement was observed in the prostate. (*C*) Subsequently, within 1 second, the first contrast enhancement is seen in the left peripheral zone (*yellow circle*). (*D–F*) The area (*circle*) continues to enhance more compared with the rest of the prostate until 40 seconds post injection. (*G*) At 40 seconds post injection, the entire prostate shows a homogeneous enhancement. (*H*) Step-section histopathology after radical prostatectomy confirmed the cancer focus (*yellow outline,* T) with Gleason score 3 + 5.

a valuable tool for the detection of cancer, evaluation of extraprostatic extension of cancer, and treatment follow-up. MR imaging of the prostate preferably is performed with an endorectal coil. On T2-weighted images the zonal anatomy is distinguished clearly. The peripheral zone displays hyperintense signal compared with the central gland because the latter is more inhomogeneous because of BPH. Prostate cancer commonly occurs as an area of low signal intensity within the brighter peripheral zone (Fig. 4A).

Currently, MR imaging plays no role as a screening imaging modality in patients who have suspected prostate cancer. It is costly and time-consuming and only a few scientific papers have been published regarding this topic. In patients who have at least two negative TRUS-guided biopsy sessions, however, MR imaging plays an important role [51].

T2-weighted MR imaging obtained accuracies of 67% to 72%, with relatively high sensitivities (54% to 81%), whereas specificities were low (46%–61%) in localizing tumors [52–55]. Functional MR imaging techniques, such as dynamic contrast-enhanced MR imaging (DCE-MRI) (Fig. 4B–C) and proton magnetic resonance spectroscopic imaging (MRSI), can be applied to increase the localization performance. Two meta-analyses on local staging by MR imaging found combined maximum sensitivities and specificities of 71% to 74%, whereas sensitivity was 62% to 69% at a specificity of 80% [56,57]. Significant improvement of anatomic details, extracapsular extension accuracy, and specificity is found when a combined endorectal-pelvic phased-array coil setup is used [58]. The use of an endorectal coil and high field strength (ie, 3 tesla [T]) resulted in

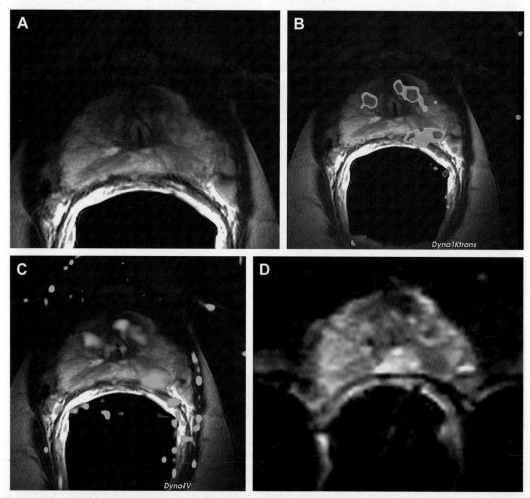

Fig. 4. A 63-year-old man who had stage T2a prostate cancer. (*A*) Axial T2-weighted image demonstrates two low signal intensity areas in the left and right peripheral zone. DCE-MRI demonstrated (*B*) increased permeability and (*C*) extravascular extracellular space in the left peripheral zone. Whole-mount section histopathology confirmed this cancer nodule. (*D*) ADC map at the same level as in Fig. 4A shows a significant reduction in ADC in the left peripheral zone. This area corresponded with prostate cancer.

high staging accuracies (82%–94%) with moderate to substantial observer agreement [59]. In addition, minimal capsular invasion could be detected.

Proton magnetic resonance spectroscopic imaging

MRSI is a unique method that can provide information on prostate metabolism. It provides quantitative data based on the citrate, choline, and creatine levels and the ratios between these metabolites. A high level of citrate is an important marker in healthy or benign prostate tissue. Thus, reduced levels of citrate and increased levels of choline are indicative of prostate cancer. A commonly used marker for cancer tissue is the ratio of (choline + creatine)/citrate. This allows MRSI to be used for tumor localization, characterization, treatment planning, and therapy evaluation. The addition of MRSI to T2-weighted MR imaging increases the localization specificity up to 91% [53]. At 1.5 T, an endorectal coil is needed for signal reception to acquire high-quality spectra. At 3 T, however, a matrix of external radiofrequency surface coils alone was able to discriminate cancer from healthy tissue accurately in the peripheral zone and central gland [60].

Dynamic contrast-enhanced MR imaging

DCE-MRI is a method that provides information about microvascularity and angiogenesis. This technique is reported an effective tool in visualizing the pharmacokinetics of gadolinium uptake in the prostate. Therefore, data reflecting tissue perfusion, microvessel permeability, and extracellular leakage space can be obtained. Insights into these physiologic processes are obtained qualitatively by characterizing kinetic enhancement curves or quantitatively by applying complex compartmental modeling techniques. The addition of DCE-MRI to T2-weighted imaging resulted in an increase of the area under the receiver-operating curve for localizing prostate cancer from 0.68 with anatomic T2-weighted MR imaging to 0.91 [61].

Diffusion-weighted imaging

Diffusion is a 3-D physical process important in many physiologic functions. Only recently, this technique has been introduced in prostate MR imaging as a result of the introduction of ultrafast echo-planar sequences. The apparent diffusion coefficient (ADC) values of malignant tissue are lower than in the healthy peripheral zone (Fig. 4D), probably caused by increased cellular density [62]. The ADC value of the healthy peripheral zone also is higher compared with the central gland because of the higher water content in the prostatic luminal space. The clinical value of diffusion-weighted imaging in prostate cancer has to be investigated.

Positron emission tomography

The usefulness of PET scanning with 18-fluorine–labeled deoxyglucose (FDG) in detecting prostate cancer is compromised by the low uptake of FDG by prostate cancer cells and significant overlap with marker uptake by BPH, fibrosis, and inflammation. Generally, FDG-PET is not recommended for evaluation of the prostate.

Carbon-11–labeled choline (^{11}C-choline) accumulates in prostatic cells and has an advantage, unlike FDG, in that it is not excreted via the urinary tract and thereby does interfere with the visualization of the prostate. Furthermore, the prostate is the only organ in the pelvis to accumulate ^{11}C-choline. Drawbacks are the high costs of ^{11}C-choline and its short, 20-minute half-life.

Scrotum

The spectrum of conditions that affect the scrotum and its contents ranges from incidental findings to pathologic events that require expeditious diagnosis and immediate treatment. Imaging of the scrotum is indicated when there is an acute situation with pain and swelling. The most important aim of imaging in these patients is to rule in or out testicular torsion and testicular cancer that warrant emergency surgery.

Anatomy of the scrotum

Around the time of birth, and occasionally during the first weeks thereafter, the testes descend into the scrotum through the processus vaginalis. The normal adult testis is ovoid, measuring 3 to 5 cm in length and 2 to 3 cm in transverse and anteroposterior dimensions, and is enveloped by the tunica vaginalis [63]. The tunica vaginalis is a potential space formed from the processus vaginalis, an outpouching of the fetal peritoneum that descends into the scrotum along with the testis. An inner visceral layer covers the testis and epididymis whereas an outer parietal layer lines the scrotum. These two layers join at the posterolateral aspect of the testis, where they attach to the scrotal wall. The testis also is fixed at its lower pole by the gubernaculum. The median raphe separates the scrotum into two compartments.

The tunica albuginea, a dense fibrous capsule deep to the tunica vaginalis, extends multiple septa toward the mediastinum testis, which divide the testis into lobules that contain the seminiferous tubules. Spermatogenesis occurs within these tubules. The seminiferous tubules converge toward the mediastinum testis to form the rete testis. The spermatozoa then move into the head of the epididymis and subsequently pass toward the tail of the epididymis where they reach the vas deferens.

The vas deferens and the testicular artery, deferential artery, cremasteric artery, and pampiniform plexus form the spermatic cord.

The main blood flow to the testicle is via the testicular artery, with branches off the deferential and cremasteric arteries. These arteries course through the spermatic cord, along with their corresponding veins and nerves. The testicular artery pierces the tunica albuginea, forming capsular arteries that, in turn, form recurrent rami that course centrifugally toward the mediastinum. The venous drainage of the testes is provided by the pampiniform plexus.

Cryptorchidism

Failure of the intra-abdominal testes to descend into the scrotal sac is known as cryptorchidism. Identification and localization of an undescended testis is of great importance, because abdominal testes are prone to malignant degeneration. The cryptorchid testis may be located at any point along the route of descent. An undescended testis is present at birth in 3.5% of newborns and this decreases to below 1% at 1 year of age. The incidence of an undescended testis is higher in premature infants [64].

US is useful only for identifying undescended testes in the inguinal canal (the most frequent location: 70% of cases) or the prescrotal region just beyond the external inguinal ring (20%) and should be the initial imaging procedure. The cryptorchid testis usually is smaller and iso- or hypoechoic relative to the normally descended testis. US has an accuracy of approximately 90% in localizing an undescended testis [65]. When it is situated in the abdomen, shadowing from bowel gas might impair its visualization at US. The testis can be identified if the mediastinum testis is seen; however, this infrequently is the case.

In cases where US cannot locate the testis, MR imaging should be performed. MR imaging, however, which is highly accurate (94%) for locating testes in the inguinal canal, also may fail to detect abdominally located testes [66]. In these cases, laparoscopic surgery may be required.

Acute scrotal pain

Causes of acute scrotal pain are multiple; the most common causes are testicular torsion, torsion of the testicular appendages, and epididymo-orchitis.

Testicular torsion

Testicular torsion, or twisting of the spermatic cord, causes first venous and eventually arterial flow obstruction. The extent of testicular ischemia depends on the degree of twisting (180°–720°) and the duration of the torsion. Testicular salvage is more likely in patients treated within 4 to 6 hours after the onset of torsion. On the basis of the surgical findings, two types of testicular torsion are recognized: extravaginal and intravaginal. Extravaginal torsion is seen mainly in newborns. The testis usually is necrotic at birth and the hemiscrotum is swollen and discolored. Intravaginal torsion can occur at any age but is more common in adolescents.

Differentiation between testicular torsion and epididymo-orchitis is a clinical challenge, because scrotal pain, swelling, and redness or tenderness are clinical symptoms common to these two entities.

The US appearance of testicular torsion depends on the duration and degree of the torsion. Grayscale images are nonspecific for testicular torsion and often appear normal if the torsion has just occurred [67]. Testicular swelling and decreased echogenicity are the findings encountered most commonly 4 to 6 hours after the onset of torsion (Fig. 5). After 24 hours (a late or missed torsion), the echogenicity of the testis becomes heterogeneous, a sign of loss of viability. Normal testicular echogenicity and lack of scrotal wall thickening or hydrocele are strong predictors of testicular viability. The epididymal head may be enlarged because of involvement of the deferential artery [68]. Unilateral diminished or absent flow is the most accurate sign of testicular torsion. Power Doppler US is more sensitive (97%) than color Doppler US (88%) for the detection of intratesticular blood flow, a result of increased depiction of intratesticular vessels [69,70]. Alternatively, the presence of blood flow does not exclude torsion [68] because some false-negative results with color Doppler US are attributed to an incomplete torsion of the spermatic cord when the systolic value still is recorded whereas the diastolic one is absent or reduced. Other false-negative results are secondary to the reactive hyperemia of the tunica vaginalis, which is interpreted wrongly as blood flow into the capsular arteries.

A preliminary study on DCE-MRI in the diagnosis of testicular torsion reported a sensitivity and specificity of 93% and 100%, respectively. It cannot be used, however, to rule out intermittent torsion [71].

Torsion of the testicular appendages

Appendage torsion makes up 5% of cases of the acute scrotum. Patients present with a focally tender area in the upper pole of the testis. The classic finding at physical examination is a small firm nodule that is palpable on the superior aspect of the testis and exhibits bluish discoloration through the overlying skin; this is called the "blue dot" sign.

The diagnosis of torsion of the appendages of the testis and epididymis is not difficult using scrotal MR imaging, in contrast with that using color Doppler US, which is difficult without the blue dot sign on physical examination and absence of

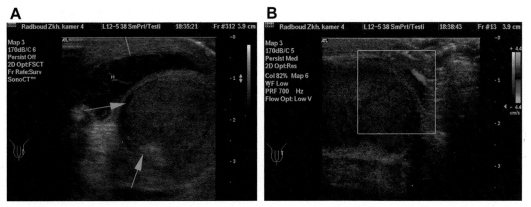

Fig. 5. A 12-year-old boy who had testicular torsion of the left testicle. He presented with worsening left testicular pain. (*A*) Testicular US illustrates an enlarged left testicle, which is diffusely hypoechoic (*arrows*). The scrotal wall is thickened. (*B*) Doppler examination demonstrates an avascular left testicle and increased flow in the scrotal wall. These findings are consistent with a left testicular torsion.

a hydrocele [72,73]. The characteristic MR imaging finding is an oval paratesticular nodule, which shows hyperintensity on T2-weighted images and no contrast enhancement around the upper pole of the epididymis or in the vicinity of the testis [71,72].

Epididymo-orchitis

Epididymo-orchitis mainly is of infectious origin. It usually originates in the bladder or prostate gland, subsequently spreads through the vas deferens and the lymphatics of the spermatic cord to the epididymis, and eventually reaches the testis, causing epididymo-orchitis. Isolated orchitis is rare. In adolescents, epididymo-orchitis mostly is caused by sexually transmitted disease (chlamydia).

US findings demonstrate the hypoechoic appearance of the enlarged epididymis. In cases of testicular inflammation, the testis can appear hypoechoic,

enlarged, and inhomogeneous. In most cases, scrotal wall thickening and reactive hydrocele are present [74]. These gray-scale findings are nonspecific, however. Increased blood flow to the testis and epididymis aids to establish the diagnosis of inflammation correctly (diagnostic accuracy: 98%) (Fig. 6) [75–77].

On MR imaging, the characteristic findings of epididymitis are epididymal enlargement, intermediate T1 and T2 signal intensity, and postcontrast enhancement of the epididymis and the spermatic cord [77,78].

Scrotal masses

The initial determination of a scrotal mass as intratesticular or extratesticular is important, because malignant extratesticular masses are rare, whereas intratesticular solid masses must be considered malignant until proved otherwise.

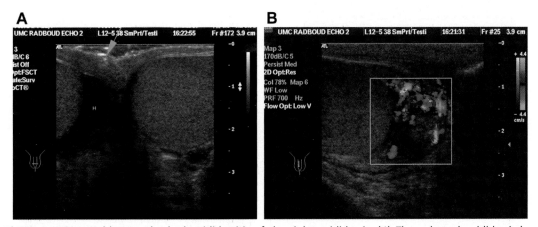

Fig. 6. An 18-year-old man who had epididymitis of the right epididymis. (*A*) The enlarged epididymis has a hypoechoic appearance. A reactive hydrocele and scrotal wall thickening is visible. (*B*) Color Doppler examination demonstrates increased flow.

Extratesticular

Inguinal hernias Inguinal hernias occur because of protrusion of peritoneal contents, usually omentum or bowel, through a patent processus vaginalis. Fluid- or air-filled loops of bowel with peristalsis in the scrotal sac are diagnostic of an inguinal hernia. Hyperechoic areas on US likely represent omentum [79]. The overall accuracy in finding a hernia of any kind by clinical evaluation, US, and MR imaging is 80% to 92%, 89% to 94%, and 95%, respectively [80–82].

Hydrocele Normally, a small amount of fluid may be seen within the tunica vaginalis sac; however, larger amounts are termed hydroceles (Fig. 7). The fluid within a hydrocele may be simple (serous) or complex (hematocele, pyocele) in appearance. A simple hydrocele may be idiopathic or in the neonate be the result of a persistent communication between the scrotum and peritoneal cavity via a patent processus vaginalis, which usually resolves (80%) by 1.5 years of age.

Spermatocele Spermatocele, a common type of extratesticular cyst, represents cystic dilation of tubules of the efferent ductules in the head of the epididymis. Clinical examination reveals a soft, freely movable transilluminating mass separate from and superior to the testicle. In general, US seldom is needed to confirm the clinical diagnosis. It is a useful and simple procedure, however, in patients who have inconclusive clinical findings. On US, a spermatocele is observed as a well-defined hypoechoic lesion usually measuring 1 to 2 cm and demonstrating posterior acoustic enhancement.

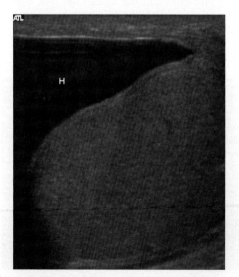

Fig. 7. A 47-year-old man who had a simple hydrocele. Scrotal US showing normal testicle and hydrocele (H).

Varicocele Varicocele (idiopathic or primary) represents abnormal dilation and tortuosity of the veins of the pampiniform plexus within the spermatic cord, caused by incompetent valves of the internal spermatic vein. The condition is more common on the left and is idiopathic in 15% of men between 15 and 25 years of age. Approximately one third of men who have varicocele are infertile. Secondary varicoceles result from increased pressure on the spermatic vein produced by disease processes, such as hydronephrosis, cirrhosis, or an abdominal neoplasm. A neoplasm most likely is the cause of nondecompressible varicocele in men over 40 years of age. Therefore, noncompressible varicoceles on the left or right in an patients should prompt evaluation of the retroperitoneum to exclude a retroperitoneal mass.

Gray-scale US can establish the diagnosis if the vessels of the pampiniform plexus are enlarged (ie, greater than 2–3 mm in diameter). In all inconclusive cases, color Doppler represents a significant diagnostic improvement. If a varicocele is present, a retrograde flow in the vessels of the pampiniform plexus is observed. This retrograde flow does not occur at rest or in healthy subjects. The sensitivity and specificity of Doppler for varicocele detection approaches 100% [83].

Intratesticular

Testicular germ cell tumors Although differential diagnosis must be established with any other intratesticular mass or disease, any scrotal complaint at young age needs to be investigated thoroughly to rule out testicular germ cell cancer (TGCC). Although TGCC accounts for only 1% of all cancers in male patients, it is the most common malignancy among 15- to 34-year-old men [84].

The most common sign of TGCC is a painless unilateral mass in the scrotum, which is inseparable from the testis. The vast majority (95%) of TGCC are of germ cell origin. TGCCs are divided into seminoma and nonseminoma types. Serum tumor markers are especially helpful to differentiate the various germ cell tumors from each other and from other malignancies [84].

The first step in diagnosing testicular cancer usually is made by self-examination. US confirms the presence of a testicular mass and can explore the contralateral testis [85]. US also is able to distinguish intra- from extratesticular lesions. The homogeneous echo texture of the normal testicular tissue represents an excellent background for the detection of intratesticular lesions. Small tumors are displayed as focal lesions, whereas larger tumors may destroy the entire testicular structure. Tumor borders may be smooth or irregular. Most testicular tumors are hypoechogenic, although they also may be displayed as hyper- or mixed echogenic lesions [86] (Fig. 8). The sensitivity of US in detecting testicular tumors is almost 100%. Furthermore, US is able to detect microlithiasis. Microlithiasis requires cautious follow-up, because it can be associated with TGCC [87].

As soon as the diagnosis of germ cell cancer has been confirmed pathologically, further staging examinations are warranted to examine the extent of disease. Staging is of utmost importance as it is the cornerstone of further treatment after orchiectomy. The staging system used most commonly for dissemination is the Royal Marsden Hospital Classification system [88]. Today, CT scanning of the chest and abdomen is the standard initial staging technique.

Imaging in clinical stage I testicular germ cell cancer Patients who have clinical stage I tumors have disease that is confined to the testis. Approximately 30% of the clinical stage I nonseminomas, however, are understaged by radiologic imaging and are found to have metastatic disease at retroperitoneal surgery.

The abdominal CT scan offers a sensitivity of 30% to 35% in the evaluation of retroperitoneal lymph nodes in the landing zone by using a threshold of 1 cm. Lowering this threshold results in increased sensitivity but decreased specificity (with a criterion of 4 mm, the sensitivity increases to 93%, but the specificity decreases to 58%) [89]. Alternative imaging methods, like PET and MR imaging, add little to the management of clinical stage I nonseminoma germ cell tumor (NSGCT). Examining the role of PET in clinical stage I NSGCT, by combining three retrospective trials, shows a sensitivity of 42% and a negative predictive value of 68% [90–92]. The accuracy of MR imaging is in line with that of CT scanning [93,94].

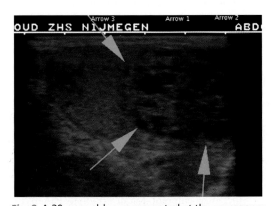

Fig. 8. A 29-year-old man presented at the emergency room with a palpable mass in the right testicle. Testicular US revealed a hypoechoic mass with cystic components in the right testicle. Histopathology revealed an embryonal cell carcinoma.

Currently, the value of intravenous ferumoxtran–enhanced MR imaging has been evaluated. Ferumoxtran is a contrast agent, which consists of ultrasmall iron-oxide particles. This technique yields a higher sensitivity and specificity when compared with unenhanced MR imaging (sensitivity: 88.2% versus 70.5%, specificity: 92% versus 68%). Although the results are encouraging, the precise role of this tool in clinical stage I TGCC remains to be determined [95].

Imaging in advanced staged testicular germ cell cancer The most common sites for metastases are via the lymphatic system to the retroperitoneal nodes and via the hematogenous route to the lungs and less commonly to the liver, brain, and bone. In general, advanced stage disease is treated primarily with chemotherapy. Today, CT is the standard initial staging method. Although FDG-PET has the potential to improve clinical staging, more studies are warranted to establish its definitive value.

After the completion of chemotherapy, residual tumorous lesions are found in up to 15% of patients who have seminomas and up to 20% of patients who have nonseminomas [96]. Furthermore, 40% of the nonseminomatous residual masses contain mature teratoma (premalignantdisease). The key to success is complete surgical removal of these masses. A major challenge is to find the optimal method for differentiating patients who have postchemotherapy (pre-)malignant residual mass from those who have fibrotic lesions. Again, CT scanning and establishment of the change in size of the mass is the standard for assessing residual masses. PET is of incremental value in assessing residual seminomatous disease. A study of 56 scans by De Santis and colleagues [97] reveals that PET had a sensitivity, specificity, positive predictive value, and negative predictive value of 100%, 80%, 100%, 96%, respectively, versus 74%, 70%, 37%, and 90% for CT scanning. They conclude that FDG-PET is the best predictor of viable residual seminoma in postchemotherapy masses. In contrast, in nonseminomas, there is no real additive value as PET cannot differentiate between fibrosis and mature teratoma [92].

Follow-up of testicular germ cell cancer Because most recurrences after curative therapy occur in the first 2 years, follow-up should be most frequent and intensive during this time. Follow-up protocols vary by institution and by type, disease stage, and treatment of the primary disease. After treatment, all patients are followed-up with regular outpatient visits, including physical examination and serum tumor marker assessments, and with performing chest radiographs and CT scanning.

Summary

Prostate

TRUS-guided biopsy remains the imaging modality of choice in detecting prostate cancer. Application of contrast-enhanced targeted or elastography targeted biopsy significantly increases the per core biopsy rate compared with systematic biopsy. Contrast-enhanced targeted biopsy detected a significantly higher mean Gleason score per biopsy. The role of TRUS in recurrence detection remains limited. MR imaging of the prostate is the best modality for localization and staging of prostate cancer and for the detection of recurrent disease. DCE-MRI and MRSI result in a significantly higher prostate cancer localization rate. Endorectal MR imaging at 3 T increased the local staging performance significantly.

Scrotum

US is the mainstay for imaging of the scrotum. It is used primarily for determining the location and nature of palpable lesions, to demonstrate non-palpable lesions. Scrotal US is characterized by high sensitivity in the detection of intrascrotal abnormalities and is a good mode for differentiating testicular from paratesticular lesions. Scrotal US is limited, however, in determining whether or not a focal testicular lesion is benign or malignant. The limitations of gray-scale US in the assessment of an acute scrotum and in particular of testicular torsion now have been overcome by color-coded duplex sonography and power Doppler. In malignant disease, CT is the first choice of staging of the abdomen and thorax.

References

[1] Jemal A, Siegel R, Ward E, et al. Cancer statistics, 2007. CA Cancer J Clin 2007;57(1):43–66.

[2] Krieger JN, Riley DE, Cheah PY, et al. Epidemiology of prostatitis: new evidence for a world-wide problem. World J Urol 2003;21:70–4.

[3] Kravchick S, Cytron S, Agulansky L, et al. Acute prostatitis in middle-aged men: a prospective study. BJU Int 2004;93:93–6.

[4] Griffiths GJ, Crooks AJ, Roberts EE, et al. Ultrasonic appearances associated with prostatic inflammation: a preliminary study. Clin Radiol 1984;35:343–5.

[5] Horcajada JP, Vilana R, Moreno-Martinez A, et al. Transrectal prostatic ultrasonography in acute bacterial prostatitis: findings and clinical implications. Scand J Infect Dis 2003;35:114–20.

[6] Shukla-Dave A, Hricak H, Eberhardt SC, et al. Chronic prostatitis: MR imaging and 1H MR spectroscopic imaging findings—initial observations. Radiology 2004;231:717–24.

[7] Schiebler ML, Tomaszeweski JE, Bezzi M, et al. Prostatic carcinoma and bening prostatic hyperplasia: correlation of high-resolution MR and histopathologic findings. Radiology 1989;172:111–37.

[8] Lee F, Gray JM, McLeary RD, et al. Prostatic evaluation by transrectal sonography: criteria for diagnosis of early carcinoma. Radiology 1986;158:91–5.

[9] Ellis WJ, Brawer MK. The significance of isoechoic prostatic carcinoma. J Urol 1994;152:2304–7.

[10] Hodge KK, McNeal JE, Terris MK, et al. Random systematic versus directed ultrasound guided transrectal core biopsies of the prostate. J Urol 1989;142:71–4.

[11] Vashi AR, Wojno KJ, Gillespie B, et al. A model for the number of cores per prostate biopsy based on patient age and prostate gland volume. J Urol 1998;159:920–4.

[12] Djavan B, Remzi M, Marberger M. When to biopsy and when to stop biopsying. Urol Clin North Am 2003;30:253–62, viii.

[13] Presti JC Jr. Prostate biopsy: how many cores are enough? Urol Oncol 2003;21:135–40.

[14] Eichler K, Hempel S, Wilby J, et al. Diagnostic value of systematic biopsy methods in the investigation of prostate cancer: a systematic review. J Urol 2006;175:1605–12.

[15] Jang TL, Han M, Roehl KA, et al. More favorable tumor features and progression-free survival rates in a longitudinal prostate cancer screening study: PSA era and threshold-specific effects. Urology 2006;67:343–8.

[16] Ekici S, Ozen H, Agildere M, et al. A comparison of transrectal ultrasonography and endorectal magnetic resonance imaging in the local staging of prostatic carcinoma. BJU Int 1999;83:796–800.

[17] May F, Treumann T, Dettmar P, et al. Limited value of endorectal magnetic resonance imaging and transrectal ultrasonography in the staging of clinically localized prostate cancer. BJU Int 2001;87:66–9.

[18] Garg S, Fortling B, Chadwick D, et al. Staging of prostate cancer using 3-dimensional transrectal ultrasound images: a pilot study. J Urol 1999;162:1318–21.

[19] Strasser H, Frauscher F, Klauser A, et al. Three-dimensional transrectal ultrasound instaging of localised prostate cancer. AUA Poster presentation 2003.

[20] Mitterberger M, Pinggera GM, Pallwein L, et al. The value of three-dimensional transrectal ultrasonography in staging prostate cancer. BJU Int 2007;100:47–50.

[21] Freedland SJ, Sutter ME, Dorey F, et al. Defining the ideal cutpoint for determining PSA recurrence after radical prostatectomy. Prostate-specific antigen. Urology 2003;61:365–9.

[22] Boccon-Gibod L, Djavan WB, Hammerer P, et al. Management of prostate-specific antigen relapse

in prostate cancer: a European Consensus. Int J Clin Pract 2004;58:382–90.

[23] Parra RO, Wolf RM, Huben RP. The use of transrectal ultrasound in the detection and evaluation of local pelvic recurrences after a radical urological pelvic operation. J Urol 1990;144:707–9.

[24] Foster LS, Jajodia P, Fournier G Jr, et al. The value of prostate specific antigen and transrectal ultrasound guided biopsy in detecting prostatic fossa recurrences following radical prostatectomy. J Urol 1993;149:1024–8.

[25] Salomon CG, Flisak ME, Olson MC, et al. Radical prostatectomy: transrectal sonographic evaluation to assess for local recurrence. Radiology 1993;189:713–9.

[26] Leventis AK, Shariat SF, Slawin KM. Local recurrence after radical prostatectomy: correlation of US features with prostatic fossa biopsy findings. Radiology 2001;219:432–9.

[27] Wasserman NF, Kapoor DA, Hildebrandt WC, et al. Transrectal US in evaluation of patients after radical prostatectomy. Part II. Transrectal US and biopsy findings in the presence of residual and early recurrent prostatic cancer. Radiology 1992;185:367–72.

[28] Connolly JA, Shinohara K, Presti JC Jr, et al. Local recurrence after radical prostatectomy: characteristics in size, location, and relationship to prostate-specific antigen and surgical margins. Urology 1996;47:225–31.

[29] Saleem MD, Sanders H, Abu EN, et al. Factors predicting cancer detection in biopsy of the prostatic fossa after radical prostatectomy. Urology 1998;51:283–6.

[30] Scattoni V, Roscigno M, Raber M, et al. Multiple vesico-urethral biopsies following radical prostatectomy: the predictive roles of TRUS, DRE, PSA and the pathological stage. Eur Urol 2003;44:407–14.

[31] Naya Y, Okihara K, Evans RB, et al. Efficacy of prostatic fossa biopsy in detecting local recurrence after radical prostatectomy. Urology 2005;66:350–5.

[32] Tang J, Li S, Li J, et al. Correlation between prostate cancer grade and vascularity on color doppler imaging: preliminary findings. J Clin Ultrasound 2003;31:61–8.

[33] Heijmink SW, Barentsz JO. Contrast-enhanced versus systematic transrectal ultrasound-guided prostate cancer detection: an overview of techniques and a systematic review. Eur J Radiol 2007;63:310–6.

[34] Okihara K, Kojima M, Nakanouchi T, et al. Transrectal power Doppler imaging in the detection of prostate cancer. BJU Int 2000;85:1053–7.

[35] Ismail M, Petersen RO, Alexander AA, et al. Color Doppler imaging in predicting the biologic behavior of prostate cancer: correlation with disease-free survival. Urology 1997;50:906–12.

[36] Sauvain JL, Palascak P, Bourscheid D, et al. Value of power doppler and 3D vascular sonography as a method for diagnosis and staging of prostate cancer. Eur Urol 2003;44:21–30.

[37] Sudakoff GS, Smith R, Vogelzang NJ, et al. Color Doppler imaging and transrectal sonography of the prostatic fossa after radical prostatectomy: early experience. AJR Am J Roentgenol 1996;167:883–8.

[38] Tamsel S, Killi R, Apaydin E, et al. The potential value of power Doppler ultrasound imaging compared with grey-scale ultrasound findings in the diagnosis of local recurrence after radical prostatectomy. Clin Radiol 2006;61:325–30.

[39] Halpern EJ, Rosenberg M, Gomella LG. Prostate cancer: contrast-enhanced us for detection. Radiology 2001;219:219–25.

[40] Mitterberger M, Pinggera GM, Horninger W, et al. Comparison of contrast enhanced color doppler targeted biopsy to conventional systematic biopsy: impact on gleason score. J Urol 2007;178:464–8 [discussion: 468].

[41] Pelzer A, Bektic J, Berger AP, et al. Prostate cancer detection in men with prostate specific antigen 4 to 10 ng/ml using a combined approach of contrast enhanced color Doppler targeted and systematic biopsy. J Urol 2005;173:1926–9.

[42] Heijmink SW, van Moerkerk H, Kiemeney LA, et al. A comparison of the diagnostic performance of systematic versus ultrasound-guided biopsies of prostate cancer. Eur Radiol 2006;16:927–38.

[43] Jakobsen JA, Oyen R, Thomsen HS, et al. Safety of ultrasound contrast agents. Eur Radiol 2005;15:941–5.

[44] Ophir J, Cespedes I, Ponnekanti H, et al. Elastography: a quantitative method for imaging the elasticity of biological tissues. Ultrason Imaging 1991;13:111–34.

[45] Phipps S, Yang TH, Habib FK, et al. Measurement of tissue mechanical characteristics to distinguish between benign and malignant prostatic disease. Urology 2005;66:447–50.

[46] Konig K, Scheipers U, Pesavento A, et al. Initial experiences with real-time elastography guided biopsies of the prostate. J Urol 2005;174:115–7.

[47] Pallwein L, Mitterberger M, Pinggera G, et al. Sonoelastography of the prostate: comparison with systematic biopsy findings in 492 patients. Eur J Radiol 2007;[epub ahead of print].

[48] Pallwein L, Mitterberger M, Struve P, et al. Comparison of sonoelastography guided biopsy with systematic biopsy: impact on prostate cancer detection. Eur Radiol 2007;17:2278–85.

[49] Albertsen PC, Hanley JA, Harlan LC, et al. The positive yield of imaging studies in the evaluation of men with newly diagnosed prostate cancer: a population based analysis. J Urol 2000;163:1138–43.

[50] Harisinghani MG, Barentsz J, Hahn PF, et al. Noninvasive detection of clinically occult lymph-node metastases in prostate cancer. N Engl J Med 2003;19:2491–9.

[51] Beyersdorff D, Taupitz M, Winkelmann B, et al. Patients with a history of elevated prostate-specific antigen levels and negative transrectal US-guided quadrant or sextant biopsy results: value of MR imaging. Radiology 2002;224:701–6.

[52] Jager GJ, Ruijter ET, van de Kaa CA, et al. Local staging of prostate cancer with endorectal MR imaging: correlation with histopathology. AJR Am J Roentgenol 1996;166:845–52.

[53] Scheidler J, Hricak H, Vigneron DB, et al. Prostate cancer: localization with three-dimensional proton MR spectroscopic imaging–clinicopathologic study. Radiology 1999;213:473–80.

[54] Testa C, Schiavina R, Lodi R, et al. Prostate cancer: sextant localization with MR imaging, MR spectroscopy, and 11C-Choline PET/CT. Radiology 2007;244(3):797–806.

[55] Haider MA, van der Kwast TH, Tanguay J, et al. Combined T2-weighted and diffusion-weighted MRI for localization of prostate cancer. AJR Am J Roentgenol 2007;189(2):323–8.

[56] Sonnad SS, Langlotz CP, Schwartz JS. Accuracy of MR imaging for staging prostate cancer: a meta-analysis to examine the effect of technologic change. Acad Radiol 2001;8:149–57.

[57] Engelbrecht MR, Jager GJ, Laheij RJ, et al. Local staging of prostate cancer using magnetic resonance imaging: a meta-analysis. Eur Radiol 2002;12:2294–302.

[58] Futterer JJ, Engelbrecht MR, Jager GJ, et al. Prostate cancer: comparison of local staging accuracy of pelvic phased-array coil alone versus integrated endorectal-pelvic phased-array coils. Local staging accuracy of prostate cancer using endorectal coil MR imaging. Eur Radiol 2007;17:1055–65.

[59] Futterer JJ, Heijmink SW, Scheenen TW, et al. Prostate cancer: local staging at 3-T endorectal MR imaging–early experience. Radiology 2006;238:184–91.

[60] Scheenen TW, Heijmink SW, Roell SA, et al. Three-dimensional proton MR spectroscopy of human prostate at 3 T without endorectal coil: feasibility. Radiology 2007;[epub ahead of print].

[61] Futterer JJ, Heijmink SW, Scheenen TW, et al. Prostate cancer localization with dynamic contrast-enhanced MR imaging and proton MR spectroscopic imaging. Radiology 2006;241:449–58.

[62] Anderson AW, Xie J, Pizzonia J, et al. Effects of cell volume fraction changes on apparent diffusion in human cells. Magn Reson Imaging 2000;18:689–95.

[63] Wein AJ, Kavoussi LR, Novick AC, et al, editors. Campbell-Walsh urology. 8th edition. Philadelphia: Saunders; 2007.

[64] Nguyen HT, Coakley F, Hricak H. Cryptorchidism: strategies in detection. Eur Radiol 1999;9:336–43.

[65] Weiss R, Carter AR, Rosenfield AT. High-resolution real-time ultrasound in the localization of the undescended testis. J Urol 1986;135:936–8.

[66] Muglia V, Tucci S Jr, Elias J Jr, et al. Magnetic resonance imaging of scrotal diseases: when it makes the difference. Urology 2002;59:419–23.

[67] Horstman WG. Scrotal imaging. Urol Clin North Am 1997;24:653–71.

[68] Berman JM, Beidle TR, Kunberger LE, et al. Sonographic evaluation of acute intrascrotal pathology. AJR Am J Roentgenol 1996;166:857–61.

[69] Barth RA, Shortliffe LD. Normal pediatric testis: comparison of power Doppler and color Doppler US in the detection of blood flow. Radiology 1997;204:389–93.

[70] Luker GD, Siegel MJ. Scrotal US in pediatric patients: comparison of power and standard color Doppler US. Radiology 1996;198:381–5.

[71] Terai A, Yoshimura K, Ichioka K, et al. Dynamic contrast-enhanced subtraction magnetic resonance imaging in diagnostics of testicular torsion. Urology 2006;67:1278–82.

[72] Cohen HL, Shapiro MA, Haller JO, et al. Torsion of the testicular appendage sonographic diagnosis. J Ultrasound Med 1992;11:81–3.

[73] Strauss S, Faingold R, Manor H. Torsion of the testicular appendagesonographic appearance. J Ultrasound Med 1997;16:189–92.

[74] Aso C, Enriquez G, Fite M, et al. Gray-scale and color Doppler sonography of scrotal disorders in children: an update. Radiographics 2005;25:1197–214.

[75] Burks DD, Markey BJ, Burkhard TK, et al. Suspected testicular torsion and ischemia: evaluation with color Doppler sonography. Radiology 1990;175:815–21.

[76] Middleton WD, Siegel BA, Melson GL, et al. Acute scrotal disorders: prospective comparison of color Doppler US and testicular scintigraphy. Radiology 1990;177:177–81.

[77] Andipa E, Liberopoulos K, Asvestis C. Magnetic resonance imaging and ultrasound evaluation of penile and testicular masses. World J Urol 2004;22:382–91.

[78] Sica GT, Teeger S. MR imaging of scrotal, testicular, and penile diseases. Magn Reson Imaging Clin N Am 1996;4:545–63.

[79] Jamadar DA, Jacobson JA, Morag Y, et al. Sonography of inguinal region hernias. AJR Am J Roentgenol 2006;187:185–90.

[80] Lilly MC, Arregui ME. Ultrasound of the inguinal floor for evaluation of hernias. Surg Endosc 2002;16:659–62.

[81] Kraft BM, Kolb H, Kuckuk B, et al. Diagnosis and classification of inguinal hernias. Surg Endosc 2003;17:2021–4.

[82] van den Berg JC, de Valois JC, Go PM, et al. Detection of groin hernia with physical examination, ultrasound, and MRI compared with laparoscopic findings. Invest Radiol 1999;34:739–43.

[83] Tessler FN, Tublin ME, Rifkin MD. Ultrasound assessment of testicular and paratesticular masses. J Clin Ultrasound 1996;24:423–36.

[84] Garner MJ, Turner MC, Ghadirian P, et al. Epidemiology of testicular cancer: an overview. Int J Cancer 2005;116:331–9.

[85] Hricak H. Imaging of the scrotum. Textbook and atlas. New York: Raven press; 1995. p. 49–93.

[86] Schwerk WB, Schwerk WN, Rodeck G. Testicular tumors: prospective analysis of real-time US patterns and abdominal staging. Radiology 1987;164:369–74.

[87] Backus ML, Mack LA, Middleton WD, et al. Testicular microlithiasis: imaging appearances and pathologic correlation. Radiology 1994; 192:781–5.

[88] Peckham MJ, Barrett A, McEwlain TJ, et al. Non-seminoma germ cell tumours (malignant teratomas) of the testis. Br J Urol 1981;53: 162–72.

[89] Hilton S, Herr HW, Teitcher JB, et al. CT detection of retroperitoneal lymph node metastases in patients with clinical stage I testicular nonseminomatous germ cell cancer: assessment of size and distribution criteria. AJR Am J Roentgenol 1997;169:521–5.

[90] Albers P, Bender H, Yilmaz H, et al. Positron emission tomography in the clinical staging of patients with Stage I and II testicular germ cell tumors. Urology 1999;53:808–11.

[91] Muller-Mattheis V, Reinhardt M, Gerharz CD, et al. [Positron emission tomography with [18 F]-2-fluoro-2-deoxy-D-glucose (18FDG-PET) in diagnosis of retroperitoneal lymph node metastases of testicular tumors]. Urologe A 1998;37: 609–20 [in German].

[92] Spermon JR, De Geus-Oei LF, Kieinmeney LA, et al. The role of (18)fluoro-2-deoxyglucose positron emission tomography in initial staging and re-staging after chemotherapy for testicular germ cell tumours. BJU Int 2002;89: 549–56.

[93] Ellis JH, Bies JR, Kopecky KK, et al. Comparison of NMR and CT imaging in the evaluation of metastatic retroperitoneal lymphadenopathy from testicular carcinoma. J Comput Assist Tomogr 1984;8:709–19.

[94] Hogeboom WR, Hoekstra HJ, Mooyaart EL, et al. The role of magnetic resonance imaging and computed tomography in the treatment evaluation of retroperitoneal lymph-node metastases of non-seminomatous testicular tumors. Eur J Radiol 1991;13:31–6.

[95] Harisinghani MG, Saksena M, Ross RW, et al. A pilot study of lymphotrophic nanoparticle-enhanced magnetic resonance imaging technique in early stage testicular cancer: a new method for noninvasive lymph node evaluation. Urology 2005;66:1066–71.

[96] Flechon A, Bompas E, Biron P, et al. Management of post-chemotherapy residual masses in advanced seminoma. J Urol 2002;168: 1975–9.

[97] De Santis M, Becherer A, Bokemeyer C, et al. 2-18fluoro-deoxy-D-glucose positron emission tomography is a reliable predictor for viable tumor in postchemotherapy seminoma: an update of the prospective multicentric SEMPET trial. J Clin Oncol 2004;22:1034–9.

RADIOLOGIC
CLINICS
OF NORTH AMERICA

Radiol Clin N Am 46 (2008) 149–166

MR Imaging–Guided Interventions in the Genitourinary Tract: An Evolving Concept

Fiona M. Fennessy, MD, PhD*, Kemal Tuncali, MD,
Paul R. Morrison, MSc, Clare M. Tempany, MD

MR imaging–guided interventions are a well-established form of routine patient care in many centers around the world. There are many different approaches, depending on magnet design and clinical need. The rationale behind this is based initially on MR imaging providing excellent inherent tissue contrast, without ionizing radiation risk for patients. MR imaging–guided minimally invasive therapeutic procedures have major advantages over conventional surgical procedures. In the genitourinary tract, MR imaging guidance can play a role in tumor detection, localization, and staging and can provide accurate image guidance for minimally invasive procedures for the confirmation of pathology, tumor treatment, and treatment monitoring. Depending on the body part accessed,

This work was supported in part by National Institutes of Health grant U41RR019703.
Department of Radiology, Harvard Medical School/Brigham and Women's Hospital, 75 Francis Street, Boston, MA 02115, USA
* Corresponding author.
E-mail address: ffennessy@partners.org (F.M. Fennessy).

doi:10.1016/j.rcl.2008.01.004

a customizable magnet bore configuration and magnetic resonance (MR)-compatible devices can be made available. The advent of molecular and metabolic imaging and the use of higher strength magnets likely will improve diagnostic accuracy and allow patient-specific targeted therapy, designed to maximize disease control and minimize side effects.

Genital tract: female

One of the most unique and exciting MR-guided interventional procedures in the female pelvis is MR-guided focused ultrasound surgery (MRgFUS). In addition, MR is used to guide other interventions and therapies, such as biopsies and gynecologic tumor treatments. The latter have been done in several centers, guiding the placement of radiation catheters for delivery of high-dose radiation in cervical or endometrial cancer [1].

Magnetic resonance–guided focused ultrasound surgery for treating uterine fibroids

Uterine fibroids are the most common female pelvic tumor, occurring in approximately 25% of women [2]. Although many patients remain asymptomatic, others suffer from symptoms, such as pelvic pain, menorrhagia, dysmenorrhagia, dyspareunia, urinary frequency, and infertility. Ultrasound (US) usually is the first diagnostic imaging modality of choice for fibroids, demonstrating a well-defined, usually hypoechoic mass. Providing good inherent tissue contrast, MR imaging is the optimal modality for fibroid detection, accurate localization, and volumetrics.

A wide spectrum of treatment options for uterine fibroids exists, ranging from expectant waiting to medical management to myomectomy to hysterectomy. Women, however, increasingly are seeking less invasive treatment options, perhaps motivated by fertility preservation and the possibility of reduced postprocedure recovery time. A good example of a less invasive choice is uterine artery embolization, a procedure that has demonstrated significant growth and interest since its introduction in 1995 [3]. Only MRgFUS, however, is completely noninvasive. Approved by the United States Food and Drug Administration (FDA) in October 2004, much of the worldwide experience with MRgFUS has been with treatment of uterine fibroids, with more than 3500 patients treated to date.

Fundamentals of magnetic resonance–guided focused ultrasound surgery

The potential surgical application of focused ultrasound surgery (FUS) was first demonstrated in 1942 [4]. Since then, it has been evaluated extensively in animal [5,6] and human [7] brains and in the kidney, prostate, liver, bladder [8–11], and eye [12] within clinical trials. Clinical acceptance, however, was hampered because of the difficulty in controlling the focal spot position, defining the beam target precisely, and coping with the lack of feedback about thermal damage.

MR imaging can satisfy the requirements of FUS, having excellent anatomic resolution and high sensitivity for tumor visualization, thereby offering accurate planning of the tissue to be targeted. By exploiting the temperature dependence of the water proton resonant frequency [13], MR-based temperature mapping is possible. This allows for targeting of the beam during subthreshold US exposures [14] and online estimation of the ablated volume [15,16]. Phase imaging is used to estimate the temperature-dependent proton resonant-frequency shift using a fast spoiled gradient-recalled-echo sequence (SPGR) [17]. Therefore, obtaining temperature-sensitive MR images before, during, and after each sonication can monitor tissue temperature elevations, including any slight elevations in normal adjacent surrounding tissue, thereby preventing damage.

Magnetic resonance–guided focused ultrasound surgery equipment for fibroid treatment

Sonications are performed using an MR-compatible focused US system that is built into a table that docks with a compatible MR scanner. The system consists of a focused piezoelectric phased-array transducer (208 elements, frequency 0.96–1.14 MHz) that is located within the specially designed table surrounded by a water tank. A thin plastic membrane covers the water tank and allows the US beam to propagate into the tissue. Patients lie in a prone position in the magnet, with the anterior abdominal wall positioned over the water tank. The location of the focal spot is controlled electronically by the transducer array that controls the volume of coagulation necrosis.

Patient selection for magnetic resonance–guided focused ultrasound surgery of uterine fibroids

The FDA has approved this procedure for premenopausal women who have symptomatic uterine fibroids and who have no desire for future pregnancy. This treatment is not indicated for pregnant women, postmenopausal women, or those who have contraindications to contrast-enhanced MR imaging. If multiple fibroids are present, clinical symptomatology and accessibility to the target fibroids are reviewed and a target fibroid is selected. The anterior abdominal wall is evaluated for extensive scarring. Those women who have such scarring are excluded from treatment because of the risk for skin burns [18].

Treatment planning

Immediately before treatment, T2-weighted fast spin-echo images in three orthogonal planes are obtained to plan the beam path to the targeted lesion. The MR images are analyzed to evaluate the area to be treated for possible obstructions. Although patients who have extensive anterior abdominal wall scarring in the beam path generally are excluded at screening, it may be possible, however, to treat women who have abdominal wall scarring that is not extensive by angling the beam path, ensuring that the scar is not traversed (Fig. 1). Filling of the urinary bladder by Foley catheter clamping also may help in moving the uterus and selected fibroid into a position away from the abdominal wall scar. Coursing bowel loops lying anterior to the uterus at the level of the uterine fibroid also may cause treatment-planning difficulties. Placement of a gel spacing device may allow the bowel loops to be displaced out of the treatment field, thereby enlarging the acoustic window and allowing for greater treatment volume (Fig. 2).

Clinical trials in the treatment of uterine fibroids with magnetic resonance–guided focused ultrasound surgery

Multicenter clinical trials investigating the use of MRgFUS in the treatment of uterine fibroids, which subsequently resulted in device labeling by the FDA, were performed at five medical centers across the United States in addition to centers in the United Kingdom, Germany, and Israel. Follow-up of many patients is ongoing.

Enrollment for phase I/II began in 1999 to assess the safety and feasibility of MRgFUS in the treatment of fibroids. Eligible patients underwent MRgFUS followed by hysterectomy, and subsequent pathologic examination of the uterus and fibroid showed that MRgFUS did result in hemorrhagic necrosis in the area of nonperfusion on the post-treatment MR [19,20].

Phase III of the clinical trial involved treatment of larger volumes of fibroids in women who had symptomatic uterine fibroids who otherwise would have opted for hysterectomy (Fig. 3). To date, the longest-term follow-up—in 359 patients—is up to 24 months [21]. These patients reported durable symptom relief. Those who had a greater nonperfused treatment volume fared better, with fewer of these patients undergoing additional fibroid treatment. These findings concur with those of Fennessy and colleagues [22], where greater clinical outcome was found in those treated with a modified treatment protocol that allowed for greater nonperfused fibroid volumes post treatment.

Cryotherapy for uterine fibroids

MR-guided cryotherapy is a minimally invasive procedure. It involves a percutaneous approach in an

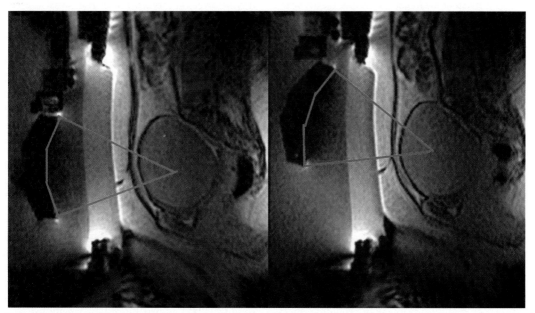

Fig. 1. Linear scar through the subcutaneous tissue lies between the transducer and the fibroid, on the sagittal localizer image on the left. The sagittal localizer image on the right is obtained after tilting the transducer superiorly, without moving the patient, allowing treatment planning that will not course through the anterior abdominal subcutaneous tissue scar. (*Reproduced from* Fennessy FM, Tempany CM. A review of magnetic resonance imaging-guided focused ultrasound surgery of uterine fibroids. Top Magn Reson Imaging 2006;17(3): 173–9; with permission.)

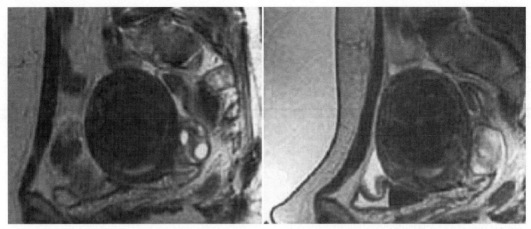

Fig. 2. The sagittal localizer image on the left demonstrates bowel loops coursing between the anterior abdominal wall and the uterine fibroid. After placement of a spacer device (sagittal localizer image on the right) under the anterior abdominal wall, the bowel loops are displaced, allowing for treatment through a larger acoustic window. (*Reproduced from* Fennessy FM, Tempany CM. A review of magnetic resonance imaging-guided focused ultrasound surgery of uterine fibroids. Top Magn Reson Imaging 2006;17(3):173–9; with permission.)

interventional setting with multiple (1 to 5) needle-like 17-G cryotherapy probes. Each probe creates a tear-drop shaped volume of frozen tissue about its tip (approximately 2.5-mm diameter); the simultaneous use of multiple probes gives a larger volume of treated tissue in the same time frame as treating with a single probe. The freeze is provided by pressurized argon gas that circulates within the probe. Typical treatments involve a cycling of the gas that delivers a freeze-thaw-freeze to destroy tissue, with each stage of the cycle 10 to 15 minutes in duration. MR imaging–guided cryotherapy has been evolving through experiment and clinical use during the past 20 years to target a range of tumors in various organ systems [23]. Compared with US that has shadow artifacts, visibility of the ice ball for monitoring is not as limited.

There are several promising reports of MR imaging–guided cryotherapy to treat symptomatic patients who have uterine fibroids [24–27]. During cryotherapy, the ice appeared as a signal void in the image as a result of the short MR relaxation time of the solid ice, giving a clear demarcation between frozen and unfrozen tissue. Though all reported relief from deleterious symptoms, short-term clinical outcome, however, is reported in only 8 of 9 treated patients, who demonstrated on average, 65% volume reduction in uterine size [25].

One of these studies [26] was performed transvaginally, with the investigators proposing that such an approach had the advantage of providing direct access, especially for submucosal tumors. Procedures usually are performed with epidural anesthesia in a horizontally open MR imaging scanner with multiple 2- to 3-mm cryotherapy probes (Fig. 4). Gradient-echo and T2-weighted spin-

echo sequences were used to guide probe placement and monitor the treatment cycle of freeze-thaw-freeze (Fig. 5).

Percutaneous ablation of fibroids is a nascent procedure and not practiced widely. This method of ablation has found a place in treating other parts of the body but not necessarily treating uterine fibroids, possibly because of the recent emergence of other minimally invasive procedures, such as uterine artery embolization, or noninvasive procedures, such as MRgFUS.

Genital tract: male

The leading cause of cancer death in men over 50, prostate cancer, affects one man in six in his lifetime. The American Cancer Society estimates that in 2007 in the United States, 218,890 new cases of prostate cancer will be diagnosed, and approximately 27,050 men will die of the disease [28]. There is only a 33% 5-year survival rate in men who have metastatic disease [29], making early tumor detection and localized treatment a necessity.

MR imaging–guided prostate biopsy

Early diagnosis and cancer localization within the prostate gland usually are found through digital examination and scrum prostate-specific antigen (PSA) measurement, followed by transrectal ultrasound (TRUS)-guided biopsy. Image-guided prostate biopsy with ultrasound (US) has become a universally accepted tool [30], but because of a low sensitivity and specificity for tumor detection [31], interest continues in the development of a more accurate technique. In addition, for men

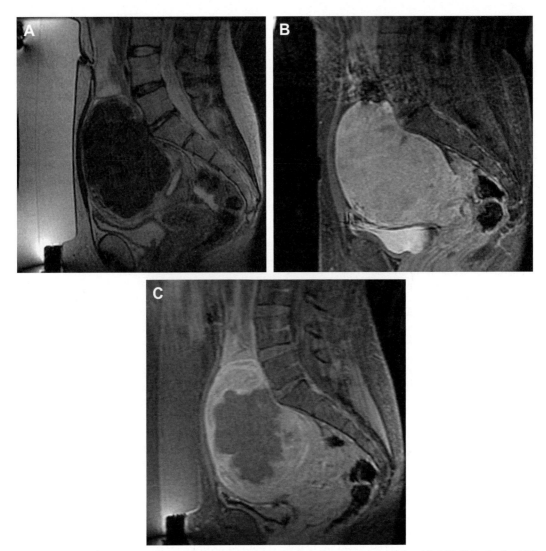

Fig. 3. Imaging of a uterine fibroid pretreatment (*A, B*) and post-treatment (*C*) with MRgFUS. Sagittal T2-weighted image (*A*), obtained with the patient in the prone position overlying the US transducer, demonstrates a large solitary uterine fibroid of low-signal intensity. Sagittal SPGR post gadolinium (*B*) demonstrates homogenous enhancement of the fibroid. After treatment, sagittal SPGR post gadolinium (*C*) demonstrates a new large nonperfused area within the fibroid, consistent with treatment-induced necrosis.

who have increasing PSA levels and repeatedly negative TRUS-guided prostate biopsies (the concern being that a sampling error may result in a false-negative biopsy), for those in whom a transrectal biopsy is not possible, or for those who are reluctant to undergo transrectal biopsy because of its recognized complications, such as infection, hematuria, hematospermia, and rectal bleeding [32–34], an alternative approach may be necessary.

MR imaging can outline prostate architecture and substructure. Although the specificity for diagnosis may be limited, MR imaging can demonstrate suspicious nodules in the peripheral zone, the most common site for prostate cancer. On T2-weighted images, tumor is demonstrated most commonly

by focal or diffuse regions of decreased signal intensity relative to the high-signal-intensity normal peripheral zone. MR imaging is used most routinely for staging men who have known cancer. The reported accuracy of prostate cancer detection and staging on MR images varies widely, with reports of accuracy ranging from 54% to 93%, likely because of differences in techniques and interobserver variability [35–38].

Its role in detection and characterization, particularly in the initial diagnosis of high-risk patients or those who have previous negative biopsy findings but persistently high PSA levels, is increasing as techniques such as MR spectroscopy imaging (MRSI) and dynamic contrast enhancement

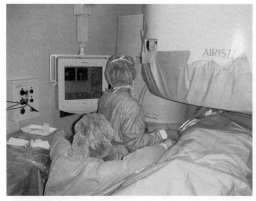

Fig. 4. Photograph demonstrating the set-up for percutaneous MR imaging–guided cryotherapy for uterine fibroids in an open horizontal 0.3-T AIRIS II (Hitachi, Tokyo, Japan) scanner. (*Courtesy of* Yusuke Sakuhara, MD, Department of Radiology, Hokkaido University Hospital, Sapporo, Japan.)

become more widely available. The ultimate role and application in clinical practice, however, remain controversial [35]. MR imaging contributes significant incremental value to TRUS-guided biopsy and digital rectal examination in cancer detection and localization in the prostate [39]. It offers an excellent second-line alternative to those who have failed to obtain a diagnosis with conventional methods.

MR imaging–guided prostate biopsy: technique

Two basic strategies have been explored for MR imaging–guided prostate biopsy. The first is coregistration of previously acquired diagnostic MR images to TRUS images, localizing suspected tumor lesions on MR and correlating these locations to the

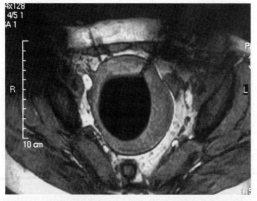

Fig. 5. Axial T2-weighted spin-echo sequence demonstrating a probe in the left anterolateral aspect of a uterine fibroid. The diffuse low-signal intensity in the fibroid represents the ice-ball. (*Courtesy of* Yusuke Sakuhara, MD, Department of Radiology, Hokkaido University Hospital, Sapporo, Japan.)

US [40]. The second strategy is stereotactic needle interventions within diagnostic MR scanners using careful patient positioning. By implementing surgical navigation software originally developed for neurosurgery [41,42] and adapting the technical capabilities of MR imaging–guided prostate brachytherapy in an open configuration magnet [43], biopsy of suspected tumor foci in the peripheral zone is made possible (Fig. 6) [44]. In addition, the feasibility of transrectal needle access to prostate tumors has been assessed in a closed-bore 1.5-T magnet [45–48] in a small number of patients, which potentially could provide for additional functional and spectroscopic imaging in comparison with a 0.5-T scanner. The procedure requires the use of a specialized device that consists of a needle guide and support system. The same guidance also has been used recently in a 3-T system [49]. Larger studies of clinical usefulness, however, are necessary. With progress in biologic imaging of the prostate gland, it is likely that MR imaging guidance will play an increasing role in the diagnosis and treatment of prostate cancer.

MR imaging–guided prostate biopsy: the future

The move toward targeted interventions, for diagnosis and treatment, underscores the need for precise image-guided needle placement. Based on a patient's anatomy and lesion detection in pretreatment MR imaging, a graphic planning interface that allows desired needle trajectories to be specified, through MR-compatible robotic assistance, recently has been described [50]. Avoiding the limitations of a fixed-needle template is a positive move forward for tissue sampling and treatment. As the field of prostate imaging moves to higher strength magnets, namely 3 T, the biopsy devices are reconfigured to allow sampling in a closed-bore environment. A recent study of prostate biopsy using 3-T MR imaging guidance described it as a promising tool for detecting and sampling cancerous regions in patients who have known prostate cancer [49]; however, the role (even at 3 T) of MR imaging–guided prostate biopsy as a screening tool in patients who have elevated PSA levels and recent previous negative biopsy remains to be determined.

MR imaging–guided brachytherapy for prostate cancer

Established options for the management of localized prostate cancer include one or a combination of the following: radical prostatectomy, external beam radiation therapy, brachytherapy, or watchful waiting. In radiation therapy, the goal is to achieve the prescribed dose throughout the prostate gland

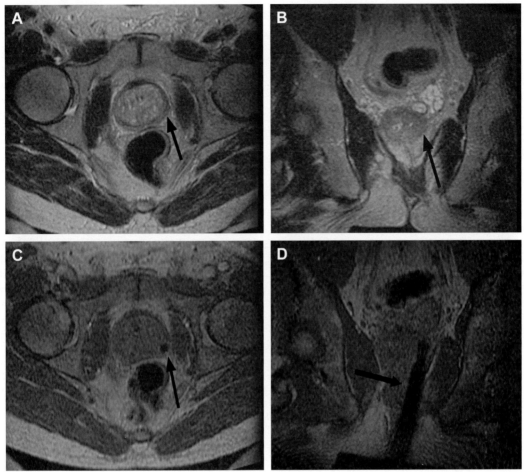

Fig. 6. Imaging before and during MR imaging–guided prostate biopsy. Axial (*A*) and coronal (*B*) T2-weighted spin-echo sequence outline areas to be biopsied. In this example, an area in the left midgland is demonstrated (*arrow*), reformatted to the same spatial location as the corresponding real-time axial (*C*) and coronal images (*D*) taken during needle insertion. The biopsy needle is seen in cross section as a circle of low-signal intensity (*arrow*) on the axial gradient-echo real-time image (*C*) and as a longitudinal area of low-signal intensity (*arrow*) on the coronal gradient-echo real-time image (*D*).

while minimizing toxicity to adjacent structures and minimizing morbidity from the procedure. Prostate brachytherapy is one of the more popular radiation methods in the prostate and involves the percutaneous placement of I-125 radiation seeds into the gland under image guidance. This is done most commonly with TRUS. It also can be done with MR guidance and the goal in both procedures is to optimize seed placement and allow maximal dose to the prostate peripheral zone tumor and minimal dose to the urethra and rectum.

Imaging-guided radiation therapy, therefore, allows directed tumor treatment, decreasing the chances of disease spreading outside the gland, while healthy prostate tissue and its neighboring structures are not overdosed. This is extremely important for structures such as the urethra, in which over-radiation may cause stricture and fistualization that

can be avoided with good image guidance [51,52]. Radiation dose fall-off is sharp at the rectal wall and at the urethra. Unlike external beam radiotherapy, there is no entrance or exit dose. Brachytherapy, therefore, has the potential to achieve superior tumor control with decreased morbidity and side effects. It is not, however, without its own set of complications, such as rectal irritation and ulceration, incontinence, and impotence resulting from inadvertent delivery of radiation dosing to the rectum, bladder, and urethra.

Patient selection

Low-risk prostate cancer patients who have a high probability of organ-confined disease are screened appropriately with an endorectal coil MR for potential treatment with brachytherapy monotherapy. Most centers include patients who have stage T1-T2a (according to the American Joint Committee on Cancer/International Union Against Cancer 1997 staging), PSA level of 10 ng/mL or less, and a Gleason score of 6 or lower. The few contraindications to the procedure include prior transurethral resection of the prostate or morbid obesity (equipment cannot sustain the weight).

Procedure

MR-guided prostate brachytherapy using open configuration 0.5-T and 1.5-T scanners are described [43,45]. Using the open 0.5-T magnet, patients are placed supine between the two magnets in the lithotomy position under general anesthesia. A Foley catheter is inserted, the skin is prepared and draped in a sterile fashion, and a template for needle guidance is placed against the perineum. A rectal obturator then is placed and T2-weighted images are acquired in the axial, coronal, and sagittal planes and used to outline the urethra, peripheral zone, and anterior rectal wall. Surgical simulation software outlines these areas, and the targeted volume is calculated using designated planning software [53]. Seed number and depth of catheter insertion are calculated.

While gradient-echo MR images are obtained in real time [44], seed-loaded catheters then are positioned in the prostate gland (Fig. 7). The images are compared to their intended locations, according to the radiation therapist plan. Dose-volume histograms of the urethra, anterior rectal wall, and target volume are obtained before final deployment of seeds. Six weeks after the procedure, CT imaging (to identify the seeds accurately) and MR imaging (for prostate anatomic correlation) are fused to calculate the final dose distribution to the gland and surrounding tissues.

Although open-bore magnets offer good patient accessibility and allow satisfactory prostate tumor and anatomic depiction, higher-quality MR intervention images in a closed 1.5-T system also have been investigated [45]. This system uses a customized perineal template, an endorectal imaging coil, and a lockable positioning arm. Patients are placed in the left lateral decubitus position. Although patient accessibility with this technique may be limited because of the closed-bore configuration and the 60-cm diameter bore, the investigators found that dependence on deformable registration between image sets (high-field 1.5-T diagnostic images and low-field–strength interventional images) was reduced.

Outcomes

Short-term toxicity after MR-guided brachytherapy is rare, with no gastrointestinal or sexual dysfunction reported during the first month after treatment [54]. Within 24 hours of removal of the Foley catheter, acute urinary retention was reported in 12% of men, which was self-limited to within 1 to 3 weeks of treatment. Prostatic volume and transitional zone volume, determined by MR imaging, and number of brachy therapy seeds placed were found to be significant predictors of acute urinary retention.

The long-term genitourinary and rectal toxicity was compared between those who received MR-guided brachytherapy alone and those who received combined MR-guided brachytherapy and external beam radiation therapy [55]. The 4-year estimates of rectal bleeding requiring coagulation for patients who underwent MR-guided brachytherapy compared with patients who received combined-modality therapy were 8% versus 30%. The 4-year estimate of freedom from radiation cystitis was 100% versus 95% for patients who received MR-guided brachytherapy alone and patients who received combined-modality therapy, respectively. In a separate study evaluating the long-term toxicity in patients who received MR-guided brachytherapy as a salvage procedure for radiation therapy failure [56], the 4-year estimate of grade 3 or 4 gastrointestinal or genitourinary toxicity was reported at 30% of all patients, with 13% requiring an intervention, such as a colostomy or urostomy for fistula repair.

Supplemental external beam radiotherapy, in addition to brachytherapy seed implantation, has been given to patients who have intermediate- to high-risk prostate cancer (according to the D'Amico risk stratification for prostate cancer) [57]. This combination of radiation therapy has demonstrated good long-term results [58,59], resulting in a 15-year biochemical relapse-free survival equal to 80.3% for intermediate-risk disease and 67.2% for high-risk disease.

Brachytherapy: the future

The current manual method of needle placement, using a fixed-needle template guide, constrains needle orientation. The manual method also makes use of manual computation and transcription of needle coordinates that are prone to human error. The future points toward a system that incorporates an interactive planning interface with MR-compatible robotic assistance. Such a device, which serves as a dynamic guide for precise needle placement, has been developed [60]. Likely the future direction for percutaneous MR imaging–guided prostatic interventions, this MR-compatible robotic device has been integrated with a software planning interface, allowing physicians to specify desired needle trajectories based on MR imaging anatomy.

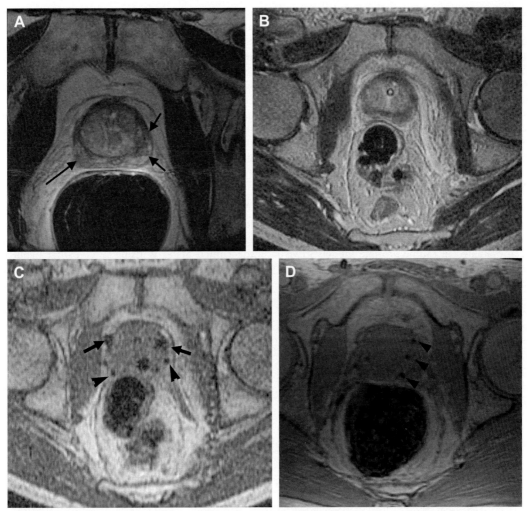

Fig. 7. Pre-, intra-, and postoperative MR imaging–guided brachytherapy in prostate cancer. Preoperative 1.5-T (*A*) axial T2-weighted spin-echo image through the prostate base, demonstrating low signal intensity in the peripheral zone (*arrows*), previously demonstrated to be tumor. Intraoperative 0.5-T (*B*) axial T2-weighted spin-echo T2 weighted spin-echo image through the same area. Intraoperative axial gradient-echo MR images (*C*) obtained in real time during needle and seed placement in the prostate base. The larger round areas represent the needles (*arrows*), before deployment, and the small round areas represent the deployed seeds (*arrowheads*). A postoperative axial SPGR (*D*) through the prostate base demonstrates multiple round areas of low signal in the peripheral zone (*arrowheads*), consistent with deployed seeds.

Focused ultrasound surgery in the prostate

As discussed previously regarding the female genital tract, there is growing interest in MRgFUS because of its many potential applications as a minimally invasive therapy. US-guided FUS (USgFUS) has been used predominantly in Europe for the treatment of prostate cancer. Limitations include difficulty in treating the anterior prostate or small-volume prostates, and lack of long-term follow-up.

Literature describing the results of USgFUS for prostate cancer suggests that USgFUS treatment is a valuable option for well-differentiated and moderately differentiated tumors and for local recurrence after external-beam radiation therapy [61–63]. USgFUS treatment is whole-gland therapy, without selective tumor-directed targeted treatment, that should allow for minimal disruption of normal function. USgFUS arguably is limited by the lack of direct temperature and thermal dose measurements during thermocoagulation. Without the latter, the energy delivery cannot be controlled or monitored nor can the thermal dose be measured accurately.

To address these challenges, MR imaging–compatible prostate applications have been developed for hyperthermia [64], and phased-array applicators for thermal ablation [65]. Insightec (Haifa, Israel) has developed a MRgFUS system for prostate treatment (Fig. 8). A major potential advantage of MR imaging guidance is its ability to map functional changes in prostate tissue, with the possibility of 3-D tumor mapping before and during treatment. Overall, noninvasive thermal ablation using MR imaging guidance should improve prostate treatment significantly and its application should increase in the near future.

MR imaging–guided catheter-based ultrasound thermal therapy of the prostate

In a similar mode, catheter-based US devices (in interstitial and transurethral configurations) have been evaluated in canine prostate models in vivo and found to produce spatially selective regions of thermal destruction in the prostate [66–68]. Transurethral US devices with tubular transducers have been developed, which can coagulate sectors of the prostate using preshaped angular patterns [69,70]. Devices with finer spatial control using planar [71,72] or curvilinear transducers [73] can be rotated slowly using a computer-controlled, MR-compatible stepper motor while under MR imaging guidance and feedback (Fig. 9). The feasibility of MR imaging–guided interstitial US thermal therapy of the prostate has been evaluated in an in vivo canine prostate model [66]. MR

imaging–compatible, multielement interstitial US applicators were used. The applicators were inserted transperineally into the prostate with the energy directed ventrally away from the rectum. This study demonstrated a large volume of ablated tissue within the prostate and, importantly, demonstrated contiguous zones of thermal coagulation. At least in an animal model and using MR guidance, transurethral and interstitial treatment strategies have, therefore, demonstrated significant potential for thermal ablation of localized prostate cancer.

Urinary tract

Renal cell carcinoma (RCC) is the sixth leading cause of cancer death [74], and its incidence in the United States is rising [75]. Partial nephrectomy, a nephron-sparing surgical method, has replaced radical nephrectomy for the treatment of small RCC. Less invasive methods also have emerged that can be performed laparoscopically (partial nephrectomy and cryosurgery) or percutaneously (radiofrequency ablation [RFA] and cryoablation). Image-guided percutaneous ablations have the potential to replace others as the least invasive and least costly [76] of all nephron-sparing treatments clinically available, particularly in patients who are poor surgical candidates because of comorbid disease and patients who have renal insufficiency, solitary kidney, or multiple RCC.

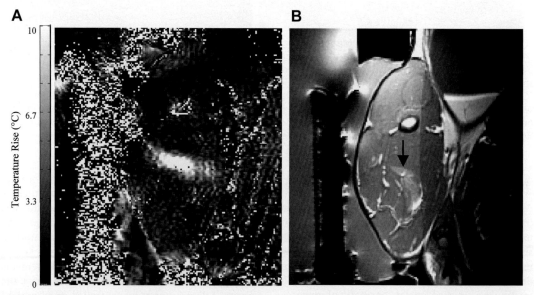

Fig. 8. (A) MR imaging–based temperature image during a sonication (130 W for 30 seconds) into rabbit thigh muscle during a test of an MR imaging–compatible transrectal phased array applicator for MRgFUS of prostate. (B) The thermal lesion (*arrow*) seen in T2-weighted imaging. The bright region to the right of the lesion is a tissue fascia layer. (*From* Sokka SD, Hynynen K. The feasibility of MRI-guided whole prostate ablation with a linear aperiodic intracavitary ultrasound phased array. Phys Med Biol 2000;45:3373–83; with permission.)

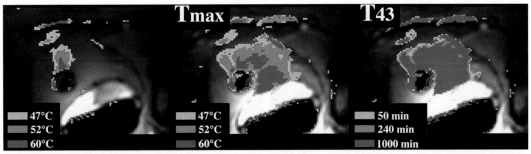

Fig. 9. MR imaging–guided catheter-based US thermal therapy of the prostate: real-time temperature image (*left*), maximum temperature image (*middle*), and thermal dose (*right*) of the prostate during catheter-based US thermal therapy. The transurethral catheter, with a rotating curvilinear transducer array, is depicted as the round low-signal intensity structure within the prostate gland [69]. (*Courtesy of* Kim Butts Pauly, PhD, Viola Rieke, MD, and Graham Sommer, PhD, Stanford University School of Medicine, Stanford, CA; and Chris Diederich, PhD, UCSF, San Francisco, CA.)

MR imaging–guided radiofrequency ablation in the kidney

RFA is a focal thermal tumor therapy method in which tissue is heated by an electric current. The current is present with a high density surrounding a percutaneously placed electrode that is driven by an electrical generator. The circuit is completed by the placement of grounding pads on a patient. The electrode is placed interstitially and intended to be activated to create a volume of coagulative necrosis in place of the tumor.

Many reports of successful treatment of renal tumors with percutaneous RFA have been published [77–85]. Real-time monitoring of RFA, however, is not possible with CT or US because the thermal ablation zone is not visible with these imaging modalities. RFA can be monitored with MR imaging [86,87] but with limitations. Radiofrequency energy has to be interrupted during MR imaging because of the significant interference it causes otherwise. Furthermore, the temperature-sensitive, very short repetition time/echo time gradient-echo sequences typically are not suitable for detailed visualization of retroperitoneal anatomy.

Specific to MR imaging–guided RFA in the kidney, the first report was an in vivo study in porcine kidney [88]. The procedures were performed in a 0.2-T open magnet and demonstrated the suitability of MR imaging for guiding needle placement and the benefit of its inherent soft-tissue sensitivity where the electrode could be placed and the thermal lesion observed. Clinical studies of MR imaging–guided RFA in the kidney subsequently reported the safety and efficacy of the procedure [87,89] in tumors less than 4 cm in diameter. No recurrences at 25 months' post procedure were reported.

Overall, RFA is a feasible therapeutic modality for kidney lesions, under MR imaging, CT, or US guidance [90]. Although RFA is performed more routinely under CT guidance, many practices turn to MR imaging for the assessment and long-term follow-up of treated patients [91–93].

MR imaging–guided percutaneous cryotherapy of renal tumors

Cryoablation, a focal thermal tumor therapy method which uses extreme cold to establish coagulative necrosis, has several advantages over RFA. While RFA may require the need to perform multiple overlapping ablations of larger tumors, with percutaneous cryoablation, larger tumors can be treated simultaneously with the placement of multiple applicators [94,95]. Evidence suggests that renal tumors more likely are treated in one session with cryoablation compared to RFA [96]. Lower doses of medications are required for intravenous conscious sedation suggesting that percutaneous cryoablation of renal tumors is associated with less intraprocedural pain than with percutaneous RFA [97].

US monitoring of cryoablation is limited by an inability to image the entire ice ball because of acoustic shadowing from the edge closest to the US probe [98]. Cryoablation of renal tumors can be monitored with CT because the ice ball is readily apparent as a hypoattenuating structure in the renal parenchyma [94,95,98–103]. There are two main limitations with CT, however. One is that the portion of the ice ball in the perinephric fat, a hyperattenuating region, provides only a modest contrast-to-noise ratio [104,105] compared to surrounding fat, and the ablation zone edge is not demarcated clearly in fatty tissue (Fig. 10A). This limits its use for real-time monitoring of the effect of ablation on adjacent critical structures, such as bowel, ureter, pancreas, and adrenal gland. Another is that the streak artifact created by the applicators with CT imaging can interfere with ice ball visibility (Fig. 10B).

Since the initial clinical reports of MR imaging–guided percutaneous cryoablation of renal tumors

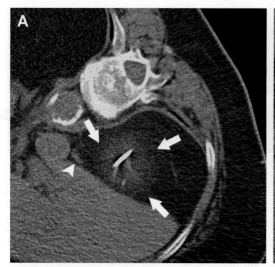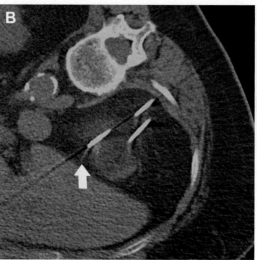

Fig. 10. CT–guided percutaneous cryotherapy of renal yumors. A 77-year-old woman who had RCC of the right kidney upper pole. Unenhanced transverse CT images obtained during percutaneous cryoablation performed in the right lateral decubitus position show that (*A*) low contrast-to-noise ratio and poor edge definition of ice ball (*arrows*) in the perinephric fat renders assessment for overlap of ablation zone with adjacent adrenal gland (*arrowhead*) difficult, and (*B*) streak artifact from applicator interferes with visualization of portion of the ice ball (*arrow*).

[98,100] in 2001, several investigators have shown the feasibility and safety of the procedure [106–112], all demonstrating the advantages of MR imaging monitoring during percutaneous cryoablation procedures.

MR imaging depicts the ice ball as a signal void region with high contrast-to-noise ratio compared to surrounding tissues, with sharp edge definition in multiple planes and with minimal applicator artifact (**Fig. 11**). Ice ball volume on intraprocedural MR imaging correlates well with volume of cryonecrosis on postprocedural MR imaging [113]. Because the ice ball is well depicted on all pulse sequences, the ablation can be monitored using pulse sequences that display tumor or adjacent critical structures best [111]. If images demonstrate incomplete coverage of tumor, additional applicators may be placed to improve coverage [111,112]. Alternatively, if the ice ball edge approaches adjacent critical structures, the freezing can be stopped [111]. Applicators can be controlled individually. Additional maneuvers to reduce risk for injury to surrounding bowel, such as water instillation described for CT-guided ablations [114], also can be performed during MR imaging–guided cryoablations [111]. A noninvasive method of external manual displacement of bowel during MR imaging–guided cryoablation of renal tumors also is described—a maneuver unique to cryoablation procedures performed in an open-configuration interventional MR imaging unit [115].

Limitations of MR imaging–guided cryoablation include the high cost of MR imaging units and its limited availability, generally long procedure times, smaller gantry sizes compared to CT scanners, and inability to detect ST-T segment changes of cardiac ischemia on an EKG in the magnetic environment during procedures.

In summary, image-guided percutaneous ablative therapies have the potential to replace conventional surgical treatment of small RCC. Compared with other image-guided ablative therapies, with its vast advantages and minimal limitations, MR imaging–guided percutaneous cryoablation is well poised to play an important role in the management of renal tumors.

The future

Recent developments in MR imaging paralleling those in computer-assisted surgery have set up an ideal environment for MR-compatible robotic systems and manipulators. Materials used in mechatronic devices inside the magnet ideally should have a magnetic susceptibility similar to that of human tissue and be electrical insulators to avoid image distortion. Although image quality is reduced because of reduction in static field strength, interventional open-bore magnets have fewer spatial constraints. Alternatively, closed MR scanners can impose severe constraints on procedural manipulations, despite their imaging advantage of higher field strengths. New wide- and short-bore 1.5-T magnets (Espree, Siemens, Erlangen, Germany) will expand the use of interventional MR imaging. Emerging use of 3-T magnets for interventions will bring about improved monitoring of thermal therapies. Much research is

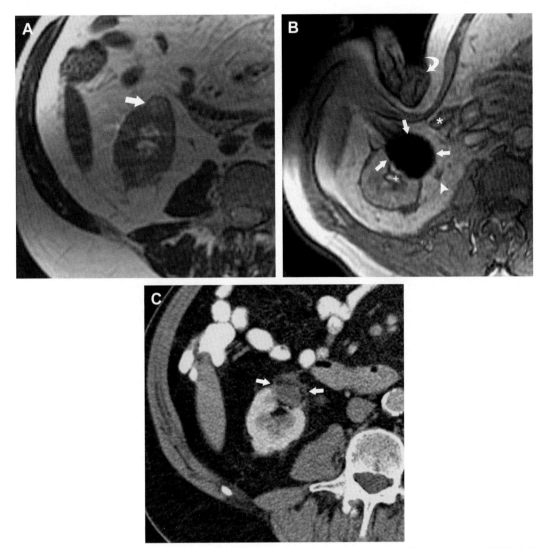

Fig. 11. MR imaging–guided percutaneous cryotherapy of renal tumor. A 70-year-old man who had RCC of the right kidney lower pole treated with MR imaging–guided percutaneous cryoablation. (*A*) Transverse T2-weighted fast recovery fast spin–echo sequence image obtained before treatment in 1.5-T MR image shows a small exophytic renal mass in the lower pole of the right kidney anteriorly (*arrow*). (*B*) Intraprocedural transverse gradient-echo image obtained in 0.5-T open configuration interventional MR imaging shows that sharp edge definition of signal void ice ball (*arrows*) contributes to monitoring of tumor coverage and assessment of proximity to adjacent ureter (*arrowhead*), renal collecting system (+), and colon (*), which is being displaced by an interventionalist's hand (*curved arrow*). (*C*) An 18-month follow-up contrast-enhanced transverse CT image shows no enhancement in the involuted ablation zone (*arrows*).

underway evaluating material selection, position detection sensors, different actuation models and techniques, and design strategies [116]. Once the engineering hurdle is overcome, systems must undergo clinical validation before introduction into the commercial realm.

Summary

MR imaging has become part of routine care in many places around the world, for tumor detection,

localization, and staging. In the genitourinary tract, MR imaging guidance is playing an increasing role in minimally invasive procedures for confirmation of tumor pathology and for tumor treatment and treatment monitoring. It offers inherent ability for tumor detection and biopsy guidance and, currently, MR-guided ablative therapies are an increasing and real alternative to more invasive surgical options. As the capabilities of MR imaging expand and newer imaging modalities become more accessible (PET imaging, for example), the need for nonrigid registration of multiple modalities will be necessary. A combination of functional imaging and high-resolution tumor detail in the genitourinary tract, in a patient-specific treatment environment, should increase demand and the use of semi-invasive or noninvasive technology. Clearly, the pressure is on to provide MR-compatible devices and methodology that easily integrate with imaging and are supportive of patients' clinical needs.

References

[1] Stewart AJ, Viswanathan AN. Current controversies in high-dose-rate versus low-dose-rate brachytherapy for cervical cancer. Cancer 2006;107(5):908–15.

[2] Stewart EA. Uterine fibroids. Lancet 2001;357: 293–8.

[3] Ravina J, Herbreteau D, Ciraru-Vigneron N, et al. Arterial embolisation to treat uterine myomata. Lancet 1995;346:671–2.

[4] Lynn JG, Zwemer RL, Chick AJ, et al. A new method for the generation and use of focused ultrasound in experimental biology. J Gen Physiol 1942;26:179–93.

[5] Fry WJ, Barnard JW, Fry FJ. Ultrasonically produced localized selective lesions in the central nervous system. Am J Phys Med 1955; 34:413–23.

[6] Lele PP. A simple method for production of trackless focal lesions with focused ultrasound: physical factors. J Physiol 1962;160:494–512.

[7] Heimburger RF. Ultrasound augmentation of central nervous system tumor therapy. Indiana Med 1995;78:469–76.

[8] Gelet A, Chapelon JY, Bouvier R, et al. Local control of prostate cancer by transrectal high intensity focused ultrasound therapy: preliminary results. J Urol 1999;161:156–62.

[9] Paterson RF, Barret E, Siqueira TM Jr, et al. Laparoscopic partial kidney ablation with high intensity focused ultrasound. J Urol 2003; 169(1):347–51.

[10] Yang R, Sanghvi NT, Rescorla FJ, et al. Extracorporeal liver ablation using sonography-guided high-intensity focused ultrasound. Invest Radiol 1992;27(10):796–803.

[11] Watkin NA, Morris SB, Rivens IH, et al. A feasibility study for the non-invasive treatment of superficial bladder tumours with focused ultrasound. Br J Urol 1996;78(5):715–21.

[12] Lizzi FL, Deng CX, Lee P, et al. A comparison of ultrasonic beams for thermal treatment of ocular tumors. Eur J Ultrasound 1999;9(1):71–8.

[13] Ishihara Y, Calderon A, Watanabe H, et al. A precise and fast temperature mapping using water proton chemical shift. Magn Reson Med 1995;34(6):814–23.

[14] Hynynen K, Vykhodtseva NI, Chung AH, et al. Thermal effects of focused ultrasound on the brain: determination with MR imaging. Radiology 1997;204(1):247–53.

[15] Chung AH, Jolesz FA, Hynynen K. Thermal dosimetry of a focused ultrasound beam in vivo by magnetic resonance imaging. Med Phys 1999;26(9):2017–26.

[16] McDannold N, Tempany CM, Fennessy FM, et al. Uterine leiomyomas: MR imaging-based thermometry and thermal dosimetry during focused ultrasound thermal ablation. Radiology 2006;240(1):263–72.

[17] Chung AH, Hynynen K, Colucci V, et al. Optimization of spoiled gradient-echo phase imaging for in vivo localization of focused ultrasound beam. Magn Reson Med 1996; 36(5):745–52.

[18] Leon-Villapalos J, Kaniorou-Larai M, Dziewulski P. Full thickness abdominal burn following magnetic resonance guided focused ultrasound therapy. Burns 2005;31(8):1054–5.

[19] Tempany CM, Stewart EA, McDannold N, et al. MR imaging-guided focused ultrasound surgery of uterine leiomyomas: a feasibility study. Radiology 2003;226(3):897–905.

[20] Stewart EA, Gedroyc WM, Tempany CM, et al. Focused ultrasound treatment of uterine fibroid tumors: safety and feasibility of a noninvasive thermoablative technique. Am J Obstet Gynecol 2003;189(1):48–54.

[21] Stewart EA, Gostout B, Rabinovici J, et al. Sustained relief of leiomyoma symptoms by using focused ultrasound surgery. Obstet Gynecol 2007;110(2 Pt 1):279–87.

[22] Fennessy FM, Tempany C, McDannold N, et al. Uterine leiomyomas: MR imaging-guided focused ultrasound surgery–results of different treatment protocols. Radiology 2007;243(3): 885–93.

[23] Morrison PR, Silverman SG, Tuncali K, et al. MRI guided cryotherapy. J Magn Reson Imaging 2008;27(2):410–20.

[24] Sewell PE, Arriola RM, Robinette L, et al. Real-time I-MR-imaging-guided cryoablation of uterine fibroids. J Vasc Interv Radiol 2001; 12(7):891–3.

[25] Cowan BD, Sewell PE, Howard JC, et al. Interventional magnetic resonance imaging cryotherapy of uterine fibroid tumors: preliminary observation. Am J Obstet Gynecol 2002; 186(6):1183–7.

[26] Dohi M, Harada J, Mogami T, et al. MR-guided transvaginal cryotherapy of uterine fibroids with a horizontal open MRI system: initial experience. Radiat Med 2004;22(6):391–7.

[27] Sakuhara Y, Shimizu T, Kodama Y, et al. Magnetic resonance-guided percutaneous cryoablation of uterine fibroids: early clinical experiences. Cardiovasc Intervent Radiol 2006; 29(4):552–8.

[28] American Cancer Society. Cancer facts and figures 2007. Publication no. 500807. Atlanta (GA): American Cancer Society; 2006.

[29] American Cancer Society. Cancer facts and figures. Publication no. 500807. Atlanta (GA): American Cancer Society; 2008.

[30] Lee F, Gray JM, McLeary RD, et al. Prostatic evaluation by transrectal sonography: criteria for diagnosis of early carcinoma. Radiology 1986; 158:91–5.

[31] Terris MK. Sensitivity and specificity of sextant biopsies in the detection of prostate cancer; preliminary report. Urology 1999;54:486–9.

[32] Aus G, Hermansson CG, Hugosson J, et al. Transrectal ultrasound examination of the prostate: complications and acceptance by patients. Br J Urol 1993;71:457–9.

[33] Collins GN, Lloyd SN, Hehir M, et al. Multiple transrectal ultrasound-guided prostatic biopsies: true morbidity and patient acceptance. Br J Urol 1993;71:460–3.

[34] Rodriguez LV, Terris MK. Risks and complications of transrectal ultrasound guided prostate needle biopsy: a prospective review of the literature. J Urol 1998;160:2115–20.

[35] Rifkin MD, Zerhouni EA, Gatsonis CA, et al. Comparison of magnetic resonance imaging and ultrasonography in staging early prostate cancer: results of a multi-institutional cooperative trial. N Engl J Med 1990;323:621–6.

[36] Schnall MD, Pollack HM. Magnetic resonance imaging of the prostate gland. Urol Radiol 1990;12(2):109–14.

[37] Cornud F, Flam T, Chauveinc L, et al. Extraprostatic spread of clinically localized prostate cancer: factors predictive of pT3 tumor and of positive endorectal MR imaging examination results. Radiology 2002;224(1):203–10.

[38] Outwater EK, Petersen RO, Siegelman ES, et al. Prostate carcinoma: assessment of diagnostic criteria for capsular penetration on endorectal coil MR images. Radiology 1994;193(2): 333–9.

[39] Mullerad M, Hricak H, Kuroiwa K, et al. Comparison of endorectal magnetic resonance imaging, guided prostate biopsy and digital rectal examination in the preoperative anatomical localization of prostate cancer. J Urol 2005; 174:2158–63.

[40] Perrotti M, Han KR, Epstein RE, et al. Prospective evaluation of endorectal magnetic resonance imaging to detect tumor foci in men with prior negative prostatic biopsy: a pilot study. J Urol 1999;162:1314–7.

[41] Hata N, Morrison PR, Kettenbach J, et al. Computer-assisted intra-operative MRI monitoring of interstitial laser therapy in the brain: a case report. SPIE J Biomed Optics 1998;3: 302–11.

[42] Gering D, Nabavi A, Kikinis R, et al. An integrated visualization system for surgical planning and guidance using image fusion and interventional imaging. Medical Image Computing and Computer-Assisted Intervention (MICCAI), Cambridge, England September 22, 1999.

[43] D'Amico AV, Cormack R, Tempany CM, et al. Real-time magnetic resonance image-guided interstitial brachytherapy in the treatment of select patients with clinically localized prostate cancer. Int J Radiat Oncol Biol Phys 1998;42: 507–15.

[44] Hata N, Jinzaki M, Kacher D, et al. MR imaging-guided prostate biopsy with surgical navigation software; device validation and feasibility. Radiology 2001;220:263–8.

[45] Susil RC, Camphausen K, Choyke P, et al. System for prostate brachytherapy and biopsy in a standard 1.5 T MRI scanner. Magn Reson Med 2004;52(3):683–7.

[46] Susil RC, Menard C, Kreiger A, et al. Transrectal prostate biopsy and fiducial marker placement in a standard 1.5T magnetic resonance imaging scanner. J Urol 2006;175(1):113–20.

[47] Beyersdorff D, Winkel A, Hamm B, et al. MR imaging-guided prostate biopsy with a closed MR unit at 1.5 T: initial results. Radiology 2005;234(2):576–81.

[48] Kreiger A, Susil RC, Menard C, et al. Design of a novel MRI compatible manipulator for image guided prostate interventions. IEEE Trans Biomed Eng 2005;52(2):306–13.

[49] Singh AK, Kreiger A, Lattouf JB. Patient selection determines the prostate cancer yield of dynamic contrast-enhanced magnetic resonance imaging-guided transrectal biopsies in a closed 3-Tesla scanner. BJU Int 2008; 101(12):181–5.

[50] DiMaio SP, Pieper S, Chinzei K, et al. Robot-assisted needle placement in open MRI: system architecture, integration and validation. Comput Aided Surg 2007;12(1):15–24.

[51] Lee WR, Hall MC, McQuellon RP, et al. A prospective quality-of-life study in men with clinically localized prostate carcinoma treated with radical prostatectomy, external beam radiotherapy, or interstitial brachytherapy. Int J Radiat Oncol Biol Phys 2001;51(3):614–23.

[52] Zelefsky MJ, Yamada Y, Marion C, et al. Improved conformality and decreased toxicity with intraoperative computer-optimized transperineal ultrasound-guided prostate brachytherapy. Int J Radiat Oncol Biol Phys 2003; 55(4):956–63.

[53] Kooy HM, Cormack RA, Mathiowitz RV, et al. A software system for interventional magnetic resonance image-guided prostate brachytherapy. Comput Aided Surg 2000;5(6):401–13.

[54] D'Amico AV, Cormack R, Kumar S, et al. Real-time magnetic resonance imaging-guided brachytherapy in the treatment of selected patients with clinically localized prostate cancer. J Endourol 2000;14:367–70.

[55] Albert M, Tempany CM, Schultz, et al. Late genitourinary and gastrointestinal toxicity after

magnetic resonance image-guided prostate brachytherapy with or without neoadjuvant external beam radiation therapy. Cancer 2003; 98(5):949–54.

[56] Nguyen PL, Chen MH, D'Amico AV, et al. Magnetic resonance image-guided salvage brachytherapy after radiation in select men who initially presented with favorable-risk prostate cancer: a prospective phase 2 study. Cancer 2007;110(7):1485–92.

[57] D'Amico AV, Moul J, Carroll PR, et al. Cancer-specific mortality after surgery or radiation for patients with clinically localized prostate cancer managed during the prostate-specific antigen era. J Clin Oncol 2003;21(11):2163–72.

[58] Sylvester JE, Grimm PD, Blasko JC, et al. 5-Year biochemical relapse free survival in clinical Stage T1-T3 prostate cancer following combined external beam radiotherapy and brachytherapy; Seattle experience. Int J Radiat Oncol Biol Phys 2007;67(1):57–64.

[59] Lawton CA, DeSilvo M, Lee WR, et al. Results of a phase II trial of transrectal ultrasound-guided permanent radioactive implantation of the prostate for definitive management of localized adenocarcinoma of the prostate (radiation therapy oncology group 98-05). Int J Radiat Oncol Biol Phys 2007;67(1):39–47.

[60] Chinzei K, Miller K. Towards MRI guided surgical manipulator. Med Sci Monit 2001;7: 153–63.

[61] Poissonier L, Chapelon JY, Rouviere O, et al. Control of prostate cancer by transrectal HIFU in 227 patients. Eur Urol 2007;51(2):381–7.

[62] Uchida T, Ohkusa H, Nagata Y, et al. Treatment of localized prostate cancer using high-intensity focused ultrasound. BJU Int 2006;97(1):56–61.

[63] Ficarra V, Antoniolli SZ, Novara G, et al. Short-term outcome after high-intensity focused ultrasound in the treatment of patients with high-risk prostate cancer. BJU Int 2006;98(6): 1193–8.

[64] Smith NB, Buchanan MT, Hynynen K. Transrectal ultrasound applicator for prostate heating monitored using MRI thermometry. Int J Radiat Oncol Biol Phys 1999;43(1):217–25.

[65] Sokka SD, Hynynen KH. The feasibility of MRI-guided whole prostate ablation with a linear aperiodic intracavitary ultrasound and phased array. Phys Med Biol 2000;45(11): 3378–83.

[66] Nau WH, Diederich CJ, Ross AB, et al. MRI-guided interstitial ultrasound thermal therapy of the prostate: a feasibility study in the canine model. Med Phys 2005;32(3):733–43.

[67] Pauly KB, Diederich CJ, Rieke V, et al. Magnetic resonance-guided high-intensity ultrasound ablation of the prostate. Top Magn Reson Imaging 2006;17(3):195–207.

[68] Diederich CJ, Nau WH, Ross AB, et al. Catheter-based ultrasound applicators for selective thermal ablation: progress towards MRI-guided applications in prostate. Int J Hyperthermia 2004;20(7):739–56.

[69] Diederich CJ, Stafford RJ, Nau WH, et al. Transurethral ultrasound applicators with directional heating patterns for prostate thermal therapy: in vivo evaluation using magnetic resonance thermometry. Med Phys 2004; 31(2):405–13.

[70] Hazle JD, Diederich CJ, Kangasniemi M, et al. MRI-guided thermal therapy of transplanted tumors in the canine prostate using a directional transurethral ultrasound applicator. J Magn Reson Imaging 2002;15(4):409–17.

[71] Chopra R, Burtnyk M, Haider MA, et al. Method for MRI-guided conformal thermal therapy of prostate with planar transurethral ultrasound heating applicators. Phys Med Biol 2005; 50(21):4957–75.

[72] Ross AB, Diederich CJ, Nau WH, et al. Highly directional transurethral ultrasound applicators with rotational control for MRI guided prostatic thermal therapy. Phys Med Biol 2004;49(1): 189–204.

[73] Ross AB, Diederich CJ, Nau WH, et al. Curvilinear transurethral ultrasound applicator for selective prostate thermal therapy. Med Phys 2005;32(6):1555–65.

[74] Godley PA, Ataga KI. Renal cell carcinoma. Curr Opin Oncol 2000;12:260–4.

[75] Chow WH, Devesa SS, Warren JL, et al. Rising incidence of renal cell cancer in the United States. JAMA 1999;281:1628–31.

[76] Link RE, Permpongkosol S, Gupta A, et al. Cost analysis of open, laparoscopic, and percutaneous treatment options for nephron-sparing surgery. J Endourol 2006;20:782–9.

[77] Gervais DA, McGovern FJ, Wood BJ, et al. Radio-frequency ablation of renal cell carcinoma: early clinical experience. Radiology 2000;217: 665–72.

[78] Ogan K, Jacomides L, Dolmatch BL, et al. Percutaneous radiofrequency ablation of renal tumors: technique, limitations, and morbidity. Urology 2002;60:954–8.

[79] Farrell MA, Charboneau WJ, DiMarco DS, et al. Imaging-guided radiofrequency ablation of solid renal tumors. AJR 2003;180:1509–13.

[80] Mayo-Smith WW, Dupuy DE, Parikh PM, et al. Imaging-guided percutaneous radiofrequency ablation of solid renal masses: technique and outcomes of 38 treatment sessions in 32 consecutive patients. AJR 2003; 180:1503–8.

[81] Roy-Choudhury SH, Cast JE, Cooksey G, et al. Early experience with percutaneous radiofrequency ablation of small solid renal masses. AJR 2003;180:1055–61.

[82] Su LM, Jarrett TW, Chan DYS, et al. Percutaneous computed tomography-guided radiofrequency ablation of renal masses in high surgical risk patients: preliminary results. Urology 2003;61:26–33.

[83] Zagoria RJ, Hawkins AD, Clark PE, et al. Percutaneous CT-guided radiofrequency ablation of renal neoplasms: factors influencing success. AJR 2004;183:201–7.

[84] Gervais DA, McGovern FJ, Arellano RS, et al. Radiofrequency ablation of renal cell carcinoma: part 1, indications, results, and role in patient management over 6-year period and ablation of 100 tumors. AJR 2005;185: 64–71.

[85] Varkarakis IM, Allaf ME, Inagaki T, et al. Percutaneous radiofrequency ablation of renal masses: results at a 2-year mean followup. J Urol 2005;174:456–60.

[86] Lewin JS, Connell CF, Duerk JL, et al. Interactive MRI-guided radiofrequency interstitial thermal ablation of abdominal tumors: clinical trial for evaluation of safety and feasibility. JMRI 1998;8:40–7.

[87] Lewin JS, Nour SG, Connell CF, et al. Phase II clinical trial of interactive MR imaging-guided interstitial radiofrequency thermal ablation of primary kidney tumors: initial experience. Radiology 2004;232(3):835–45.

[88] Merkle EM, Shonk JR, Duerk JL, et al. MR-guided RF thermal ablation of the kidney in a porcine model. AJR Am J Roentgenol 1999; 173(3):645–51.

[89] Boss A, Clasen S, Kuczyk M, et al. Magnetic resonance-guided percutaneous radiofrequency ablation of renal cell carcinomas: a pilot clinical study. Invest Radiol 2005;40(9): 583–90.

[90] Boss A, Clasen S, Kuczyk M, et al. Image-guided radiofrequency ablation of renal cell carcinoma. Eur Radiol 2007;17(3):725–33.

[91] Merkle EM, Nour SG, Lewin JS. MR imaging follow-up after percutaneous radiofrequency ablation of renal cell carcinoma: findings in 18 patients during first 6 months. Radiology 2005;235(3):1065–71.

[92] Memarsadeghi M, Schmook T, Remzi M, et al. Percutaneous radiofrequency ablation of renal tumors: midterm results in 16 patients. Eur J Radiol 2006;59(2):183–9.

[93] Kawamoto S, Permpongkosol S, Bluemke DA, et al. Sequential changes after radiofrequency ablation and cryoablation of renal neoplasms: role of CT and MR imaging. Radiographics 2007;27(2):343–55.

[94] Atwell TD, Farrell MA, Callstrom MR, et al. Percutaneous cryoablation of 40 solid renal tumors with US guidance and CT monitoring: initial experience. Radiology 2007;243: 276–83.

[95] Atwell TD, Farrell MA, Callstrom MR, et al. Percutaneous cryoablation of large renal masses: technical feasibility and short-term outcome. AJR 2007;188:1195–200.

[96] Matina SF, Ahrarb K, Cadedduc JA, et al. Residual and recurrent disease following renal energy ablative therapy: a multi-institutional study. J Urol 2006;176:1973–7.

[97] Allaf ME, Varkarakis IM, Bhayani SB, et al. Pain control requirements for percutaneous ablation of renal tumors: cryoablation versus radiofrequency ablation—initial observations. Radiology 2005;237:366–70.

[98] Tacke J, Speetzen R, Heschel I, et al. Imaging of interstitial cryotherapy—an in vitro comparison of ultrasound, computed tomography, and magnetic resonance imaging. Cryobiology 1999;38:250–9.

[99] Saliken J, McKinnon J, Gray R. CT for monitoring cryotherapy. AJR 1996;166:853–5.

[100] Sandison GA, Loye MP, Rewcastle JC, et al. X-ray CT monitoring of iceball growth and thermal distribution during cryosurgery. Phys Med Biol 1998;43:3309–24.

[101] Gupta A, Allaf ME, Kavoussi LR, et al. Computerized tomography guided percutaneous renal cryoablation with the patient under conscious sedation: initial clinical experience. J Urol 2006;175:447–53.

[102] Permpongkosol S, Link RE, Kavoussi LR, et al. Percutaneous computerized tomography guided cryoablation for localized renal cell carcinoma: factors influencing success. J Urol 2006;176:1963–8.

[103] Littrup PJ, Ahmed A, Aoun HD, et al. CT-guided percutaneous cryotherapy of renal masses. J Vasc Interv Radiol 2007;18:383–92.

[104] Harada J, Dohi M, Mogami T, et al. Initial experience of percutaneous renal cryosurgery under the guidance of a horizontal open MRI system. Radiat Med 2001;19:291–6.

[105] Shingleton WB, Sewell J, Patrick E. Percutaneous renal tumor cryoablation with magnetic resonance imaging guidance. J Urol 2001;165: 773–6.

[106] Shingleton WB, Sewell PE. Percutaneous renal cryoablation of renal tumors in patients with von Hippel-Lindau disease. J Urol 2002;167: 1268–70.

[107] Shingleton WB, Sewell PE. Percutaneous cryoablation of renal cell carcinoma in a transplanted kidney. BJU International 2002;90: 137–8.

[108] Sewell PE, Howard JC, Shingleton WB, et al. Interventional magnetic resonance image-guided percutaneous cryoablation of renal tumors. South Med J 2003;96:708–10.

[109] Shingleton WB, Sewell PE. Cryoablation of renal tumours in patients with solitary kidneys. BJU International 2003;92:237–9.

[110] Kodama Y, Abo D, Sakuhara Y, et al. MR-guided percutaneous cryoablation for bilateral multiple renal cell carcinoma. Radiat Med 2005;23:303–7.

[111] Silverman SG, Tuncali K, vanSonnenberg E, et al. Renal tumors: MR imaging guided percutaneous cryotherapy–initial experience in 23 patients. Radiology 2005;236:716–24.

[112] Miki K, Shimomura T, Yamada H, et al. Percutaneous cryoablation of renal cell carcinoma guided by horizontal open magnetic resonance imaging. Int J Urol 2006;13:880–4.

[113] Silverman SG, Tuncali K, Adams DF, et al. MR imaging-guided percutaneous cryotherapy of liver tumors: initial experience. Radiology 2000;217:657–64.

[114] Farrell MA, Charboneau JW, Callstrom MR, et al. Paranephric water instillation: a technique to prevent bowel injury during percutaneous renal radiofrequency ablation. AJR 2003;181:1315–7.

[115] Tuncali K, Morrison PR, Tatli S, et al. MRI-guided percutaneous cryoablation of renal tumors: use of external manual displacement of adjacent bowel loops. Eur J Radiol 2006;59:198–202.

[116] Elhawary H, Zivanovic A, Davies B, et al. A review of magnetic resonance imaging compatible manipulators in surgery. Proc Inst Mech Eng [H] 2006;220(3):413–24.

RADIOLOGIC
CLINICS
OF NORTH AMERICA

Radiol Clin N Am 46 (2008) 167–173

Index

Note: Page numbers of article titles are in **boldface** type.